Competency Exam Prep & Review for Nursing Assistants

Fourth Edition

Barbara Acello, MS, RN

THOMSON

DELMAR LEARNING

Australia • Canada • Mexico • Singapore • Spain • United Kingdom • United States

THOMSON

DELMAR LEARNING

Competency Exam Prep & Review for Nursing Assistants, Fourth Edition
by Barbara Acello, MS, RN

Vice President, Health Care Business Unit:
William Brottmiller

Director of Learning Solutions:
Matthew Kane

Managing Editor:
Marah Bellegarde

Acquisitions Editor:
Matthew Seeley

Product Manager:
Jadin Babin-Kavanaugh

Editorial Assistant:
Ncole Bruno

Marketing Director:
Jennifer McAvey

Marketing Manager:
Michele McTighe

Production Director:
Carolyn Miller

Production Manager:
Barbara A. Bullock

Content Project Manager:
Anne Sherman

Library of Congress Cataloging-in-Publication Data

Acello, Barbara.
  Competency exam prep & review for nursing assistants / Barbara Acello.—4th ed.
    p. ; cm.
  Includes index.
  ISBN 1-4018-8904-2
  1. Nurses' aides—Outlines, syllabi, etc.
2. Nurses' aides—Examinations, questions, etc. I. Title. II. Title: Competency exam prep and review for nursing assistants.
  [DNLM: 1. Nurses' Aides--Examination Questions. 2. Nurses' Aides--Outlines. 3. Clinical Competence—Examination Questions. 4. Clinical Competence—Outlines. 5. Nursing Care—methods—Examination Questions. 6. Nursing Care—methods—Outlines. WY 18.2 A173c 2007]
  RT84.K37 2007
  610.7306'98—dc22
                                    2006017441

Notice to the Reader

Brief Contents

Contents

Chapter 11   Nutrition and Fluid Needs   186

Chapter 12   Elimination Needs   203

Chapter 13   Vital Signs, Height, and Weight   218

Appendices   241

Index   429

Performance Procedures

Preface

INTRODUCTION

This textbook was developed to comply with the guidelines set by the Department of Health and Human Services in compliance with Public Law 100-203, referred to as the Omnibus Reconciliation Act of 1987 (OBRA). This law requires that nursing assistants (nurse aides) have, at a minimum, 75 hours of education and successfully complete a competency evaluation program.

This textbook was designed to serve as a guide to the competency evaluation program. Included in this course is the content required to successfully complete the written and manual skills components of the examination.

Cardiopulmonary resuscitation (CPR) is not included in this curriculum. It is strongly recommended that the CPR and Clearing Obstructed Airway components be taught by a certified CPR instructor.

ORGANIZATION OF TEXT CONTENT

Chapters 1 through 7 serve as the core module. By OBRA standards, study of this initial material must consist of at least 16 hours. The author feels that 16 hours can provide only an overview of the content of chapters 1 through 7. Reinforcement of the content in these chapters can be given in succeeding lessons.

This manual is a very basic, "need-to-know" text. It is assumed that the instructor will draw upon professional experiences involving patient care to provide the "nice-to-know" content. Throughout the entire content of this textbook, the intent of the OBRA law is supported. This ensures that residents in long-term care facilities are treated with care, dignity, and respect, while assisting residents to attain and main-tain the highest possible level of independence.

Forty-nine basic nursing procedures are included in this text. These procedures are included in the competency examination evaluation program in many states. The procedures were selected based on the OBRA guidelines, as well as suggestions by the manuscript reviewers. There are common steps at the beginning and end of all nursing procedures. These steps are listed on the inside covers of this text to emphasize the importance of handwashing, communication, safety, and respecting the resident's right to privacy. As students become proficient in clinical skills, these procedures become automatic.

This exam review can be used with other Delmar resources to create a comprehensive educational package.

Health care is constantly changing. This fourth edition of *Competency Exam Prep and Review* has been revised to ensure that all of the technical and procedural information is current. New information has been added on:

- The Health Insurance Portability and Accountability Act (HIPAA)
- HCV (hepatitis C virus)
- Necrotizing fasciitis, pseudomembranous colitis (also called *Clostridium difficile* or *C. difficile*), and shingles (herpes zoster)
- Waterless hand cleaners
- Risk of entrapment in side rails
- Low beds in resident care
- Low-bed safety for the nursing assistant
- Procedures for denture care, waterless bathing (bag bath), measuring a tympanic temperature, and measuring the blood pressure (one-step procedure)
- Guidelines for care of African American residents' hair.
- Appendix B contains useful information and diagrams with information that may not be committed to memory, although the nursing assistant is responsible for knowing the content. The tables and diagrams in this section facilitate learning and comprehension.

USING DELMAR RESOURCES

Several texts and a video series were developed to meet educational needs for materials leading to the certification of nursing assistants for jobs in the long-term care industry.

Video Series

Thomson Delmar Learning's Basic Core Skills for Nursing Assistants is a series of 10 videos. The videos contain 87 segments relating to specific skills. The instructor can begin teaching skills immediately using these high-quality video demonstrations. Medical professionals developed the videos based on requests from our textbook users. The procedural steps coordinate with all Delmar competency-based texts for nursing assistants. The procedures and activities shown on the videos recognize the nursing assistant as a skilled paraprofessional who works as an important member of the interdisciplinary team under the supervision of a licensed nurse.

Geriatric long-term care is a specialized segment of the health care industry. The focus of nursing assistant education must reflect the specific health care needs of long-term care residents, the significance of establishing a personal relationship with the resident, and the vulnerability of the elderly person who is suddenly placed in an institutional environment. To that end, the videos were produced to be current in light of the OBRA legislation and accurate in reflecting the "real" environment in a long-term care facility. Special emphasis is placed on the fact that the nursing facility resident is a real person with a unique identity and a personal life history. We are highly aware that the nursing assistant is also a complex person with goals and problems that affect his or her daily approach to life. Consequently, we have tried, beyond providing guidelines for nursing procedures and a message of compassion for our residents, to develop a program that will instill a sense of pride and self-worth in the student.

Text Packages

Nursing Assisting: Essentials for Long-Term Care, 2nd edition, is a complete text for any 75- to 150-hour curriculum. This text starts with the initial 16 hours and then covers basic and intermediate procedures. It is designed to enhance learning for average and special-needs learners and for those who speak English as a second language. An instructor's manual is available, providing program management support and learning resources. Although the text may be used as a stand-alone item, a workbook was added with the second edition to meet the needs of students and instructors in programs exceeding 90 hours in length. A computerized test bank is also available. The objective of this turnkey package is to

teach the development of critical thinking skills. Learning critical thinking involves having the knowledge and skills to process information, and practicing use of this information to guide behavior and benefit residents.

Competency Exam Prep & Review for Nursing Assistants, 4th edition, can be used with the video series and all nursing assistant texts, study aids, and exam preparatory materials. This combination of learning aids is ideal for the 100- to 150-hour program.

For multicompetency programs, the instructor may choose from any of the following texts:

- *Nursing Assisting: Essentials for Long-Term Care,* 2nd edition, by Barbara Acello
- *Nursing Assistant: A Nursing Process Approach,* 9th edition, by Hegner, Caldwell and Acello
- *Assisting in Long-Term Care,* 5th edition, by Hegner and Gerlach.

The Delmar program provides a complete collection of materials for all levels of nursing assistant education, from basic to advanced. Many additional learning materials are available to assist in upgrading the basic nursing assistant to the advanced practitioner or patient care technician level.

Competency Exam Prep & Review was designed to provide exposure to test-taking using multiple-choice questions in a simulation of the certification examination. An appendix on test-taking techniques is provided to help the learner build confidence to take the certification exam and succeed. Thomson Delmar Learning has many tools available to prepare nursing assistants for the state nursing assistant and competency evaluation. The *Nurse Aide Exam Review Cards* and *Nurse Aide Exam Review Cards with Audio CD* are available in both English and Spanish. Using these items to study for the state test further improves students' ability to successfully complete the state certification examination.

Competency Exam Prep & Review for Nursing Assistants is part of the most comprehensive and flexible educational system available. It is hoped that these extensive resources will contribute to quality assurance and to job satisfaction and self-esteem for long-term care paraprofessionals. The author and publisher hope their efforts enhance the quality of life for long-term care residents.

About the Author

ABOUT THE AUTHOR

Barbara Acello is an independent nurse consultant and educator. She has many years of experience in nursing assistant education in the public and private sectors. She is an approved RN Program Director in the state of Texas and a contributor to the Texas Curriculum for Nurse Aides.

Mrs. Acello can be contacted through the Allied Health Department of Thomson Delmar Learning or by e-mail at bacello@spamcop.net.

Acknowledgments

I would like to thank Marah Bellegarde, Managing Editor at Thomson Delmar Learning, for her ongoing encouragement, assistance, and support. I also sincerely appreciate the efforts of the many unnamed individuals at Delmar who contributed to the production team effort. These individuals give much of themselves and take pride in producing quality products. I would also like to thank my copyeditor, Brooke Graves. I am always delighted when she copyedits my books—thank you for making me look good!

Last but not least, I offer sincere thanks to the instructors who have supported me and provided constructive feedback on my various projects. It is my strong desire that this book will provide the support and assistance to students who are committed to learning and mastering this material. Becoming a nursing assistant is a very special goal. Realize that to attain this goal, you must take many small steps. Each step you master takes you closer to your ultimate goal. I wish you well in your journey, and have the utmost respect for the important job you do.

A dedicated team of peer reviewers devoted many hours to reviewing this manuscript, and provided many helpful comments during the preproduction period and throughout manuscript development. Your contributions have made this a better book. Your input has been invaluable, and I sincerely appreciate your dedication, prompt turnaround, and willingness to share your knowledge and suggestions.

The author and Thomson Delmar Learning wish to thank the following reviewers:

Judith Bateman, RN, MSN, C
Instructor
Black Hawk College, Moline, IL

Susan Erue, RN, BSN, MS, PhD
Professor
Iowa Wesleyan College, Mt. Pleasant, IA

Sally Flesch, RN, BSN, MA, EDS, PhD
Professor
Black Hawk College, Moline, IL

Robin Nabity, RN
Instructor/CNA Program Coordinator
Estrella Mountain Community College, Avondale, AZ

Lucretia Moore-Peters, RN
Nursing Department Coordinator
Gretna Career College, Gretna, LA

Ann E. Sims, RN, BSN
Director of Nursing Assistant Programs
Albuquerque TVI, Albuquerque, NM

The book was designed and assembled by Interactive Composition Corporation (ICC), Portland, OR. Lori Hazzard, the project manager, has done a commendable job in taking over a thousand pages of raw manuscript and turning it into the attractive, legible book that you hold in your hands. Layout, design, and legibility are key to student mastery of the content, and ICC has done a tremendous job in ensuring a high quality finished product. I am grateful for their effort, assistance, and commitment to quality.

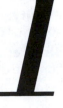

The Role and Responsibilities of the Nursing Assistant

OBJECTIVES

In this chapter you will learn about your role and responsibilities as a member of the health care team. After reading this chapter, you will be able to:

- Spell and define key terms.
- Describe the role and responsibilities of the nursing assistant.
- Describe the nursing assistant's role in the health care delivery system.
- Describe the purpose and intent of the OBRA legislation.
- Identify members of the interdisciplinary health care team.
- Describe ethics for the nursing assistant.
- Identify legal issues the nursing assistant must be aware of.
- State the purpose of the individualized resident care plan.
- Explain why individualized care is important.
- Define restorative care and explain why this type of care is important.
- Identify normal changes that occur during the aging process.

KEY TERMS

abuse: doing physical or mental harm to a resident, or threatening a resident with harm

acute illness: an illness that occurs quickly and does not last very long

aiding and abetting: seeing someone do something wrong and not reporting it

assault: trying to or threatening to touch a resident's body without permission

attitude: how you present yourself; an outward reflection of your feelings

battery: touching someone without permission

care plan: an individualized plan that lists the problems, needs, strengths, and goals for the resident and describes what care and interventions should be done

charge nurse: the person responsible for supervising the resident's care and assignments during a certain work period

chronic illness: an illness that lasts for a long time, perhaps for life

clergy: a minister of the gospel, a pastor, priest, or rabbi

client: the individual cared for in the home

continuity of care: the process by which the care of a resident continues uninterrupted, using the same methods and approaches by all caregivers to meet the resident's goals

dependability: being trustworthy; reliable

dignity: the state of being respected or held in honor or esteem

disease: a state in the body in which normal functions are disturbed and do not perform as they should

ethics: rules of moral, responsible conduct that guide a person's behavior

etiquette: being polite, courteous, and kind toward others

false imprisonment: restricting someone's movement without permission

geriatrics: related to the aged or the aging process and diseases of the elderly

health: a state in which the body functions normally and is free from disease

interdisciplinary team: a group of individuals working and cooperating to help the resident attain and maintain the highest possible level of function

invasion of privacy: failure to keep resident information confidential or exposing the resident's body during caregiving

involuntary seclusion: isolating a resident as a form of punishment

job description: a list of duties and responsibilities for a particular job

long-term care facility: a nursing home or place where people with long-standing or chronic illnesses are cared for

licensed practical nurse (LPN) or **licensed vocational nurse (LVN):** one who has completed a 12- to 18-month nursing program and passed a state licensing examination for practical nurses

neglect: failing to provide needed services or care to residents; the failure may be accidental or deliberate

negligence: carelessness; failing to give the care needed in the way you were taught

nursing assistant (NA), nurse aide (NA), nurse assistant, state registered (NASR), state tested nurse assistant (STNA): a person who works under the supervision of a licensed nurse to provide personal care and nursing-related services to persons in health care facilities

OBRA 1987: Omnibus Budget Reconciliation Act of 1987; a set of laws that govern long-term care facilities and nursing assistant practice

patient: a person in a hospital who needs care

registered nurse (RN): a person who has completed two to four years of nursing school and has passed a state licensing examination for registered nurses. The RN is responsible for assessing and planning care for residents and supervising other nursing employees.

rehabilitation center: a health care facility whose goal is to help ill or injured persons to function at their highest level of independence

resident: a person living in a nursing home or other long-term care facility

restorative care: care designed to help the resident attain and maintain the highest possible level of functioning

subacute care: highly specialized care for individuals with specific medical problems that require frequent skilled intervention. This care is delivered by highly trained personnel.

theft: taking something that does not belong to you

THE ROLE OF NURSING ASSISTANTS

Welcome to the health care field! You are about to become a member of a growing industry in which your work can give you great personal satisfaction. The most common title for this position is **nursing assistant (NA).** In some states the worker is called a **nurse aide (NA).** In others, the title **nurse assistant, state registered (NASR)** is used. Some states call this position **state tested nurse assistant (STNA).** Regardless of the title of your position, you will help others while achieving personal growth and satisfaction. The nursing assistant works in a health care setting to help the nurse give personal care to a resident, patient, or client (Figure 1-1).

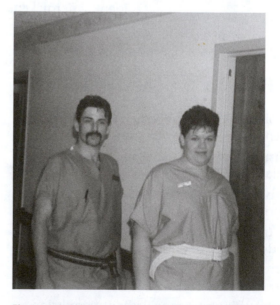

Figure 1-1 Being a nursing assistant is a rewarding career for both men and women. These assistants project a positive image. They are neat and clean, with name badges and gait belts.

HEALTH CARE FACILITIES

Health care facilities can be grouped into two categories: those that give acute care and those that give less acute care, usually for long periods. Hospitals are examples of acute care facilities, where persons usually stay for a short time. Individuals who receive care in hospitals are called **patients.** Patients in hospitals have **acute illnesses** and injuries. An acute illness is one that occurs quickly and does not last very long. Some people receive care in their own home after they are discharged from the hospital. In the home, the caregiver may be called a home health aide (HHA) or home care aide (HCA). The home health aide usually completes a nursing assistant program and learns additional home health applications of the material. The person being cared for is called the **client. Long-term care facilities** are referred to by different names, such as convalescent homes, nursing homes, care centers, care facilities, **rehabilitation centers,** skilled nursing facilities, and other names. The people who reside in these long-term care facilities are called **residents.** Many residents in long-term care facilities have **chronic illnesses.** A chronic illness is one that lasts a long time, perhaps for life. These individuals usually stay for a long time, sometimes for years. The long-term care facility is their home, and you are a visitor in it. Many residents in long-term care facilities are elderly, although younger residents may also reside in the facility because they require daily personal care. The term **geriatrics** refers to care of the elderly, so you may be called a geriatric aide. Some long-term care facilities have highly specialized units, such as those where care is provided to residents with AIDS or Alzheimer's disease, those who use ventilators for breathing, or those who require **subacute care.** This book is designed to prepare you to work in a long-term care facility.

THE OBRA LEGISLATION

OBRA 1987 means the Omnibus Budget Reconciliation Act of 1987. OBRA refers to federal laws that regulate long-term care facilities. In 1987 the OBRA legislation mandated sweeping changes in the long-term care industry. This changed the way that care is given. Before OBRA, care was provided to keep residents comfortable. The OBRA legislation requires long-term care facilities to use all resources available to help residents reach and maintain their highest level of function, both physically and mentally. The legislation also requires that care be given in a homelike environment and that residents be given choices and control over their care and routines.

Another change made by the OBRA legislation is the requirement that all states develop a process for the education and competency testing of nursing assistants. The law requires classes for nursing assistants in long-term care facilities specifically, but most health care agencies also require nursing assistant education for their employees.

The OBRA legislation requires specific content for the nursing assistant course and states that the course must be a minimum of 75 hours in length. Individual states may require additional hours. After the nursing assistant completes the class, he or she must take and successfully complete a written and performance examination to be entered on the state nursing assistant registry. Only nursing assistants who have passed the examination and are on the state registry may work in long-term care facilities. Some states allow nursing assistants to work if they are enrolled in a class and will complete their program within four months from the date of hire. In these states, you may perform only skills that you learned in class and on which you have been found proficient by the instructor.

The law also requires that the nursing assistant attend a minimum of 12 hours of continuing education classes a year, although again, individual states can require additional hours and specific subjects. These classes usually are provided by the long-term care facility. It is your responsibility to attend them to maintain your certification.

THE NURSE SUPERVISOR

As a nursing assistant, you will be supervised by a licensed nurse. The nurse may be a **registered nurse (RN),** a **licensed practical nurse (LPN),** or a **licensed vocational nurse (LVN).** The supervising nurse, sometimes called the **charge nurse,** is responsible for making your work assignment. This is the nurse of whom you will ask questions and to whom you will report information about residents. Your work assignment includes work duties, assignment of the residents you will care for, and extra jobs that must be done on your unit. The nursing assistant is a part of the nursing service department in the long-term care facility.

PERSONAL QUALIFICATIONS

Because your role as a nursing assistant involves giving personal care to others, you must have certain qualities and personal characteristics.

Important Qualities for a Nursing Assistant

Nursing assistants should:

- have a sincere interest in working with people.
- have an **attitude** of respect toward the elderly.
- believe in the **dignity** of each person.
- be able to control their emotions.
- be honest, reliable, and dependable.
- have a positive attitude toward their job and employer.
- show willingness to accept direction and change.
- have a patient, cheerful, and sensitive nature.
- have a clean and neat appearance.
- be in good health without lifting restrictions. A nursing assistant must stand and walk for long periods, and lift and move people.
- be free from communicable diseases.
- be drug- and alcohol-free.

THE RESPONSIBILITIES OF NURSING ASSISTANTS

The responsibilities of the nursing assistant usually are listed in detail in a **job description.** A job description will be given to you by your employer. The description details the particular tasks you are expected to do in that facility. These tasks may vary from one health care facility to another. Remember, everything you do is under the supervision of a nurse.

Job Description

Your job description will list the duties and tasks you are expected to do and may include such things as:

- Personal care of residents
  - helping residents with personal care, such as bathing, mouth care, grooming, dressing, toileting, and skin care
  - helping residents with equipment or devices such as hearing aids, glasses, and dentures
  - caring for residents who are dying
- Assisting residents with nutrition and hydration
  - helping residents to eat and drink
- Care of the environment
  - caring for the residents' environment
  - maintaining safety in the environment
  - helping with unit organization, cleanliness, and efficiency

- Infection control
  - practicing measures that prevent the spread of infection
- Observation and recording
  - taking and recording vital signs
  - observing and reporting abnormal signs and symptoms
  - measuring height and weight
  - keeping records required by facility policy
  - reporting any suspected or actual resident abuse or neglect
- Assisting with movement, exercise, and ambulation
  - lifting, moving, turning, and transferring residents
  - helping residents with mobility
  - helping residents with exercise programs
- Other responsibilities
  - maintaining residents' legal rights guaranteed by the Resident's Bill of Rights
  - helping residents with mental health and emotional needs
  - doing other tasks as assigned by your supervisor within the legal role of the nursing assistant

The policies of facilities vary, but generally you are expected to care for any resident in the facility. Although you may be assigned to a certain group of residents, answering call signals of all residents usually is required. Male and female nursing assistants usually are expected to care for residents of both sexes. If this concerns you, discuss the situation with the employer before accepting the job.

Dependability is an important quality of any employee of a health care facility. It is important that you remain healthy so that you can be depended on to be at work. It is your responsibility to let your employer know well in advance when you are ill and cannot report for work. You should call your supervisor personally and explain the situation. If you do not call until the beginning of your shift or if you do not call at all, replacing you will be very difficult. In some facilities, failure to call in an absence results in dismissal. Dependability also means you are responsible for doing the job that you were hired to do in the manner in which you were taught.

Dress Code

Long-term care facilities usually require nursing assistants to wear a uniform. The type of uniform will be decided by your employer. The purpose of a uniform is to maintain a professional appearance. Some facilities use different color uniforms to identify members of various departments. Another purpose of the uniform is to prevent the spread of infection. It should be worn only once and changed when you get home. The uniform often includes a name tag that lists your name and title. It is your responsibility to follow facility policy regarding the uniform code.

A neat, natural hairstyle is part of a well-groomed appearance. Your hair is like a magnet for germs. Keeping it short makes it easier to care for. Wash your hair regularly. If you have long hair, pull it back or wear it up. Avoid extreme fashion statements such as shaving the head, Mohawk hairdos, or other radical cuts, styles, or unnatural colors. Do not wear hats, scarves, or other head coverings while on duty. Males should keep facial hair neat and trimmed. Keep your fingernails short and clean. Avoid long fingernails, artificial nails, and chipped nail polish.

Keep jewelry to a minimum. Wear only simple jewelry when on duty. Avoid sharp stones and settings. Most facilities permit only a watch (with a sweep second hand) and a wedding band. Small, stud-type pierced earrings also reduce your risk of injury from an earring being pulled or caught. If you have multiple ear piercings, wear one small pair of studs in your lower earlobe. Leave the others out. For your safety, avoid hoops and wires. Avoid bracelets and necklaces unless they are used for medical identification. Do not wear sunglasses while you are on duty.

Residents in the long-term care facility are usually elderly, and many do not understand, or are afraid of, employees who have piercings and tattoos. In some communities, residents may associate piercings and tattoos with gang membership. Most facilities do not permit employees to have body piercings in areas of the body other than the ears. This includes the tongue. If you have piercings in other areas, cover them with clothing. Cover tattoos with clothing. Some facilities will not permit employees with visible tattoos to work in resident care positions.

Most facilities have policies prohibiting the use of non-work-related personal communication devices, such as cell phones and pagers. Plan to make and return phone calls during your breaks. In some facilities, employees may carry pagers or cell phones set for silent alert. However, staff should not respond to personal calls when on duty. Remember, you are being paid to work. Another concern is that some radio frequency devices will interfere with medical equipment and may jeopardize resident health and safety. The devices are fragile and easily broken. The best practice is to avoid wearing them when on duty.

Job Limitations

The nursing assistant has certain job limitations and does not perform certain tasks. These will vary from one health care facility to another, but the following tasks usually are job limitations. Nursing assistants *do not*:

- give medications.
- apply prescription creams or ointments to a resident's skin.
- give reports on residents' medical condition to family members or others.
- take orders from the doctor.
- perform any procedures they have not been taught.
- perform any tasks forbidden by state law or facility policies.

Whenever you are not sure about a task or procedure, always ask the nurse for help.

THE INTERDISCIPLINARY HEALTH CARE TEAM

A nursing assistant is a part of the very important **interdisciplinary team.** The goal of the entire staff of the long-term care facility is to provide the best care possible for residents. This requires the cooperation of staff in all departments. We each may think the service we provide is the most important, but we cannot care for the residents unless all of us are doing our jobs. Care provided in the long-term care facility is designed to help residents maintain the highest level of functioning possible considering each person's individual condition. Many individuals work together for the residents' benefit. Every member of the team contributes to the residents' care.

Members of the Interdisciplinary Team

The following individuals make up the interdisciplinary team:

- resident, family, or legal guardian
- physician
- nursing staff

- staff members from the various therapy departments, including physical, occupational, speech, respiratory, and activity therapy
- social workers
- dietary staff
- housekeeping, maintenance, and laundry staff
- office, administrative, and clerical workers
- **clergy**
- other staff from within or outside the nursing facility as required to help meet the residents' needs

ETHICS FOR THE NURSING ASSISTANT

Ethics is part of a moral code that guides the behavior of the health care worker. Ethics involves making judgments about what is right and what is wrong. An ethical nursing assistant is one who:

- promotes health, independence, safety, and quality of life for each resident.
- respects each resident as an individual and treats all residents with respect.
- understands and follows all the principles covered by the Residents' Bill of Rights.
- respects each resident's private space and treats the resident's personal belongings with care.
- keeps information about residents confidential.
- respects residents' right to privacy.
- maintains a positive attitude toward the facility.
- functions as a member of the health care team working within the limits of the job description, facility policies, and state laws.
- acts as a responsible employee at all times.
- performs procedures only in the manner taught and does not take shortcuts.
- accepts no money, tips, or favors for service to residents.
- considers each resident's needs to be important.
- demonstrates **etiquette;** that is, exhibits a polite, courteous, and kind attitude to residents, visitors, and other staff members.

LEGAL ISSUES FOR THE NURSING ASSISTANT

Laws are rules passed by governmental agencies and are to be obeyed by everyone. If you do not obey the law, you could be found liable. If you do things in the manner in which you were taught, you will be following the law. Situations to *avoid* are as follows:

- **Negligence** involves being careless and failing to give care in the way you were taught.
- **Theft** is taking something that does not belong to you.
- **Aiding and abetting** involves seeing someone doing something wrong or stealing something and not reporting it.
- **False imprisonment** is restricting someone's movement without permission; for example, applying restraints without proper authorization.
- **Involuntary seclusion** is isolating a resident as a form of punishment.
- **Assault** means trying to or threatening to touch a resident's body without permission.
- **Battery** means touching a resident without permission.
- **Invasion of privacy** involves failure to keep resident information confidential or exposing the resident's body when care is being given.
- **Abuse** means doing physical or mental harm to the resident, or threatening the resident with harm.
- **Neglect** consists of failing to provide needed services or care to residents; the failure may be accidental or deliberate.

THE CARE PLAN

Within 21 days of admission to a long-term care facility, a comprehensive, written **care plan** is developed. A temporary care plan is usually started to provide guidelines for care until the resident is thoroughly assessed by the interdisciplinary team and the comprehensive care plan is completed. The comprehensive care plan is developed in a staff conference to which the resident and family members of the resident's choosing are invited. The resident's strengths are used as a basis to overcome problems and needs. Long- and short-term goals are defined and agreed upon by everyone present. The care plan lists approaches to help the resident meet the goals within a set period of time and states who is responsible for each approach.

The care plan assures that the resident will have **continuity of care.** All staff members are expected to use the care plan as the basis of the care they give, so that everyone works toward the same goals and uses the same approaches. As a nursing assistant, you are responsible for knowing what your job is and how it relates to the care plan (Figure 1-2).

NURSING ASSISTANT CARE PLAN

DIETARY

Diabetic _____ Calorie ☐

Dining Room: (Bkfst) (Lunch) (Dinner)

Room: Bkfst. Lunch Dinner

Feeder Room: Bkfst. Lunch Dinner

Set Tray Up ☒

Feed ☐

Tube Feeding ☐

Adaptive Equipment

Regular
Diet

House supplement 2p+HS
Nourishment/Supplement/HS Snack

Measure:

Intake ☒

Output ☒

ELIMINATION

Toilet q 2 hrs. ☒

Bedpan/Urinal ☐

Incontinence Bowel ☐

Incontinence Bladder ☐

Catheter

Foley ☐

Supra Pubic ☐

Condom ☐

Leg Bag ☐

Catheter Strap ☐

Ostomy ☐

RESTRAINTS

Vest: When _____ ☐

Waist (soft) When in Chair ☐

Mitts _____ ☐

Geri Chair ☐

Roller Bar: When in W/C ☐

Lap Belt ☐

Other *Self release belt* ☒

Restrain at All Times ☐

SIDERAILS

At All Times ☐

At Night Only ☒

Signed Release: ☐

Do not use any restraint not checked above.
Observe q 30 minutes and release q 2 hours x's
10 minutes for care/exercise.

BATHING

Tub ☐

Shower ☒

Bed ☐

Day: M (T) W (T) F (S) S

AM ☐   PM ☒

Shampoo

Beauty Shop ☐

Staff ☒

AM/PM Care

Self ☒

Staff ☐

Shave by Noon, Remove Facial
Hair. Finger Nail Care on
Bath/Shower Day. Toe Nail Care
as Directed by Nurse.

HEARING

Hard of Hearing:

Right ☐   Left ☒

Hearing Aid:

Right ☐   Left ☒

Look at Resident While
Speaking to Them.

FREQUENCY OF VITAL SIGNS

Weight *weekly*

TPR *monthly*

B/P *monthly*

POSITIONING

Turn q 2 hours ☒

Range of Motion with Cares ☒

Special Mattress/Device

Sheepskin

Positioning Equip.

_____

Braces/Splints/Cones

(L) *Hand splint.*

Follow Turning Schedule.

DRESSING

Self ☐

Assist ☒

Supervise ☐

Total ☐

Adult Brief ☐

Lap robe ☐

All Residents to Wear
Underwear.

SIGHT

Blind:

Right ☐   Left ☐

Poor Vision ☐

Glasses ☒

Contact Lens ☐

Clean Glasses or Contact
Lens with A.M. Care.

ORAL CARE

Self ☐

Assist ☒

Own Teeth ☐

No Teeth ☐

Dentures:

Upper ☒

Lower ☐

Partial ☐

Oral Care in A.M., at
Bedtime and PRN.

MOBILITY

Independent ☐

Cane ☐

Walker ☒

Wheelchair ☒

Own ☐

Other ☐

No Weight Bearing:

Right ☐   Left ☐

Partial Weight Bearing

Right ☐   Left ☐

Gait Belt ☒

Transfer ☐

Hoyer Lift ☐

No. of Assist for Transfers

_____

Other _____

Special Instructions:

*ABL Goals: Wash face,
hands, + chest. Will
put on blouse + button it.
Mobility Goals: Ambulate c̄ gait belt,
Walker, and minimum assist to
dining room for lunch each day.
Encourage independence c̄ selfcare.
Allow the resident to struggle slightly.
but not to the point of frustration.
Praise her efforts, then assist her in
completing the task.*

Room No.: *203-2*   Date: *1/4/97*

Resident: *Wallace, Eleanor*

Figure 1-2 Become familiar with and follow each resident's care plan.

Ask your supervisor about anything you do not understand. If you notice that certain approaches are not working, or if you discover something else that works but is not listed on the care plan, inform the nurse. The care plan is updated quarterly, and whenever there is a change in the resident's condition.

An important nursing assistant responsibility is to notice any changes in residents and report those changes to the nurse, even if they seem minor. When observing and reporting, you must be accurate. Reporting too much is better than forgetting to report something.

INDIVIDUALIZED CARE

The long-term care facility is home to many different types of residents. Because patients stay in hospitals for shorter periods, many residents come to the long-term care facility to complete their recovery. You may find one entire facility that specializes in a certain type of care. Some facilities have separate areas or units that provide specialized care. Many long-term care facilities do not specialize; they admit persons with any condition. The reasons for admission to the long-term care facility may vary widely, but each resident needs individualized care.

Although residents' ages may vary, most residents will be elderly. People are living longer than ever before. As one ages, resistance to disease, stress, and injury decreases. Therefore, the elderly are more likely to require help in meeting their personal needs. Treat each resident as an individual. Remember the following when giving individualized care:

- Each resident is a separate person with different wants and needs.
- Help residents to become and remain independent.
- Maintain dignity by treating residents appropriately for their age.
- Promote self-worth and dignity by allowing residents to do as much as possible and promoting and encouraging independence.
- Offer choices whenever possible. This helps residents maintain a sense of control and adds to self-esteem.
- If a resident cannot complete a skill independently, compliment him or her for the part he or she was able to complete. Finish the task without complaint.
- Allow residents who are completely unable to perform self-care to direct you in their care. Directing the care verbally gives the resident a sense of control and improves self-esteem.

- Be involved with the resident's family, and be aware of activity programs that include family members.
- Schedule care to allow residents to participate in activity programs.
- Assist residents to meet their physical, psychosocial, and spiritual needs by using the approaches listed on the care plan.

RESTORATIVE CARE

Restorative care is care given to help each resident become as independent as possible, considering the limitations of his or her medical condition. Restorative care is highly individualized based on each resident's strengths and needs. When providing restorative care, we look at the whole person, not just the disease or diagnosis. The goal of this type of care is to help residents function at the highest level possible. This includes physical function, mental function, and psychosocial well-being. The care plan will guide you on what restorative measures to take and how to do them. Maintain a restorative attitude by believing that restorative approaches will help residents. Maintaining a restorative attitude takes patience. It takes time for residents to learn new skills. Even learning new ways to do previously learned skills does not happen immediately. Patience and a consistent approach from all caregivers will help residents learn new skills and regain abilities lost due to illness or injury. Doing things for residents that they can do for themselves does not help. Over time, residents lose the ability to perform certain activities if they do not practice them consistently. The nursing assistant's role here is to offer support and encouragement, and allow enough time for the resident to complete tasks independently. If the resident is having difficulty, suggest easier ways of doing the task. If you are not sure, consult the care plan or the nurse. Over the long term, providing restorative care is very beneficial to residents physically and helps them develop healthy self-esteem.

BODY SYSTEMS

The human body is made up of tiny cells. Similar cells group together to form organs. Similar organs group together to form systems. There are 10 body systems:

- integumentary system
- skeletal system

- muscular system
- endocrine system
- reproductive system
- digestive system
- cardiovascular (circulatory) system
- respiratory system
- urinary system
- nervous system

All systems must function normally for the person to be healthy. One might think that if one system was weak, the other, stronger systems, would make up for it. In fact, the reverse is true. One weak system will affect the resident's entire body and state of health.

NORMAL AGING PROCESS

Because many residents in a long-term care facility are elderly, having a general understanding of the normal aging process is important. All nursing care is given to help residents reach their highest state of health, well-being, and independence. When in good **health,** the body functions properly. In **disease,** the body is not functioning as it should.

Body Systems and Normal Aging

All parts of the body are affected by the normal aging process. When studying the body, we look at it as a group of systems that work together. A body system is a group of organs working together to do a particular job. A brief overview of body systems and how the aging process affects each follows.

Integumentary system.   The integumentary system includes the skin, hair, and nails. Sweat and oil glands are part of the exocrine glands.

- Changes in normal aging:
  - Skin becomes fragile, tears easily, and loses fatty tissue under skin.
  - Hair thins and grays.
  - Nails thicken and harden.
  - Less natural oil and sweat are produced.
  - Circulation to the skin decreases.

- Results of normal aging:
  - Skin is less sensitive to heat.
  - Skin is less resistant to injury.
  - Skin bruises and tears more readily.
  - Skin becomes drier.
  - Tissues heal slowly.

  - Changes in skin and other systems make body regulation of temperature more difficult. Elderly persons often complain of feeling cold.

- Nursing assistant responsibilities:
  - Protect residents' skin from injury by padding side rails, arms of chairs, and so on. Long-sleeved clothing also helps protect the skin.
  - Keep residents' skin clean, dry, and free from secretions and excretions.
  - Use lotions as needed to keep skin supple.
  - Report any injuries or changes in the appearance of the skin to the nurse.
  - Know your facility policy for providing nail care. Some facilities do not allow nursing assistants to trim nails. Most facilities require nursing assistants to clean nails, but some do not allow the use of sharp objects, such as nail files.
  - Prevent pressure ulcers from developing.

Skeletal system.   The skeletal system includes the bones and joints.

- Changes in normal aging:
  - Bones become porous and brittle.
  - The spine becomes less flexible and stable, and is more easily injured.
  - Joints become less flexible.

- Results of normal aging:
  - Fractures occur easily.
  - Loss of height occurs.

- Nursing assistant responsibilities:
  - Monitor the resident's nutrition to be sure that the diet is balanced.
  - Provide a safe environment to prevent injury.
  - Assist the resident to use devices to make ambulation easier, if ordered.

Muscular system.
- Changes in normal aging:
  - Muscles lose strength and bulk.
  - Ligaments become less flexible.

- Results of normal aging:
  - Slower movements.
  - Less strength.
  - Posture may become stooped.

- Nursing assistant responsibilities:
  - Help the resident exercise to prevent contractures, or deformities of the joints.
  - Perform range-of-motion exercises as directed by the care plan.
  - Be patient with residents. Avoid completing tasks for residents just to save time.

Endocrine system.

- Changes in normal aging:
  - Production of estrogen, progesterone, and testosterone decreases.
  - Insulin production becomes less efficient.

- Results of normal aging:
  - Weight gain.
  - Diabetes mellitus.

- Nursing assistant responsibilities:
  - Monitor the resident for signs and symptoms of diabetes mellitus.
  - If the resident is diabetic, monitor for signs and symptoms of hyperglycemia and hypoglycemia.
  - Monitor weight monthly, or as stated on the care plan.

Reproductive system.

- Changes in normal aging:
  Females:
  - Ovulation and menstruation cease.
  - Vaginal walls become thinner and drier.

  Males:
  - Scrotum enlarges and becomes less firm.
  - Prostate gland may enlarge.

- Results of normal aging:
  Females:
  - Increased risk of injury and infection.

  Males:
  - Difficulty with urination.

- Nursing assistant responsibilities:
  - Assist with cleanliness and personal hygiene by providing proper perineal care.
  - Monitor for signs and symptoms of infection, and report to the nurse.

  - In males, monitor for urinary dribbling, urine retention, difficulty with starting flow of urine, and frequency of urination.

Digestive system. The digestive system includes the stomach, intestines, and other organs that help digest food.

- Changes in normal aging:
  - Digestive system gradually slows.
  - Appetite decreases.
  - Sense of thirst decreases.
  - Chewing ability often decreases due to loss of teeth and dental problems.
  - Loss of primary tastebuds of sweet and salt.

- Results of normal aging:
  - Constipation may occur.
  - Residents may consume less food and not take in enough nutrients and fluids in the diet.
  - Residents may increase condiment use at meals.

- Nursing assistant responsibilities:
  - Monitor residents' bowel movements and record them according to facility policy.
  - Report signs of constipation to the nurse.
  - Report dental caries and unusual mouth odors.
  - Check dentures for proper fit.
  - Season food according to resident preference and diet order.
  - Monitor resident food intake and record it according to facility policy.
  - Offer substitutes if residents do not eat food items on their trays.
  - Eliminate unpleasant sights, odors, and sounds when residents are eating.
  - Make mealtime pleasant and encourage residents to eat. Help them if necessary.
  - Report to the nurse if the resident eats less than 75 percent of a meal.
  - Report changes in weight to the nurse.
  - Pass snacks and supplements; assist and encourage residents to consume them, and record the percentage.

Cardiovascular system. The cardiovascular system includes the heart and blood vessels. The circulatory system is composed of the blood vessels. The immune system is part of the circulatory system.

- Changes in normal aging:

  — Cardiac output is reduced.

  — Blood vessels become less elastic.

  — Inner walls of blood vessels become narrow.

  — Heart disease is common in the elderly.

  — The immune system weakens with age.

- Results of normal aging:

  — Residents may need to rest more frequently.

  — Exercise is necessary to stimulate circulation.

  — Blood pressure may be elevated.

  — Heart rate decreases.

  — Fluid may collect in tissues, especially in the lower legs and feet.

  — Elderly and chronically ill residents are at increased risk of infection.

- Nursing assistant responsibilities:

  — Monitor vital signs as instructed by the nurse.

  — Report blue color of the skin immediately, especially in the lips and nailbeds.

  — Report swollen areas to the nurse.

  — Provide adequate rest periods between activities.

  — Help and encourage the resident to exercise in the manner stated on the care plan.

  — Follow facility policies and practices to prevent the spread of infection.

Respiratory system. The respiratory system includes the lungs and air passages.

- Changes in normal aging:

  — Exchange of oxygen and carbon dioxide decreases.

  — Lungs lose some elasticity.

  — Breathing capacity decreases.

  — Deep breathing becomes more difficult.

- Results of normal aging:

  — Respiratory infections are more likely.

  — Respiratory changes may make an elderly person more tired.

- Nursing assistant responsibilities:

  — Report difficulty breathing to the nurse immediately.

  — Know positions that promote good air exchange.

  — Monitor for and report shortness of breath on exertion.

  — Encourage residents to breathe deeply.

Urinary system. The urinary system includes the kidneys and bladder. Common words for the elimination process performed by this system are *urination* or *voiding*.

- Changes in normal aging:

  — Kidney function is reduced.

  — Bladder elasticity decreases.

  — Men often have prostate enlargement.

- Results of normal aging:

  — Bladder emptying is less efficient.

  — More urinary infections occur.

  — Need to empty the bladder is often urgent and frequent.

  — Coughing and sneezing may cause women to be unable to control urine passage.

  — Men may have trouble urinating.

- Nursing assistant responsibilities:

  — Report changes in color, consistency, amount, and odor of urine.

  — Report painful or burning urination.

  — Toilet residents according to the schedule on the care plan.

  — In mentally confused residents, monitor behavior for clues of the need to toilet.

  — Do not scold residents if accidents occur.

  — Keep residents clean, dry, and odor-free.

  — Assist with bowel and bladder evaluations and programs.

Central nervous system. The central nervous system includes the brain and spinal cord. The nervous system involves nerve endings.

- Changes in normal aging:

  — Nerve cells are lost.

  — Reaction time to stimuli becomes slower.

  — Blood flow to the brain decreases.

  — Diseases of these systems may cause physical or mental disability.

- Results of normal aging:

  — More time is needed when caring for many elderly residents.

  — Residents may need more time to make choices.

- Nursing assistant responsibilities:

  — Keep the environment safe and free from hazards.

  — Know seizure precautions to follow.

  — Monitor water temperature with a thermometer before bathing a resident.

  — Be patient and allow the resident adequate time to perform activities.

The senses. The eyes, ears, nose, and tastebuds of the mouth are part of the sensory system.

- Changes in normal aging:

  — All senses gradually slow down.

  — Vision and hearing acuity decreases.

- Results of normal aging:

  — Vision, hearing, and agility are reduced.

  — Irritations on skin and feet may go unnoticed due to less sensation or feeling.

- Nursing assistant responsibilities:

  — Know how to communicate with residents who have vision and hearing impairments.

  — Be patient and allow enough time for residents to answer questions.

  — Keep the environment safe and hazard-free.

  — Report observations about resident skin condition to the nurse.

Becoming aware of these normal changes in the aging process is important. The changes that occur in these body systems will affect the manner of care needed for each resident. For your convenience, aging changes are summarized in Table 1-1.

TABLE 1-1 Aging Changes

Body System	Aging Changes
Circulatory	■ Heart rate slows, causing a slower pulse and less efficient circulation. Residents have less energy and slower responses. They tire easily. ■ Blood vessels lose elasticity and develop calcium deposits, causing vessels to narrow. ■ Blood pressure increases because of changes to the blood vessel walls. ■ Heart rate takes longer to return to normal after exercise. ■ Veins enlarge, causing blood vessels close to the skin surface to become more prominent. ■ Immune system weakens; susceptibility to infection increases.
Respiratory	■ Lung capacity decreases as a result of muscular rigidity in the lungs. ■ The ability to cough effectively is reduced; this results in pooling of secretions and fluid in the lungs, increasing the risk of infection and choking. ■ Shortness of breath on exertion as a result of aging changes in lungs. ■ Gas exchange in the lungs is less effective, resulting in decreased oxygenation.
Integumentary	■ Skin thins and loses elasticity; wrinkles appear; skin becomes irritated and breaks, cuts, and tears easily. ■ Increased fragility of blood vessels that nourish the skin causes bruising, senile purpura, and skin tears. ■ Reduced blood flow in vessels that nourish the skin results in delayed healing. ■ Reduced secretion from oil glands that supply the skin causes dryness and itching. ■ Decreased perspiration results in impaired ability to regulate temperature. ■ Subcutaneous fat diminishes, resulting in less protection and increased sensitivity to cold. ■ Blood supply to the feet and legs is reduced, increasing risk of injury and ulcers, feeling of coldness. ■ Fingernail and toenail growth slows and nails become brittle. ■ Hair thins and turns gray.

(continues)

Urinary	■ Bladder capacity decreases, increasing the frequency of urination.
	■ Kidney function increases at rest, causing increased urination at night.
	■ Weakening of bladder muscles, causing leaking of urine or inability to empty the bladder completely.
	■ Enlargement of the prostate gland in the male, causing frequency of urination, dribbling, urinary obstruction, and urinary retention.
Digestive (Gastrointestinal)	■ Saliva production in the mouth decreases, causing difficulty with digestion of starches.
	■ Tastebuds on the tongue decrease, beginning with sweet and salt; changes in tastebuds may result in appetite changes and increase in condiment use.
	■ Gag reflex is less effective, increasing the risk of choking.
	■ Movement of food into the stomach through the esophagus is slower.
	■ Digestion of food in the stomach slows, so food remains there longer before moving to the small intestine.
	■ Indigestion and slower absorption of fat is caused by decreased digestive enzymes.
	■ Food movement through the large intestine is slower, resulting in constipation.
Endocrine	■ Delayed release of insulin increases blood sugar level; incidence of diabetes increases greatly with age.
	■ Metabolism rate and body function slow, reducing the amount of calories needed for the body to function normally. This increases the risk of overweight and obesity.
Reproductive	Changes in the Male
	■ Hormone production decreases, decreasing size of testes and lowering sperm count.
	■ More time is required for an erection.
	Changes in the Female
	■ Fewer female hormones are produced.
	■ Vagina becomes shorter and narrower.
	■ Vaginal secretions decrease.
	■ Breast tissue decreases and the muscles supporting the breasts weaken.
Nervous	■ Tasks involving speed, balance, coordination, and fine motor activities take longer because of slowed transmission of nerve impulses.
	■ Balance and coordination problems result from deterioration in the nerve terminals that provide information to the brain about body movement and position.
	■ Visual changes result from decreased flexibility in the lens in the eye.
	■ Dryness and itching of the eyes result from decreased secretion of fluids.
	■ Difficulty hearing is due to a decrease in the nerves and blood supply to the ears.
	■ Risk of injury increases because of decreased ability to feel pressure and temperature changes.
	■ Decreased blood flow to the brain may result in mental confusion and memory loss.
Muscular	■ Loss of elasticity of muscles and decrease in size of muscle mass result in reduced strength, endurance, muscle tone, and delayed reaction time.
	■ Decreased strength, stamina, endurance, reaction time, and coordination.
	■ Poor posture, including leaning forward or slumping over because of weakness in back muscles. This changes the center of gravity, increasing the risk of falls.
	■ Bones lose minerals, become brittle, porous, and break more easily.
	■ Spine becomes less stable and flexible, increasing the risk of injury.
	■ Degenerative changes in the joints cause limited movement, stiffness, and pain.
Skeletal	■ Loss of height, spinal curvature may develop or worsen.
	■ Intervertebral disks shrink, increasing pain and risk of injury and reducing flexibility of spine.

Generalizations Relating to Normal Aging

You have already learned that each resident is an individual. However, some general statements are true about normal aging:

- All body systems are affected.
- Resistance to injury and disease decreases.

- People age at different rates.
- All body systems gradually slow down.
- The aging process is affected by lifestyle, heredity, and nutrition; mental, physical, and emotional health; and attitude.

KEY POINTS IN THIS CHAPTER

▲ The nursing assistant provides personal care while working under the supervision of a nurse.

▲ The person living in a long-term care facility is a resident.

▲ A nursing assistant is part of the nursing service team.

▲ Good health, honesty, dependability, and sincere desire to work with people are required qualities of a nursing assistant.

▲ The job description is a list of tasks and duties you are expected to perform as a nursing assistant.

▲ Your assignment is made by the nurse and may include working with any resident, male or female.

▲ Cooperation with all members of the health care team is an important part of your role.

▲ The care plan is a written plan that describes strengths, weaknesses, interventions, and goals for each resident and directs resident care.

▲ Each resident is an individual and must be treated with respect and dignity.

▲ All body systems gradually slow down.

REVIEW QUIZ

1. Nursing assistants may also be called:
   a. practical nurses.
   b. nurse aides.
   c. nurse helpers.
   d. registered nurses.

2. Persons who live in long-term care facilities are called:
   a. clients.   c. residents.
   b. patients.   d. retired.

3. Which term means care of the elderly?
   a. resident   c. nursing
   b. medical   d. geriatrics

4. Who is the nursing assistant's supervisor?
   a. licensed nurse   c. administrator
   b. physician   d. therapist

5. Which department in the long-term care facility is the nursing assistant a part of?
   a. administration   c. dietary
   b. nursing   d. housekeeping

6. Which of the following qualifications are necessary for the nursing assistant?
   a. excellent grades in college
   b. large and strong body
   c. being a female
   d. honesty and reliability

7. The responsibilities of a nursing assistant are listed in a:
   a. job description.
   b. policy manual.
   c. procedure manual.
   d. résumé.

8. Some tasks and duties a nursing assistant is expected to do include:
   a. taking doctors' orders.
   b. giving medications.
   c. helping residents with personal care.
   d. preparing and cooking meals.

9. Male and female nursing assistants:
   a. usually work on separate units of the facility.
   b. work with nursing assistants of the same sex.
   c. are expected to care for residents of either sex.
   d. care only for residents of the same sex as the nursing assistant.

10. Part of the uniform you will wear daily includes:
    a. a cap or hat.   c. sterile gloves.
    b. an isolation gown. d. a name tag.

11. What should you do if you are not certain about a task assigned to you?
    a. Ask the nurse for help.
    b. Ask another nursing assistant to do it.

c. Forget about doing the task.

d. Do the task anyway.

12. Which of the following are not members of the interdisciplinary team in the long-term care facility?

   a. nursing staff

   b. dietary personnel

   c. social workers

   d. hospital workers

13. A written plan listing strengths, needs, goals, interventions, and who is responsible for assisting with specific tasks in the care of the resident is the:

   a. assignment sheet.

   b. care plan.

   c. job description.

   d. team report.

14. Which of the following statements is true regarding the normal aging process?

   a. All body systems slow down with aging.

   b. All elderly residents age at the same rate.

   c. The nervous system is the only system that is visibly affected by aging.

   d. The reproductive system stops functioning with age.

15. Ethical behavior for the nursing assistant means to:

   a. practice good body mechanics.

   b. cooperate with others.

   c. know what is right and what is wrong.

   d. call the facility when ill.

16. Mrs. Huynh has asked for pain medication. The nurse is very busy. You should:

   a. offer to take the medication to Mrs. Huynh.

   b. inform the nurse that Mrs. Huynh is requesting pain medication.

   c. do nothing and tell the nurse later.

   d. tell Mrs. Huynh that the nurse is too busy to give her the medicine.

17. The nursing assistant who is assigned to care for Mr. Redman is off the unit on break. Mr. Redman's call signal is on. You should:

   a. ignore the signal.

   b. tell Mr. Redman that his assigned nursing assistant will do what he asks when she returns to the unit.

   c. answer the signal and find out what the resident wants.

   d. inform the nurse that Mr. Redman has his call signal on.

18. A resident speaks with you about a financial matter. She says that she does not want her son to know that she has money in a savings account at Capital Bank. You should:

   a. tell the resident's son about the account.

   b. tell the other nursing assistants about the bank account.

   c. advise the resident to tell her doctor about the account and ask for his advice.

   d. say nothing about the bank account.

19. Mrs. Burns tells you that you are her "favorite nursing assistant." At Christmas, she puts a $20 bill in your pocket and insists that you take it. You should:

   a. thank Mrs. Burns and accept the money.

   b. tell Mrs. Burns you will do special favors for her because of the gift.

   c. advise the resident that you cannot accept money from her and that you are happy to care for her without gifts.

   d. tell Mrs. Burns that you can only accept gifts from her family because facility policy prohibits you from accepting gifts from residents.

20. You are assigned to care for Mrs. Beattie. She is in a restorative care program so that she can return to her home when she recovers from her illness and becomes more independent. Her care plan states that she is to wash her face, hands, and chest, then the nursing assistant is to complete her bath. When you hand Mrs. Beattie the washcloth, she tells you that she will not bathe herself. The resident says, "I am paying you to take care of me, so you will do it." You should:

   a. tell the resident that you are not being paid specifically to bathe her.

   b. ask Mrs. Beattie why she feels this way, and tell her why it is important that she do as much of her own care as she can.

   c. begin to wash Mrs. Beattie's face, because this is what she wants.

   d. inform Mrs. Beattie that you are too busy to bathe her, and that you have others to care for who need your help more than she does.

21. Mr. McClure is a resident who yells and complains frequently. He tells you that he will "have you fired" if you do not give him extra sugar packets for his coffee. Mr. McClure is on a diabetic diet. You know that sugar is not allowed on a diabetic diet. You should:

   a. tell the resident that the sugar is not allowed on his diet and that he has no right to threaten you.

   b. give Mr. McClure as much sugar as he wants because you need your job.

   c. offer Mr. McClure a sugar substitute, then notify the nurse of his threats.

   d. pretend that you don't hear Mr. McClure ask for more sugar and leave the room quickly.

CHAPTER 1
CROSSWORD PUZZLE

Directions: Complete the puzzle using these words found in Chapter 1.

acute	dignity	OBRA
attitude	disease	patient
care	ethics	plan
charge	geriatrics	privacy
client	health	resident
dependability	interdisciplinary	restorative
description	negligence	theft

CHAPTER 1
PUZZLE CLUES

ACROSS

1. Exposing the resident's body when giving care is a form of invasion of _____ .
4. Carelessness, failing to give care in the way you were taught.
7. Taking something that does not belong to you.
9. Your _____ is an outer reflection of your inner feelings.
11. _____ care is designed to help residents reach the highest possible level of functioning.
13. Care of the elderly is also known as _____ .
15. A listing of the nursing assistant's responsibilities can be found in the job _____ .
18. The person being cared for in a long-term care facility.
19. Being trustworthy, able to be relied upon.
20. _____ means treating a person with respect and honor.

DOWN

1. The person being cared for in the hospital.
2. Instructions for taking care of the resident are usually found on the care _____ .
3. Freedom from disease; wellness.
5. The _____ team meets to plan the care of the resident based on an assessment of strengths and needs.
6. The person being cared for in the home is usually called the _____ .
8. Your immediate supervisor is usually the _____ nurse.
10. A state of illness when the body does not function properly.
12. Omnibus Budget Reconciliation Act.
14. A hospital is an example of an _____ care facility.
16. The nursing assistant is responsible for helping the resident with personal _____ .
17. Principles, values, rules of moral, responsible conduct.

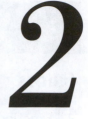

Basic Human Needs

OBJECTIVES

In this chapter you will learn the importance of basic human needs and ways you can help residents meet these needs. After reading this chapter, you will be able to:

- Spell and define key terms.
- Describe basic needs common to all people and list ways to assist residents in meeting their needs.
- Identify developmental tasks associated with the aging process.
- Explain why understanding the resident's culture is important to the nursing assistant.
- List the steps of the grieving process and describe what occurs in each step.
- Identify coping mechanisms for grief and loss.
- Describe changes that occur when a resident is dying and list nursing assistant responsibilities.
- Demonstrate postmortem care.

KEY TERMS

acceptance: the final stage in the grieving process, in which the resident is calmly waiting for death

anger: the second step in the grieving process, in which the resident is angry because of a terminal diagnosis

apathy: indifference, emptiness, lack of feeling or emotion

bargaining: the third stage in the grieving process, in which the resident attempts to buy more time

coping mechanisms: responses to stress that people use to protect feelings of self-esteem

culture: a pattern or lifestyle of a group of people

denial: refusing to accept something as the truth; also, the first stage in the grieving process, in which the resident refuses to believe the terminal diagnosis

depression: the fourth stage in the grieving process, in which the resident is very sad and is trying to deal with the loss of everything he or she has

developmental tasks: tasks that must be accomplished in each stage of life if a person is to mature in a healthy manner

grieving process: stages of grief that a dying person, family members, and others go through to move to a point of acceptance of illness and death

personal space: a comfortable distance for communication

physiological needs: physical human needs

postmortem care: care of the body after death

psychological needs (psychosocial needs): the emotional, spiritual, and mental needs of human beings

religion: a formal system of beliefs, including ceremonies and rituals that demonstrate faith

self-actualization: the state of having achieved one's full potential or ability

self-esteem: satisfaction with oneself

spiritual needs: needs concerning one's spiritual or religious beliefs

spirituality: any way that people answer the desire to be connected with the entirety or wholeness of life

stereotyping: placing all members of a group into one category and believing they are all alike

therapeutic: curing, healing, or preserving health

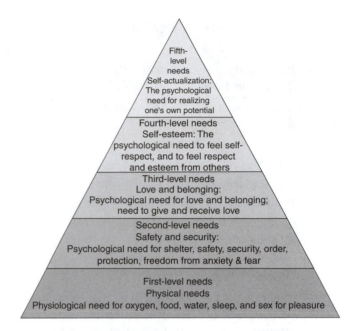

Figure 2-2 Maslow's hierarchy of needs

HUMAN NEEDS

All people have the same basic human needs, despite their age, sex, position, or status in life. Some needs, however, come first and must be satisfied before other needs become important. For example, breathing is more important than eating, although both are necessary to live. When our physical needs are met, we move up to higher levels of needs, such as safety and security, and love and belonging (Figure 2-1).

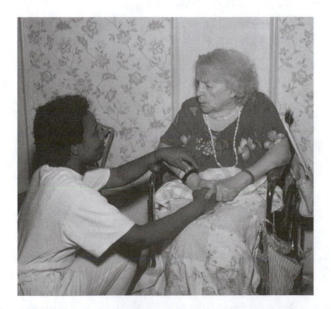

Figure 2-1 Showing sincere concern for residents is an important trait.

These basic needs are what cause people to behave as they do (Figure 2-2).

Knowledge of basic human needs will help you understand and give better care to residents. The resident who is always calling for attention may need to feel a sense of love and belonging. Many residents in the long-term care facility must have help to meet their needs.

Basic human needs can be grouped into two categories: physical and psychological. Physical needs are called **physiological.** These needs concern the body and are necessary for survival.

Other needs involve the emotional, spiritual, or mental relationships of humans. The terms to describe this emotional type of need are **psychological** or **psychosocial.**

All the basic human needs are equally important. These needs must be at least partially met for a person to be healthy. Learning about ways to meet these needs will help you give quality care to each resident. People from different countries and cultures may have different needs and customs. Be sensitive to these differences.

Physical Needs and Ways to Help Residents Meet These Needs

Assist residents to meet physical needs as follows:

- Food

  — Provide adequate lighting and a clean area before serving the meal tray. Eliminate unpleasant sights and odors.

— Make mealtime as pleasant as possible.

— Help the resident eat, if needed.

— Position the resident correctly to enable swallowing and prevent choking.

— Thicken liquids as described in the care plan.

— Help the resident with special foods.

— Feed the resident when necessary.

— Provide special utensils if the resident needs them.

— Give the resident oral hygiene before and after meals.

— Assist the resident to use the toilet before and after meals.

— Position the resident close to the table so he or she does not have to reach for food. The elbows should not be dangling in the air; they should be supported when eating, if this is the resident's preference.

— Ensure that the table height is correct, and not too high for the resident.

- Oxygen, air

    — Elevate the head of the bed for residents who have breathing problems.

    — Properly position residents in bed and chairs.

    — Make sure clothing or other garments are not too tight.

    — Assist with oxygen therapy when necessary. Check the flow meter for accuracy each time you are in the room.

    — Know how to perform the Heimlich maneuver.

- Water

    — Offer fluids frequently, especially in hot weather.

    — Keep fresh water within reach at all times.

    — Thicken liquids as described in the care plan.

    — Help the resident drink, if needed.

    — Monitor intake and output, if ordered.

- Elimination, toileting

    — Assist residents with toileting needs.

    — Provide privacy during elimination.

    — Be calm and unemotional in your response to residents who are unable to control the passage of urine or stool.

    — Assist residents with personal hygiene needs after elimination.

- Rest

    — Help with bedtime and sleep preparation.

    — Let the resident determine bedtime and routines before going to sleep.

    — Recognize any changes in sleep patterns.

    — Allow the resident to rest during the day, if desired.

- Activity and exercise

    — Encourage range-of-motion exercise during routine care and activities of daily living (ADLs).

    — Ambulate, transfer, and move residents properly.

    — Help residents to ambulate, walk, or exercise frequently as indicated on the care plan.

    — Assist residents to participate in activities of choice.

    — Remind residents of scheduled activities, plan care around them, and assist residents to activities if needed.

    — Encourage residents to be as independent as possible, as consistent with the care plan.

- Stimulation

    — Encourage involvement in facility activities.

    — Take time to listen to residents and encourage them to talk and visit.

    — Place residents in areas where they can observe activity.

    — Do not isolate residents.

    — When seating residents, arrange seating to promote socialization.

- Sexuality

    — Assist residents with hygiene, cleanliness, and grooming.

    — Encourage the use of appropriate clothing, cosmetics, and hairstyles to maintain sexual identity (Figure 2-3).

    — Compliment the resident on his or her appearance.

    — Provide privacy to couples expressing intimacy needs. Knock before entering rooms.

    — If a resident is masturbating, respond in a neutral manner. Take the resident to his or her room and provide privacy. Be nonjudgmental, and do not make the resident feel guilty or foolish. Remember, all humans need sexual satisfaction.

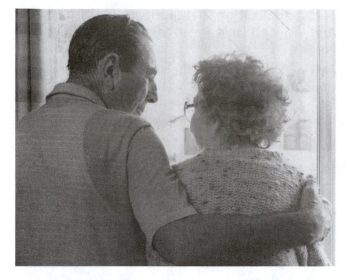

Figure 2-3 Sexuality is expressed by attractive appearance and touch. The ability to express sexuality is important to residents of all ages.

Safety and Security Needs and Ways to Help Residents Meet These Needs

Ways to help residents meet their safety and security needs are as follows:

- Safety

  — Keep the area safe and free of hazards.

  — Keep the call signal and needed personal items within reach of all residents, even those who are mentally confused.

  — Perform your job duties in the manner in which you were taught.

  — If you are unsure of how to perform a task, consult your supervisor and the facility procedure manual.

  — Know which tasks you legally can do.

  — Use lifting aids and transfer belts when indicated.

  — Follow your facility policy and residents' care plans for use of side rails and restraints.

  — Always be alert to safety. Think safety first when you enter a resident's room and last when you leave the room.

- Security

  — Respect residents' belongings and handle them with care.

  — Help residents adjust to new surroundings, other residents, and staff.

  — Reassure residents, providing physical and mental support.

  — Welcome family and friends.

  — Provide privacy. Knock on doors and wait for response before entering the room.

  — Maintain confidentiality when residents tell you something.

  — Keep the environment safe and hazard-free.

  — Make residents feel confident in your ability to do your job.

  — Keep residents' belongings safe.

Love and Belonging Needs and Ways to Help Residents Meet These Needs

You can help residents satisfy the needs for love and belonging in these ways:

- Caring about someone

  — Listen to the resident, and do not appear rushed. Encourage residents to talk of the past when appropriate.

  — Show interest in residents' family and experiences.

  — Encourage contact and visits with other residents.

  — Ask the nurse or social worker for information about the resident's past, if this information will help you care for the resident.

  — Realize that some residents may have close friends who are not family members.

- Being cared about

  — Show interest in each resident.

  — Touch residents gently to show that you care.

  — Show kindness and consideration.

  — Be kind and friendly to visitors and family members.

  — Inform and encourage family and friends to attend activities.

  — Family members may be invited to participate in the care conference, with the resident's consent.

  — Be patient and understanding when interacting with residents.

  — Treat residents as you would like your family members to be treated.

  — Allow residents to cry if needed. Offer to stay with the resident. Offer support. Occasional crying is a way to relieve built-up stress, but frequent crying may indicate a serious problem that should be reported.

  — Provide a comfortable, homelike environment.

  — Place residents' personal items in a prominent place in their rooms.

Self-Esteem and Ways to Help Residents Meet This Need

Residents' **self-esteem** is enhanced when the nursing assistant understands the following:

- Sense of identity and self-esteem

  - Call each resident by the preferred name. If you are unsure, use Mr., Mrs., or Miss.
  - Include residents in conversations and decisions about care.
  - Speak with residents when providing care.
  - Show an interest in residents' past and present activities.
  - Allow privacy when requested. Knock on doors and wait for a response before entering.
  - Allow choices whenever possible, and give residents what is requested, in keeping with the care plan.
  - If a resident's choice is against the care plan, inform the nurse.
  - Respect each resident's choice of clothing if it is appropriate and clean.
  - Respect individual differences in culture, heredity, interests, religion, and values.
  - Offer residents as much control as possible over their personal space.
  - Allow residents control over daily routines.

- Feeling important and worthwhile

  - Recognize residents' accomplishments and give praise freely.
  - Always acknowledge a resident's presence. Include the resident in your conversation with others in the room.
  - Respect each resident's property and personal items.
  - Treat residents as adults.
  - Encourage independence as much as possible.
  - Allow residents to do as much as possible.
  - Show interest in family members and past accomplishments and experiences.
  - Be courteous to family members and encourage their continued involvement and visits.
  - Treat residents with dignity and respect.
  - Develop communication skills for vision- and hearing-impaired residents.

Self-Actualization, Religion, and Spirituality, and Ways to Help Residents Meet These Needs

Self-actualization is the state of having reached one's highest potential or ability in life. It is also a feeling of being satisfied with oneself.

Assist residents to meet these needs as follows:

- Self-actualization

  - Look for each resident's strengths, and offer sincere praise.
  - Support hobbies, interests, and awareness of current events.
  - Encourage and praise accomplishments.
  - Take time to appreciate each resident's history.

- Spirituality and Religion

  - Listen to residents' concerns.
  - Respect residents' religious beliefs (Figure 2-4).
  - Do not try to impose your religious beliefs on residents.
  - Respect the resident's choice if she chooses not to participate in religious activities.
  - Plan care so that residents can be involved in religious activities.
  - Provide privacy when clergy are visiting.
  - Respect and handle religious symbols, pictures, or other objects with care.

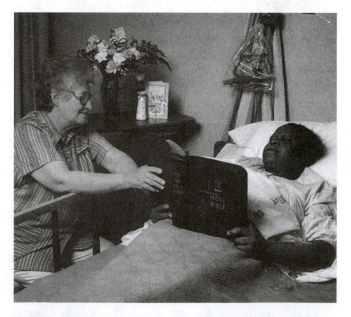

Figure 2-4 Respecting the resident's spiritual needs is an important responsibility. Spiritual needs may be greater when residents are ill.

— If the resident asks to see a member of the clergy, refer the request to the nurse.

— Provide for religious and **spiritual needs** and customs.

CULTURAL INFLUENCES ON HEALTH CARE DELIVERY

You will care for residents from many different **cultures.** A culture is a pattern or lifestyle of a group of people. Residents may come from other countries or communities. Their beliefs, values, religion, and health care and hygienic practices may be different from your own. View this as an opportunity to learn more about others. Learn as much as you can about residents' cultures. This will help you to meet their needs. Avoid **stereotyping** residents. Stereotyping means placing all members of a group into a certain category, believing they are all alike. Treat all residents as individuals, and recognize their individuality.

Culture may influence a resident's beliefs about illness and care. The best way to find out about someone's beliefs is to ask. Asking is not offensive. It shows that you want to learn, and are trying to find ways of helping the resident.

Cultural Influences on Personal Space

Personal space is a comfortable distance for communication. The preferred distance between parties varies with the culture. In the United States, a comfortable distance is about 18 to 36 inches. Residents from other cultures may be uncomfortable with this distance. Their personal space may be closer or farther away. Be sensitive to residents' needs. If they appear uncomfortable when you are close to them, move back.

People from some cultures will not permit members of the opposite sex to care for them. Saudi Arabians, for example, will not permit a male caregiver to enter the room if a female resident is alone. If you encounter this situation, consult the nurse. Avoid offending the resident.

Gestures and Eye Contact

People in the United States make eye contact when speaking. They also use gestures. In some cultures, making eye contact and using gestures are offensive. In some countries, gestures have different meanings than they do in the United States. For example, we nod the head to indicate yes and no. In India, the head motions are the opposite of those in the United States. Thus, nodding the head up and down means no. Shaking the head from side to side means yes. Monitor your body language, gestures, and eye contact carefully. If your body language makes the resident uncomfortable, avoid doing it.

Cultural Influences on Pain

Residents from other cultures may react differently to pain. In some cultures, residents are very emotional. They may cry, scream, and have dramatic reactions. In others, the resident will show no response, despite having severe pain. In some cultures, displaying pain is a sign of weakness.

Cultural Influences on Personal Hygiene

In the United States, it is normal to bathe and use deodorant daily. Women remove hair from their legs and underarms. Some cultures have different customs. They do not bathe regularly or use deodorant. Some women do not remove body hair. This may be a difficult problem for you to deal with. Do not be offended if the resident's hygiene is different from your own. Consult the care plan for instructions in caring for the resident. If you are having problems accepting cultural differences, speak with the nurse or social worker. Table 2-1 lists various cultural preferences for activities of daily living and health practices.

Cultural Influences on Clothing

In some cultures, certain garments have cultural or religious significance. Men may cover their heads. In other cultures, women keep their heads covered. Women in some cultures may not show any skin besides the face and/or hands. The resident may be very uncomfortable during bathing, or while in bed, wearing only a gown. Learn all you can about the resident's culture. Make accommodations that show you care.

Cultural Influence on Health Practices

People in some cultures believe that certain home remedies will cure their illness. Residents may believe in using wraps, rubs, teas, inhaled herbs and spices, or other folk remedies. Friends and family members may practice these remedies on residents. Some may interfere with the resident's treatment. Consult the nurse if you are unfamiliar with a cultural practice.

Cultural Influence on Choice of Food

Residents may refuse to eat certain foods because of their beliefs. Some residents believe that eating certain foods will heal their illness. Residents may refuse certain foods or food combinations because of their religious beliefs. In some religions, people fast and do not eat on certain days. Consult the nurse if a resident does not eat. The nurse may be able to make arrangements for a substitute that the resident will accept.

Language Barriers

Speak English when addressing residents. Speak slowly and gently. Show respect for the resident. If

TABLE 2-1 Culture and Personal Hygiene Preferences

Culture	Hygienic Practices/ADLs	Clothing/Jewelry	Self-Care
American Indian	Very modest. May not cut hair except for certain health practices when mourning. May save hair clippings. Some tribes do not permit outsiders to touch the hair. May perform ritualistic washing. Navajo may save fingernail clippings.	Avoid touching a medicine bag. Ask resident or family to remove it, if medically necessary. If removed, always keep it in plain sight.	Self-care is expected to the extent the resident is able. Family may participate in care.
Arab American	Very modest. Most bathe daily. Some women believe bathing during menses is harmful. Some avoid bathing when ill, believing it will interfere with their recovery. May believe that washing hair causes colds. Most females wash perineum with water after toileting.	Keep the resident's body covered as much as possible. Prefer long sleeves. Women wear long dresses and pants. Keep body covered when members of opposite sex are present. Many women cover the head with scarves. Some wear blue beads or amulets. These protect them from the evil eye. Some wear amulets when ill.	May expect families and health care workers to care for them, particularly during illness.
Central American	Very modest. Women cover legs. Women may prefer caregiver and physician of the same sex. Some bathe daily, others do not. Some women keep their heads covered. Mayan women may braid hair. Some may resist using urinal or bedpan.	Crosses, rosary beads, and other religious items may be important. Some wear red earrings to protect them from the evil eye. They believe that red is a protective color. May wear a bag of herbs around the neck. Avoid removing it, if possible.	Expect others to care for them during times of illness.
Chinese American	Very modest. Women usually prefer a caregiver of same sex. This culture has very high personal hygiene standards. Bathe daily. They may avoid washing hair when ill. Some may resist using urinal or bedpan.	Believe that wearing jade and some other articles brings them good luck and health. Avoid removing these items, if possible.	Most prefer to complete their own ADLs. Older men may expect family or staff to care for them.
Colombian	Very modest. Usually request a caregiver of same sex. This culture has very high personal hygiene standards. Bathe daily. Women may remove leg and underarm hair daily. Men shave daily.	May wear rosary beads, crosses, or religious items.	May expect family or staff to care for them when ill.

(continues)

Cuban	Very modest. Females will accept a male caregiver, but prefer caregiver of same sex. This culture has very high personal hygiene standards. Bathe and shampoo daily. May shampoo less often if ill. Women may avoid washing hair during menses. Some may resist using urinal or bedpan. Women may prefer peri care with soap and water after toileting.	May wear rosary beads, crosses, or religious items.	May expect family or staff to care for them when ill. Female family members may prefer to perform ADLs for the resident.
Filipino	Very modest. This culture has very high personal hygiene standards. Bathe and shampoo daily. Females may prefer peri care with soap and water after toileting. Some may resist using urinal or bedpan.	May wear rosary beads, crosses, or religious items.	Most prefer to complete ADLs independently. Family members may assist.
Gypsy	Very modest. Strongly believe in separation of sexes and will resist a caregiver of the opposite sex. Very high personal hygiene standards. Gypsies must keep upper and lower body separate. They use a separate washcloth, towel, and soap for the upper and lower body. Shampoo daily. Keeping the head clean is symbolic, and is believed to help keep them pure. Often request a clean pillowcase daily. Avoid touching the head and pillowcase, if possible. May refuse to use the bedpan. Avoid touching the upper body with a bedpan.	Many keep an amulet under the pillow, or wear it around the neck. Avoid moving an amulet near the foot of the bed.	Most prefer self-care. If unable, usually prefers to have family members provide care.
Haitian	Very modest. Males may refuse to wear hospital gowns, insisting on keeping the lower body covered. May believe that physicians should be male and nurses female. Hold health care workers in high regard. Most shower daily. At bedtime, females perform peri care with soap and water. Men shampoo daily, women weekly. Women may wear rollers in hair at night. May refuse to use the bedpan or urinal. Many perform peri care with soap and water after toileting.	May wear rosary beads, crosses, or religious items. Some believe in and practice voodoo.	Will follow caregivers' instructions, but most prefer self-care for ADLs. If unable, family may perform ADLs. Family may request permission before assisting.

(continues)

Continued

Iranian	Modesty and hygiene vary with age and adherence to Iranian traditions. Usually very modest. May request a caregiver of same sex. May refuse to bathe when ill. Perform perineal care with water after each urination and bowel movement. May refuse to use the bedpan.	May wear a gold charm around the neck to symbolize Islam.	If ill, may refuse to perform self-care. Some are very resistant to any suggestion of self-care.
Japanese American	Very modest. Prefer a caregiver of same sex. This culture has very high personal hygiene standards. Bathe daily, and shampoo frequently. May request a tub bath in evening.	May wear special prayer beads.	Prefer self-care for ADLs. If unable, family members may assist. May resist caregiver assistance with ADLs.
Korean	Very modest. Men and women usually prefer to wear pants; both may prefer pajama bottoms at night. Elderly may wear thermal undergarments for warmth. This culture has very high personal hygiene standards. Bathe daily, and use many washcloths. Elderly women may shampoo once or twice weekly because of dryness in hair. May perform peri care after each elimination.	May wear rosary beads, crosses, or religious items. Usually wear little jewelry.	Many elderly believe that the family is responsible for performing ADLs. Family may not ask permission; they assume this is their responsibility.
Mexican American	Very modest. Women may prefer a caregiver of same sex. Most have high hygienic standards and bathe and shampoo daily. Female may refuse to use the bedpan due to beliefs about uncleanliness.	May wear rosary beads, crosses, or religious items.	Will perform own ADLs, if asked. Many prefer family or health care workers to perform ADLs. May believe that self-care hinders recovery.
Puerto Rican	Very modest. Most prefer to wear underwear at all times. Men prefer pajama bottoms. Most bathe and shampoo daily, but may refuse bathing during illness. May refuse bedpan; prefer using commode.	May wear amulet as protection against illness and injury. Avoid removing; may require priest to bless it or pray first. May wear crosses, rosary, or other religious items.	Prefer self-care for ADLs. If unable, may prefer family members to assist.

(continues)

Russian	Sex of care provider may not be an issue except for peri care. Some may refuse to bathe when ill; otherwise bathe daily. Avoids washing hair when ill. Will use bedpan, urinal, or commode. Elderly women may request warm or thermal clothing.	Some wear religious medallions, crosses, or pictures of saints.	Some will ask family of opposite sex to leave the room during personal care. May prefer to have nursing assistant or family perform ADLs when ill.
Samoan	Very modest. Prefer to dress in street clothing if out of bed. Women may refuse clothing that exposes the thighs. Shower and shampoo frequently, as often as three times daily. Some women may refuse shampoo during menses. Toileting is very private. May refuse to use bedpan or urinal.	Some wear rosary, cross, or other religious items.	Prefer self-care for ADLs. If unable, prefer to have family assist.
Vietnamese	Very modest. Most bathe daily. Some prefer peri care after each elimination. Believe that going to bed with wet hair causes headaches.	Catholics may wear crosses, rosary, or other religious items. Buddhists may light incense.	Prefer self-care for ADLs. If unable, may prefer family members of same sex to assist.
West Indian	Very modest about private areas of body. Exposing private parts to others is shameful and embarrassing. Avoids personal care by opposite sex. Bathes or showers once or twice daily. May prefer to perform peri care in the evening, instead of bathing. May refuse showers if ill. Shampoos weekly, due to dryness, although some individuals wash hair more frequently. Will use bedpan, urinal, or commode, but demands privacy. Very strict about handwashing after toileting.	May wear religious pin, cross, or picture of saint. Avoid removing them, if possible. Residents believe that these items protect them.	Prefers self-care, but will accept ADL care from staff member of same sex, if unable. May prefer that a family member perform ADL care.

the resident does not speak English, ask if he or she has a bilingual dictionary, or some other means of communication. If not, try writing or using gestures. Some residents can read English, although they cannot speak it. Keep each communication simple and clear. Drawing pictures may be useful. Before performing a procedure, demonstrate it. Always ask if the resident understands, or say "Okay?" A smile does not necessarily mean that the resident understands. Some people smile to be polite. Caring for a resident who does not speak English will take extra time.

SPIRITUALITY

Spirituality and religion are not the same thing. **Spirituality** is any way that people answer the desire to be connected with the largeness or wholeness of life. Aspects of spirituality include:

- a belief in the goodness of people
- caring for others, and a willingness to listen to others
- an awareness of an inner, reflective life

- attention to what provides balance in our lives and makes us feel whole
- a connection to what really matters to us in life, relationships, and work
- a sense of humor
- a connection with and an appreciation of nature
- a sense of hopefulness
- peace with oneself
- personal integrity

A resident's spirituality can help him or her through difficult times in life. Spirituality is personal and is expressed in different ways. Elderly residents use their spirituality to help them cope with living in a long-term care facility, facing illness and death, and coping with loss. You use your own spirituality when caring for residents in the long-term care facility. Supporting residents' spirituality is an important responsibility.

RELIGION

Religion is a formal system of beliefs, including ceremonies and rituals that demonstrate faith. Some religions have objects of religious significance, such as rosaries and crosses. Handle religious articles with care. Respect residents' beliefs, even if you disagree with them. Support residents' beliefs by allowing them to speak openly about these beliefs and practice them. Be a willing listener. Provide privacy during prayer and when members of the clergy are visiting.

DEVELOPMENTAL TASKS

Theorists suggest that as people mature from infancy to old age, they must pass through several stages. **Developmental tasks** that help you grow psychologically must be accomplished in each stage to help you mature and move to the next stage. Realize that this theory is general. People mature in many different ways.

An understanding of the normal adult developmental tasks will help you understand the residents for whom you care. The stages and developmental tasks of the adult are grouped into four categories: early adulthood, middle adulthood, late adulthood, and old age.

Early Adulthood—20 to 40 Years
The developmental tasks in this age group are:

- establishing personal and economic independence from parents
- developing a career

- making a commitment in a relationship
- establishing a family

Middle Adulthood—40 to 65 Years
The developmental tasks in this age group are:

- expanding personal and social involvement and responsibility
- adjusting to physiological changes of middle age
- reaching and maintaining satisfaction in one's career
- observing the maturation or growing of children

Late Adulthood—65 to 75 years
The developmental tasks in this age group are:

- adjusting to decreasing strength and stamina
- adjusting to aging changes in the body
- adjusting to losses
- adjusting to chronic medical problems
- adjusting to retirement income and financial concerns
- examination of one's lifetime and accepting one's past

Old Age—75 Years Until Death
The developmental tasks in this age group are:

- adjusting to declining physical health and increasing dependency on others
- realizing and accepting one's own mortality
- dealing with chronic illness and continued loss of friends and family

GRIEF AND LOSS

When a person anticipates or experiences a loss, he or she goes through the **grieving process.** This process was first described by Dr. Elisabeth Kübler-Ross. You probably have experienced the grieving process if you have lost a pet or moved to a new school. Imagine how much more difficult it is to lose a loved one. The grieving process involves five steps: denial, anger, bargaining, depression, and acceptance (Table 2-2). Because the grieving process varies for each of us, not all persons experience each step. Some people move from one stage to another and back again. Staff, friends, and family members also go through the grieving process. The steps are not always obvious to others. Sometimes we recognize the steps in other people, but fail to recognize them in ourselves.

TABLE 2-2   Stages of Grief

Denial	Resident refuses to accept the truth.
Anger	Resident may act out feelings, directing anger toward caregivers and family.
Bargaining	Resident attempts to "make deals" for more livable time.
Depression	Resident comes to full realization that situation cannot change and feels saddened over things that will be left unfinished.
Acceptance	Resident recognizes that death is part of the natural progression of life.

Completing all the steps in the process may take a very long time. The resident may die before completing the process. During the grieving process, be honest, reassuring, and understanding. Show the resident that you care. Helping a resident die in comfort and dignity is very important.

Denial

The first stage in the grieving process is **denial.** Denial begins when a person learns of the terminal diagnosis. The resident may believe that the diagnosis is wrong. She may display false hope and tell untrue stories. During this period, the resident may refuse to participate in her care, and may not follow the directions of the physician and nursing staff. The resident and family need strong emotional support during this stage. Allow them to talk about their feelings. Do not provide false hope. Spend time with the resident. Show her that she will not be left alone.

Anger

The second stage of the grieving process is **anger.** In this stage, the resident feels angry with herself, the family, staff, the doctor, and her higher power. She may be verbally abusive and refuse care and nutrition. The resident is not angry with you personally. She is angry with her situation. Practice empathy. Let the resident know that you care and that you understand how she feels.

Bargaining

The third stage of the grieving process is **bargaining.** The resident hopes she can live to see a special event, such as a graduation or the birth of a grandchild. The resident may bargain with her higher power. She may make promises, such as attending church every Sunday, in return for more time. The resident is trying to postpone the inevitable. This stage is usually short. Spend as much time as you can with the resident to show that you sincerely care. Listen to the resident. Do not deny what she says. Avoid providing false hope.

Depression

Depression is the fourth stage in the grieving process. During this stage, the resident is dealing with the loss of everything she has. Her physical ability may decline. She may also be feeling regret for things she has said or done in the past. The resident may experience **apathy.** This is an empty feeling. She may also have no interest in others or in the environment. The resident may have decreased concentration, sleeplessness, fatigue, frequent crying, and loss of appetite. During this stage, the resident begins to separate herself from life. Avoid trying to humor or cheer her. Allow her to express her feelings. Visit as often as you can. Sit quietly and provide support.

Acceptance

The final stage in the grieving process is **acceptance.** The resident may feel empty, but peaceful. She is quietly waiting for death. The emotional pain is usually less during this stage. The resident may not want to be alone. Make her comfortable and spend as much time with her as possible. If she does not object, allow the family to assist with care. Helping care for the resident assists family members to work through the grieving process. Communication may be limited in this stage.

Coping Mechanisms

The resident in the long-term care facility has experienced many losses. An understanding of the coping mechanisms people use to deal with losses and stress in life will help you understand your residents.

Coping mechanisms are responses to stress that a person uses to protect feelings of self-esteem. Coping mechanisms develop throughout a person's life. Success or failure in gaining positive coping skills depends largely on how well the developmental tasks of earlier life have been mastered. When a person's coping ability is strained or inadequate, the following reactions may be seen:

- chronic complaining
- angry, irritable behavior
- agitation
- restlessness
- depression

- withdrawal
- weight loss or gain
- sleep disturbances

Residents who react this way may need additional emotional support. Your understanding of basic human needs, normal adult developmental tasks, and coping mechanisms will help you provide quality care for the resident. The following are other ways the nursing assistant can provide this support:

- Use **therapeutic** communication.
- Offer the resident choices whenever possible.
- Realize that angry outbursts are often the result of feelings of hopelessness, losses experienced, or unmet needs. Do not take these outbursts personally.
- Direct the resident's emotional energy in positive ways. Encourage activity programs.
- Report changes in the resident's behavior to the nurse.

DEATH AND DYING

You will be working with persons in the long-term care facility who are near death. Remember, death is a part of living. Death comes to all living things. Many persons look at death as a frightening time. Studies of people who had near-death experiences have shown that death is not unpleasant or frightening. Interviews with many elderly persons showed they have little fear of death. As a nursing assistant in a long-term care facility, dealing with death-related issues may be part of your job. Our society as a whole tends to avoid meaningful discussions of death. Discussing your own attitude toward death may help you better understand death and dying. Caring for the person when death is near and caring for the body after death will probably be part of your responsibility.

Cultural Beliefs at the Time of Death

Cultural practices and beliefs surrounding death and dying are diverse. Some families express their grief loudly. Others are calm and quiet. Most take comfort in their spiritual and religious beliefs at the time of death. Table 2-3 lists cultural and religious beliefs surrounding death and dying.

Physical Signs Indicating That Death Is Near

Some physical changes occur before a person dies. These include:

- Level of responsiveness decreases.
- The lower jaw relaxes and the mouth falls open.

- Skin becomes pale, moist, and cool.
- Lips and fingertips take on a dusky color.
- Pulse becomes rapid, weak, and thready.
- Breathing becomes slow, labored, irregular, noisy.
- Blood pressure decreases.
- Discharge of urine and feces is involuntary.
- Eyes stare, and pupils do not respond to light.
- Skin takes on a blue or dusky appearance, beginning in the lower extremities and moving upward.

Nursing care for the dying resident is a continuation of care that shows dignity and respect. Some other points to remember while caring for the dying resident are:

- Check the care plan for special instructions, or ask the nurse.
- Respect the religious beliefs of the resident and family.
- Keep the resident clean and comfortable.
- Moisten the lips and mouth as directed, and give frequent oral care.
- Touch and continue to talk to the resident as you normally would.
- Say only things you want the resident to hear. Explain all procedures before doing them. The sense of hearing may be present even if the resident does not seem aware. Do not say anything that could upset or frighten the resident.
- Support family members. Allow them to be involved in care, if appropriate.

POSTMORTEM CARE

If you are to prepare the body after death, refer to your facility's policy and procedure for **postmortem care,** or ask the nurse if you have any questions. Some facilities have a morgue to which the body is taken. In other facilities the body is left in the room until it can be transferred to a mortuary. Assist the roommate to leave the room temporarily.

When circulation stops, the blood moves into the lowest areas of the body. This process can begin within 20 minutes of death. Over time, the back of the body will appear stained if the resident is in the supine position. To reduce the risk of staining about the head and neck, elevate the head of the bed 30 degrees, to the semi-Fowler's position. Some facilities do not use ties in the morgue pack

TABLE 2-3 Cultural/Religious Beliefs Affecting Care at the Time of Death

Culture/Religion	Religious Belief
Adventist (Seventh Day, Church of God)	Some believe in divine healing, anointing with oil, and prayer. Believe in prolonging life, but may allow some to die naturally. Most do not believe in withholding care, or euthanasia. Will permit organ donation and autopsy.
American Indian	There are many different tribes, and beliefs vary with each. Some believe an owl is an omen of death. Some tribes have family members prepare the body for burial. Some tribes will not touch the dead person's belongings. Some tribes believe the dead are happy in the spirit world. Others believe the body is an empty shell. Some have extensive preparation of the body and visitation of the deceased. In some tribes, if a member dies at home, the house may be abandoned forever, or may be burned.
Armenian Church	Holy Communion may be given as a form of last rites; laying on of hands is practiced.
Baptist	Pastor, resident, and family counsel and pray. Resident may be given communion. Some practice healing and laying on of hands.
Black/African American	The deceased is highly respected. Health care providers usually prepare the body. Cremation is usually avoided. May have concerns about organ donation.
Black Muslim	Practices for washing the body, applying the shroud, and funeral rites are carefully prescribed.
Brethren	Anointing with oil is done for physical healing and spiritual guidance.
Buddhist Churches of America	The state of mind of the dying person is believed to influence rebirth. The priest is contacted to provide last rites. Chanting may be done at the bedside after death. Grieving is permitted by family. After death, the body is viewed as an empty shell. Autopsy and cremation are permitted.
Cambodian (Khmer)	Monks recite prayers. Family wants to be present at time of death and may want to care for the resident. Incense may be burned. Death is accepted in a quiet, passive manner. Family and monks may wish to prepare the body. A white cloth is used as a shroud and mourners wear white.
Central American	Catholics may want a priest to administer Sacrament of the Sick. Candles may be used if oxygen is not in use in the room. Family members may wish to prepare the body.
Chinese American	Family may prefer that resident not be told of impending death, or may prefer to inform the resident themselves. May not want to talk about the terminal illness with anyone. Some believe that dying at home is bad luck. Others believe that the spirit gets lost if the resident dies in the hospital. Family members may place special cloths and amulets on the body. Some prefer to bathe their own family members after death.
Christian Scientist	A Christian Science Practitioner may be called for spiritual support. Euthanasia is forbidden. Will not seek medical assistance to prolong life. Family responsible for disposal of the body. Most will not donate organs.
Church of God	Believes in divine healing through prayer. Speaking in tongues may be used.
Church of Jesus Christ of Latter Day Saints (LDS or Mormon)	Euthanasia forbidden. Request peaceful, dignified death. Body is dressed in white temple clothing before viewing by family members. Persons who have been married in a special temple ceremony wear undergarments that are considered sacred. The undergarments should be placed on the body after death. Cremation is discouraged. Believe in baptism for others who have died and preaching to deceased. Organ donation and autopsy permitted.

(continues)

Continued

Colombian	Catholic prayer and Anointing of the Sick common. Family may practice Catholic prayer at bedside. Family members may cry loudly or become hysterical. All family members may want to see the body before it is taken to the morgue. In Colombia, the deceased are usually buried within 24 to 36 hours. The nurse or social worker may need to inform the family that in the United States the body may not be buried this quickly.
Cuban	Family may not want resident told of impending death. This varies according to Cuban culture. Family members may stay with resident 24 hours a day during terminal phase of illness.
Eastern Orthodox	Last rites are given. Anointing of the sick is performed as a form of healing with prayer. Cremation is discouraged.
Episcopal	Last rites are available, but not mandatory. May practice prayer, communion, and confession.
Ethiopian	Friends are told of death before family so they can be present when family is informed. Female family members are never told first. Great displays of feelings are encouraged at death. They may cry loudly and hysterically. Women may tear their clothing and beat their chests. Men may cry out loud. Some families may want to say goodbye to the deceased before the body is removed from the room.
Filipino	Head of family is informed away from resident's room. Catholic priest is called to deliver Sacrament of the Sick. Do-not-resuscitate decisions may be made by the entire family. Religious objects may be placed around the resident. Family may pray at the bedside when resident is dying. After death, may cry loudly and hysterically. Family may wish to wash the body. Death is considered a very spiritual event. All family members may say goodbye before body is removed from the room.
Friends (Quaker)	Do not believe in life after death (spiritual afterlife).
Greek Orthodox	The priest should be called while the resident is still conscious. Practices last rites and administration of communion. Believe that life should be preserved until terminated by God.
Gypsy	In general, discussion of death is avoided in this culture. Eldest in authority is informed of death first. A priest may be present for body purification. Family may want the window open at the time of death and afterward so the spirit can leave the room. May ask for special personal items in room at the time of death. An older female relative may remain at the window to keep spirits out of room. The moment of death and the resident's last words are very significant. The body after death may represent a source of spiritual danger to the family. Family may want body embalmed immediately after death to remove blood. They may sit with the body around the clock after death, and will eat and drink at this location.
Haitian	Elaborate rituals after death. When death is imminent, family will cry hysterically and uncontrollably. Family members may bring religious symbols and medallions. They have a deep respect for the dead. Family members may wish to wash the body and participate in postmortem care.
Hindu	Death is the opposite of birth, but not the opposite of life. Both mark passage. Believe that unsatisfied karmic debt will pass into the next life. Believe in rebirth. Euthanasia is forbidden. Specially prescribed rites. Family, friends, and priest may chant continuously before and after death. Priest may tie a thread around wrist or neck and place water in mouth immediately after death. The thread is a blessing, and should not be removed. People in this culture express grief very loudly.

(continues)

The family washes and dresses the body and only certain persons may touch the dead. Autopsy and organ donation permitted. May prefer cremation to burial.

Hmong   Important to wear fine traditional Hmong clothing at the time of death. Family may put amulets on body, which should not be removed. The family usually prepares the body at the funeral home. The body cannot be buried with hard objects, buttons, or zippers against the body.

Iranian   Death is seen as the beginning of a spiritual relationship with God, not the end of life. Family may wish to be present at all times when resident is dying, and may cry and pray at bedside. Family may wish to wash the body.

Islam (Muslim)   Begging forgiveness and confession of sins must be done in presence of family members before death. The dying person may wish to sit and face toward Mecca. Assist with positioning in one of the Fowler's positions, if possible. Believe in judgment after death. Non-Muslim workers should avoid touching the body after death, if possible. Turn the head toward the right shoulder before rigor mortis begins so that the body can be buried with the face toward Mecca. There are five steps to prepare the body for burial. The first step involves washing of the body by a Muslim of the same sex. May offer special prayers at bedside to ease pain and suffering; however pain, suffering, and illness are viewed as God's will, and are part of paying for sin. Some have spiritual leader give resident holy water to drink prior to death to purify body. After death, arms and legs are straightened and the toes tied together with a bandage. May be opposed to autopsy.

Japanese   Resident and family may be aware of impending death, but will not speak about it. Family may wish to remain at bedside during terminal stage of illness. Cleanliness and dignity of the body are very important.

Jehovah's Witness   Euthanasia forbidden. Practice baptism and communion. May be opposed to autopsy, but acceptable if required by law. Organ donation forbidden.

Judaism (Reform, Conservative, and Orthodox)   Jews believe in the sanctity of life. Medical care is generally expected, and there are no medication restrictions. Most surgical procedures are permitted, but body parts that have been removed are traditionally saved for later burial. For most Jews, medical treatment cannot be stopped once it has been started, but members are not required to use extraordinary measures to prolong life. Expect to die with dignity. May be opposed to prolonging life if resident has irreversible brain damage. However, active euthanasia is forbidden. Traditional Jews use a burial society to care for the body after death. Society members may or may not be members of the deceased's congregation. Would prefer no autopsy, but will permit it if legally required. Embalming is generally discouraged. Burial as soon after death as possible. Cremation discouraged. For traditional Jews, mourning begins with a seven-day period called *shiva,* in which men do not shave, and family and close friends do not read the newspaper or watch television. Mourning extends over a year. Jewish practices and beliefs can be very different from family to family. Asking the resident or family members about their practices is probably best. Asking is not offensive, and shows that you care about and respect the resident's and family's wishes.

Korean   Chanting, incense, and prayer may be used. Family crying and mourning may be extreme. Family may want to spend time alone with resident after death. Some may wish to wash the body.

Lutheran   Practice prayer. Last rites optional; resident may request anointing of the sick.

Methodist   May request donation of body or body parts to medical science.

(continues)

Continued

Mexican American	Entire family may be obligated to visit the sick and dying. Pregnant women may be prohibited from visiting. Spiritual items may be important. May want to die at home because of fear that the spirit will get lost in the hospital. Crying loudly and wailing is culturally accepted and a sign of respect. A Catholic priest is called for the Sacrament of the Sick. A family member may wish to assist with postmortem care. Family will want time alone with the body before it is removed from the room.
Orthodox Presbyterian	Scripture reading and prayer. Full forgiveness is granted for any illness connected with a sin.
Puerto Rican	If death is imminent, family may stay around the clock. Some believe that all immediate family members must be present at time of death. Believe that the body must be treated with great respect.
Roman Catholic	Takes ordinary, but not extraordinary, means to prolong life. May refuse lifesaving care. Euthanasia is forbidden. Sacrament of the Sick is mandatory. Resident or family may request anointing if prognosis is poor. Autopsy, organ donation, and cremation are permitted.
Russian	Family may not want resident to know of terminal diagnosis. Depending on religion, family may wish to wash the body and dress it in special clothes.
Russian Orthodox	Practice prayer, communion, and last rites by priest. Many wear a cross necklace, which should not be removed, if at all possible. After death the arms are crossed and fingers set in the form of a cross. Clothing must be a natural fiber so the body changes to ashes sooner. May be opposed to autopsy, embalming, or cremation.
Samoan	Resident and family prefer to be told of terminal diagnosis as early as possible. Family would prefer to care for resident at home, if possible. Family members usually prefer to prepare the body.
Sikh	May recite hymns from their holy book. Believe that the soul remains alive after death. Usually do not object if workers prepare the body, but family may prefer to wash the body and dress it in new clothes. Avoid shaving or trimming beard or hair. Usually prefer cremation as soon as possible. Organ donation and autopsy permitted.
Unitarian Universalist	Cremation may be preferred to burial.
Vietnamese	DNR decisions are made by entire family. For Catholic families, religious items are kept close to resident. For Buddhist families, incense is burned. Families prefer time alone with the deceased before body is moved. The body is highly respected, and the family may prefer to wash it. Some may prefer the body left as it is.
West Indian	When death is near, close family and friends wish to remain at the bedside to pray. Family members may wish to view the body exactly as the resident was at the time of death. Most wish to be alone with the deceased.

to position the body. Follow your facility policies. If used, tie them loosely. If the ties are too tight, they will also cause permanent marks on the body.

Always use *standard precautions* (Chapter 6) when providing postmortem care. The body can be infectious after death. Handle the body very gently to prevent bruising. Respect the religious beliefs of the deceased. Beliefs vary, and people of some faiths have special religious requirements for preparation of the body.

1   Postmortem Care

1 Wash your hands.

2 Gather supplies: shroud kit with gown and identification tags, a basin of warm water, soap, washcloth, towels, swabs for oral care, linen, gown, and gloves.

3 Pull the curtains and close the door for privacy.

4 Treat the body gently and with respect.

5 Apply gloves.

6 Raise the bed to a comfortable working height.

7 Place the resident on his or her back, with a pillow beneath the head and shoulders in proper body alignment.

8 Close the eyes by gently pulling eyelids down.

9 Provide mouth care using moistened oral care swabs or sponges.

10 Place cleaned dentures in the mouth or in a labeled denture cup. The dentures should be sent to the funeral home with the body.

11 Close the mouth. A rolled-up washcloth may be placed under the chin to keep the jaw closed.

12 Remove all tubing from the body if this is your facility policy. In most facilities this is done by the nurse.

13 Bathe the body, comb hair, and straighten the arms and legs.

14 Apply clean dressings to wounds, if necessary.

15 Place a disposable pad under the buttocks.

16 Put a gown on the body.

17 Attach an identification tag to the body as indicated by facility policy.

18 Replace soiled linen and cover the body to the shoulders with a sheet.

19 Remove gloves and dispose according to facility policy.

20 Wash your hands.

21 Tidy the unit.

22 Wash your hands.

23 Provide privacy and allow family members to be alone with the resident.

24 Collect all belongings, place them in a bag, and label them correctly. Usually these are given to the family. If no family members are present, follow facility policy. Complete and sign the inventory sheet if this is your facility policy.

25 After the family leaves, wash your hands and put the shroud on the body. Wear gloves if contact with blood, body fluid, secretions, or excretions is likely.

26 Remove gloves, if worn, and dispose according to facility policy.

27 Follow facility policy to take the body to the morgue, or close the door until the funeral home staff arrives.

28 Notify the nurse when the funeral home staff arrives.

29 Assist the funeral home personnel to move the body, if necessary.

30 Strip and clean the unit according to your facility policy after the body has been removed.

KEY POINTS IN THIS CHAPTER

▲ All people have the same basic human needs, though some people may express their needs in different ways.

▲ Physical needs, called physiological needs, are needs of the body.

▲ Psychological or psychosocial needs are the emotional or mental needs of the resident.

▲ Developmental tasks at one level must be mastered before moving to the next level.

▲ The resident's culture, spirituality, and religion influence your ability to provide care.

▲ Coping mechanisms are used and developed in life to deal with stresses.

▲ The grieving process is a series of five stages that a person experiences in anticipation of a loss or after suffering a loss.

▲ A resident who is dying must be cared for with the same respect and dignity given to all other residents.

▲ The resident's body must be treated with respect after death.

REVIEW QUIZ

1. Which of the following statements is true?
   a. All people have the same basic human needs.
   b. The basic human needs of people vary according to age.
   c. Men and women have very different basic human needs.
   d. All people express their basic needs in exactly the same way.

2. What are psychological or psychosocial needs?
   a. needs having to do with the physical body
   b. mental and emotional needs
   c. need for food, air, water, and exercise
   d. elimination needs

3. Nursing assistants can help residents to meet the need for food by:
   a. keeping the head of the bed flat at mealtime.
   b. always providing privacy when residents are eating.
   c. keeping the dining area as quiet as possible.
   d. making mealtime as pleasant as possible.

4. Nursing assistants can help residents meet the need for exercise and activity by:
   a. assisting residents to the bathroom at least once a day.
   b. helping residents to ambulate and exercise according to the care plan.
   c. keeping residents in bed as much as possible.
   d. assisting residents to meals.

5. The nursing assistant can help meet residents' need for sexual expression by:
   a. dressing residents in clothing that is appropriate and attractive.
   b. encouraging residents to spend time alone.
   c. encouraging male and female communication.
   d. seating women next to men in the dining room.

6. A resident's need for love and belonging can be met by:
   a. keeping the head of the bed up when bathing the resident.
   b. making sure that equipment is working properly.
   c. showing interest and listening closely to the resident.
   d. introducing the resident to others.

7. What is your best response when the resident you are caring for begins to cry?
   a. Let the resident cry and ask if you can do something to help.
   b. Say nothing. Give the resident a tissue, leave the room, and close the door.
   c. Tell the resident, "Stop crying. Things will get better."
   d. Allow the resident to cry, but call the family immediately.

8. Calling the resident by the name he or she prefers is one way of meeting the need for:
   a. privacy.   c. identity.
   b. love.   d. spiritual growth.

9. How can the nursing assistant help the resident meet her religious needs?
   a. by insisting that the resident attend all religious services in the facility
   b. by treating religious belongings with care and respect
   c. by calling your pastor to visit with the resident
   d. by encouraging the resident to pray daily

10. A developmental task of late adulthood is:
    a. developing a career.
    b. establishing a family.
    c. making commitments in family life.
    d. accepting one's mortality.

11. Responses persons develop in life to handle stress are called:
    a. coping mechanisms.
    b. grieving processes.
    c. developmental tasks.
    d. physiological developments.

12. What is the first step in the grieving process?
    a. anger   c. depression
    b. denial   d. acceptance

13. When caring for a resident who is dying, you should:
    a. keep the room dark.
    b. keep family members away from the dying resident.
    c. continue caring for, touching, and talking to the resident.
    d. never let the resident see family members who are crying.

14. Physical signs of approaching death include all of the following *except:*
    a. decreasing responsiveness.
    b. pale skin.
    c. weak and rapid pulse.
    d. skin warm and dry.

15. Which of the following is the last sense to be lost by the dying resident?
    a. vision   c. smell
    b. hearing   d. taste

16. You are assigned to care for Mrs. Nova, a 67-year-old resident who has been in the facility for five years. She talks nonstop and tries to keep you in the room for as long as she can. Mrs. Nova uses the call signal frequently for simple requests. Which of the following best describes the need that is causing her behavior?
    a. safety and security
    b. love and belonging
    c. self-actualization
    d. physiological needs

17. Mr. Gonzales is an 87-year-old resident who is mentally confused. He is sitting in his wheelchair yelling loudly when you pass by. A few minutes later, he is quiet. You notice a large puddle of urine on the floor near the resident's chair. What is the most likely cause of the resident's yelling?
    a. He needed safety so that he would not fall on the slippery, wet floor.
    b. He was yelling for no reason.
    c. He needed to go to the bathroom.
    d. He was bored.

18. Mrs. Barnes is an alert resident who raised a large family. Her husband operated a farm and was away from home for long hours most of the time. Mrs. Barnes was the primary caregiver for her children. Now that the resident is in the long-term care facility, she is demanding and unpleasant. She is easily frustrated and yells at you because of minor irritations over which you have no control. Mrs. Barnes may be upset because she has lost control over her environment and routines. A good approach to take with this alert resident is to:
    a. give her choices.
    b. leave her alone when she is upset.
    c. follow very rigid routines.
    d. try to talk to her about her behavior.

19. Mr. Joiner is a 65-year-old resident with advanced prostate cancer. The doctor just told Mr. Joiner that his condition is terminal and that further treatment will not help. You go to the resident's room to help him to the dining room. He tells you, "The doctor told me that I am dying of cancer, but he is wrong. I do not feel sick at all." Mr. Joiner is probably experiencing:
    a. anger.   c. bargaining.
    b. acceptance.   d. denial.

20. You answer Mr. Hernandez's call signal and he yells at you for taking too long. He tells you that his breakfast was cold and that his favorite shirt is lost. You know that the call signal has been on for less than a minute, that breakfast was not cold, and that his shirt is in the laundry. He says that these things are "all your fault" and that he will report you to your supervisor because you are not taking proper care of him. You should:
    a. inform the resident that you will not take care of him if he reports you.
    b. understand that the resident is frustrated and that you should not take his comments personally.
    c. tell the resident that he is imagining things.
    d. call the family at once.

21. Mrs. Bellman has been a resident of your facility for as long as you can remember. She has a serious heart condition. When you come on duty, the nurse tells you in report that this resident is dying and that she is not responding to spoken words. When you enter Mrs. Bellman's room, you find that her bed is very wet and you must change all the linen by using the occupied bedmaking procedure. You know that:
    a. Mrs. Bellman is no longer aware of who is in the room or what is being done.
    b. you should only change the top bedding so that you do not disturb the resident.
    c. you should explain to the resident what you are going to do.
    d. the resident will not be uncomfortable despite the wet linen.

CHAPTER 2
CROSSWORD PUZZLE

Directions: Complete the puzzle using these words found in Chapter 2.

acceptance	depression	process
actualization	elimination	psychological
ambulate	esteem	safety
anger	love	security
bargaining	needs	shroud
belonging	oxygen	spiritual
coping	physiological	tasks
denial	postmortem	therapeutic

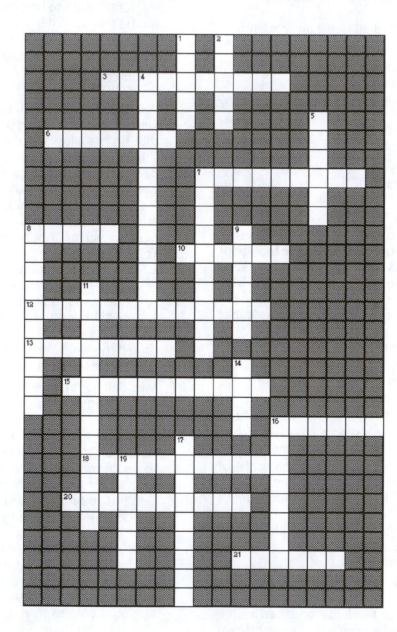

CHAPTER 2
PUZZLE CLUES

ACROSS

3. Feeling very sad and unhappy
6. There are five steps in the grieving _____ .
7. Feeling as if you are a part of something
8. The second stage of the grieving process in which the resident is mad
10. You are practicing _____ when you protect residents from injury by eliminating risks in the environment.
12. Emotional and mental needs
13. To walk
15. The process by which urine and stool pass from the body
16. The covering that is placed on the body after death
18. When residents need emotional support, it is helpful to provide _____ communication.
20. Care given to the body after death is _____ care.
21. _____ is in the air that we breathe.

DOWN

1. All humans have basic _____ for food, water, and oxygen.
2. Developmental _____ must be accomplished if a person is to mature.
4. Concerning the function of the body systems
5. Methods people have of handling stress are _____ mechanisms.
7. Attempting to make a deal with a higher power for more time to live is an example of _____ .
8. The final stage of the grieving process is _____ .
9. Refusing to accept the truth is a form of _____ .
11. Achieving one's full potential is self-_____ .
14. Deep fondness or affection
16. The assurance of feeling safe
17. Praying is a way for the resident to meet his or her _____ needs.
19. Satisfaction with oneself is self-_____ .

Rights of the Resident

OBJECTIVES

In this chapter you will learn about the importance of residents' rights. After reading this chapter, you will be able to:

- Spell and define key terms.
- List residents' rights.
- Describe ways to accommodate residents' right to make choices and explain why this is important.
- Describe your role in helping residents resolve grievances.
- List ways you can help residents participate in activities.
- Describe care that maintains the resident's dignity.

KEY TERMS

adaptive equipment: equipment or supplies used to make a task easier

confidentiality: keeping information or facts private

grievance: a complaint

infringe: to violate, remove, take away, or make difficult to attain

misappropriation of property: taking something that belongs to a resident

nontherapeutic: not relating to treatment or therapy

ombudsman: a person who acts as an advocate for residents

reasonable accommodation: considering each resident's likes, dislikes, special needs, and preferences when providing care and services

reprisal: an act performed to gain revenge or to punish another

restraint: any device or equipment used to restrict a person's freedom of movement or access to his or her own body

RESIDENTS' RIGHTS

The Resident's Bill of Rights states rights established by a federal law. All members of the health care team must respect these rights. The purpose and intent of the law is to make sure that all residents of the long-term care facility are treated with dignity and respect. The law guarantees that residents have the same rights as any other citizen. A copy of these rights is given to each person on admission (Figure 3-1).

Residents have the right to:

- have their rights explained both verbally and in writing.
- be treated with dignity and respect.

RESIDENTS' RIGHTS

- Residents have the right to exercise all their rights as citizens of the state and citizens of the United States, as well as any other rights given them by law.
- The facility must explain the rights to residents both verbally and in writing in a language that the resident understands.
- Residents cannot be discriminated against because of age, sex, race, ethnic origin, religion, or disability.

Privacy, Dignity, and Respect

- Residents have a right to privacy.
- Residents will be treated with consideration, dignity, and respect.
- The resident's likes, dislikes, and special needs and preferences must be considered in the services provided by the facility. This is called **reasonable accommodation.**
- Personal and clinical records must be kept confidential. The resident has the right to refuse to allow others to see these records unless permission is given in writing.
- Residents have the right to communicate, both verbally and in writing, with anyone of their choosing. This includes family members, other visitors, ombudsmen, attorneys, and representatives of governmental agencies.
- Residents have the right to send and receive personal mail unopened. Residents may request that staff assist them to open and read their mail when it arrives.

Safety and Security

- Residents have the right to a safe environment.
- Residents have the right to care that is free from **misappropriation of property.**

Medical Care and Treatment

- Residents have the right to choose their own physicians. They have the right to be informed of matters affecting their care and to make decisions regarding their care.
- Medical problems must be explained to a resident in a language he or she understands.

- Residents may refuse treatment. If they do refuse treatment, they have the right to be informed of the consequences of their refusal.
- Residents have a right to voice problems and complaints about their care without fear of reprisal. The facility is required to respond to these complaints.
- Residents have the right to make choices to withhold life-sustaining treatment in the event of terminal illness.
- Residents may designate someone else to make treatment decisions for them in the event they become unable to make these decisions themselves.

Freedom from Restraint, Abuse, and Misappropriation of Property

- Residents have the right to be free from abuse, neglect, and misappropriation of property. The facility is responsible for caring for the residents' health, well-being, and personal possessions.
- Drugs cannot be given for discipline or convenience of the nursing home staff. Any mood-altering drugs given must be required for the treatment of a medical condition.
- Residents cannot be punished, scolded, abused, or secluded. Their privileges cannot be taken away and they cannot be physically, mentally, or sexually abused.
- Residents cannot be restrained by physical means except for their own safety, the safety of others, in certain medical procedures, or in an emergency.

Financial Matters

- Residents have the right to manage their own financial affairs, or may choose another person to manage their money.
- Facilities must account for and properly manage resident money deposited with them.

Freedom of Association

- Residents have the right to have visitors at any reasonable hour.
- Residents do not have to talk to or see anyone they do not want to visit.
- Residents may make and receive private phone calls.

Figure 3-1 The nursing assistant must understand and respect the residents' rights.

- Married couples have the right to share a room.
- Residents have the right to organize and participate in resident and family councils.
- Residents may meet with others outside the facility.
- Residents may leave the facility for visits or shopping trips.
- Family members may meet with families of other residents in the nursing home.
- Residents have the right to plan and execute their daily activities.
- Residents have the right to vote in elections.

Work

- Residents may choose to work in the facility as part of their activity plans. They have the right to be paid the prevailing rate for the same type of work in the community. Residents may also perform certain duties without pay, if they choose to do so.

Personal Possessions

- Residents may wear their own clothing.
- Residents may bring in furnishings and personal belongings from their own homes.

Grievances

- If a resident has a problem or complaint, he has the right to speak with those in charge. The complaint may be about care or failure to receive expected services. The resident has the right to a response.
- The resident has the right to contact the ombudsman for the facility and the state survey and certification agency.

- The facility may not retaliate against residents who have complained.

Admission, Transfer, and Discharge

- The facility must advise residents about eligibility for Medicaid. If Medicaid or Medicare pays for any items or services, the resident cannot be charged additional money for these services.
- In the event of the resident's death, the facility must give an accounting of money in the resident's personal account to the person responsible for the estate.
- Residents may not be asked to give up their rights to benefits under Medicaid or Medicare.
- The facility is required to have the same policies and practices regarding services, transfer, or discharge for all individuals regardless of their source of payment.
- The facility may be required to hold a resident's bed for a specified period if the resident is hospitalized or goes on a therapeutic pass.
- The facility cannot make the resident leave or move to another room unless:
  - The health and safety of the resident or others are affected.
  - The facility cannot meet the resident's needs.
  - The resident's condition has improved so that services are no longer required.
  - The resident has not paid the bill and the facility has given the resident reasonable notice of discharge.
- Residents must be given a 30-day written notice before they can be transferred unless there are medical reasons or the life, safety, or health of the resident or others is endangered. The resident may waive the right to the 30-day waiting period if she chooses.

Figure 3-1 (*Continued*)

- receive quality care regardless of race, color, ethnic origin, sex, age, religion, marital status, sexual preference, medical condition, or physical disability.
- receive encouragement and support in making personal choices to accommodate individual needs.
- have advance notice if a change in room or roommate is necessary.

- have personal likes, dislikes, and special needs considered in the care and services given by the nursing facility.
- be respected and protected from harm, physically, mentally, and verbally.
- be free from abuse, neglect, and involuntary seclusion.
- have privacy during procedures and when requested.

- **confidentiality** about their medical condition, medical records, personal information, and other details relating to their care.
- be addressed by the preferred name.
- continuity of care.
- have personal possessions treated with respect and have them safeguarded.
- have assistance, privacy, and confidentiality in personal communication, including mail, telephone calls, and visitors.
- visits from the **ombudsman,** representatives of state agencies, family, or physician at any reasonable hour. The resident may also choose to prohibit certain people from visiting.
- complain about care and services without fear of **reprisal,** or punishment, and to expect a response.
- be informed about services available and their cost.
- refuse treatment. If treatment is refused, an explanation of the likely results of refusal must be given to the resident.
- select another person to make treatment decisions if the resident becomes incapable of making these decisions.
- be free from **nontherapeutic** chemical and physical **restraints.** If a restraint must be used, it should be the least restrictive device needed to keep the resident safe. The device should be used for the least time possible.
- wear their own clothing, keep appropriate personal possessions, and be allowed to manage and spend their own money.
- participate in care conferences and give family members permission to attend.
- exercise citizenship rights and vote in elections.
- choose the physician responsible for care.
- live in the same room with the spouse, if married.
- be informed of the procedures for filing confidential complaints and for working out complaints.
- be given information about available resources.
- organize and participate in resident and family councils.
- complain to the state survey agency.
- review state survey findings.
- participate in religious or political activities if these do not **infringe** on other residents' rights.

These rights give residents the same legal rights as any citizen. It is part of your role and responsibility to support and help residents exercise their rights. If residents are mentally confused, you are required to protect their rights if they are not able to do so themselves. The reason for this law is to promote the interests and well-being of residents in health care facilities. The long-term care facility and its staff must encourage and help residents to exercise these rights.

Ways in Which the Nursing Assistant Protects Resident Rights

Some ways that you, as a nursing assistant, can take responsibility for seeing that residents' rights are protected are to:

- Give quality care to all residents, regardless of race, color, ethnic origin, sex, age, religion, marital status, sexual preference, medical condition, or physical disability.
- Treat all residents with dignity and respect. Perform your duties to the best of your ability, and do not neglect to care for residents who are assigned to you.
- Give privacy when caring for residents. Knock on doors and wait for an answer before entering. Pull the privacy curtain and window curtain, if necessary, when doing care. Cover the sitting female resident with a blanket or lap robe so that she is not exposed.
- Give privacy to residents and visitors.
- Keep information learned about residents' medical conditions and personal situations confidential. Do not discuss information learned about phone calls, mail, or visitors. If information learned relates to the resident's care or condition, tell the nurse.
- Report changes in condition to the nurse in a timely manner.
- Call the resident by the name that the resident wants to be called.
- Protect the resident's personal possessions.
- Help the resident make phone calls, write letters, or address envelopes, if requested.
- Report injuries or suspected abuse or neglect immediately.

RESIDENTS' RIGHT TO MAKE CHOICES

It is frustrating to be physically unable to do the things you want to do. This inability affects your self-esteem. Giving a resident choices is a way to show respect for the resident's opinion and give the resident a measure of control over routines and the

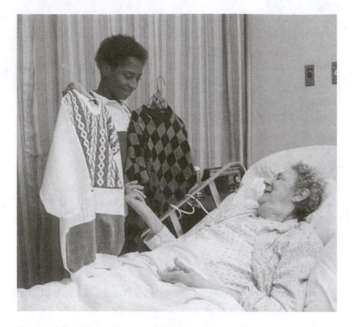

Figure 3-2 Offering the resident choices shows that you value her opinion.

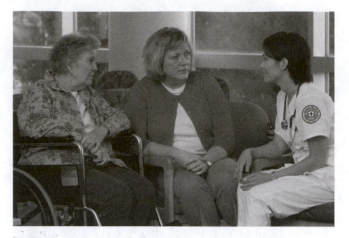

Figure 3-3 Residents have the right to voice grievances without fear of reprisal.

environment. Making choices has a positive effect on the resident's self-esteem (Figure 3-2).

The Resident's Bill of Rights gives the resident the right to make personal choices. As a nursing assistant, you have the most contact with residents in the facility. Therefore, you have the most opportunities to assist the resident to make choices. Help residents make choices in the following ways:

- Offer options whenever possible.
- Accommodate the resident's requests as to when to do certain procedures.
- Take the time to talk to residents so you can learn their personal preferences.
- Talk with the family to learn the resident's interests.
- Report resident preferences to the nurse.

A study of long-term care facilities showed that there are differences in what residents and staff feel is important. This study supports the fact that residents need to be asked what and when they want things done. Remember, this is encouraged by the Resident's Bill of Rights.

RESOLVING GRIEVANCES

A **grievance,** or complaint, may be filed when the resident feels his rights have been infringed upon. The Resident's Bill of Rights gives the resident the right to voice grievances without fear of reprisal, or punishment. The facility policies will describe how a grievance procedure is to be carried out. Usually your responsibility is to report the resident's grievance to

the nurse, making sure that what you report is accurate (Figure 3-3). Some facilities have a social worker who is responsible for helping resolve grievances. Always know and follow the procedure of your facility.

RESIDENTS' PARTICIPATION IN ACTIVITIES

The activity department of the long-term care facility has a special function. It plans recreational and social functions for the residents. Activities combat boredom and promote positive self-esteem. These functions are a form of therapy for the resident. Your role is to cooperate with the activity department. Some ways you can help the residents participate in activities are:

- Plan your work so that residents can attend activities of choice.
- Review the activity calendar and be aware of the activities planned for the day.
- Tell all residents what activities are scheduled and encourage them to attend.
- Help residents dress properly, but remember to allow the resident to do as much self-care as possible.
- Inform residents' family or friends about activities.
- Escort residents to and from activity programs if necessary.
- Talk to residents about their activities, and praise their accomplishments.

MAINTAINING RESIDENTS' DIGNITY

There are many ways you can help maintain residents' dignity. Dignity means treating a person with respect. Maintaining residents' dignity at all times is important.

Long-term care residents have had to make many difficult adjustments. Some residents have suffered many losses and may be angry and frustrated. Remember, each resident once was a younger, active person. Treat each resident as you would want a member of your family treated.

The nursing assistant can help maintain residents' dignity by:

- Calling residents by the preferred name.
- Treating all residents with respect.
- Helping residents be as independent as possible. Let the resident do as much for himself as possible, if consistent with the care plan.
- Encouraging residents to be involved in their care and make choices.

- Assisting and teaching residents to use **adaptive equipment** to enable them to be as independent as possible.
- Handling residents' personal possessions with care and security. Do not throw personal items away without permission.
- Explaining what you are going to do before you do it, and obtaining the resident's permission and cooperation.
- Becoming familiar with each resident's care plan so that you can provide individualized care.
- Being alert to safety concerns.
- Protecting residents from abuse, neglect, mistreatment, and disrespect.
- Reporting any instances of poor care, abuse, or neglect to the proper person.

KEY POINTS IN THIS CHAPTER

▲ The Resident's Bill of Rights is a law that must be respected by all members of the health care team.

▲ The Resident's Bill of Rights guarantees that residents will be treated with dignity and respect.

▲ Residents have the right to file grievances and to be given assistance in doing so.

▲ The nursing assistant must provide privacy for residents when giving personal care.

▲ The nursing assistant must cooperate with the activity department in helping residents attend activities of choice.

▲ Showing respect for residents includes handling their personal possessions carefully.

▲ Any abuse, neglect, or poor care must be reported to the appropriate staff person.

▲ Allowing residents to make decisions and personal choices is important.

REVIEW QUIZ

1. The purpose of the Resident's Bill of Rights is to:
   a. limit the cost of health care.
   b. list the cost of services provided for residents.
   c. ensure dignity and respect for residents in long-term care facilities.
   d. provide a list of rules and regulations for residents to follow.

2. Which of the following is included in the Resident's Bill of Rights?
   a. The amount of the monthly bill and due date
   b. The right to receive all needed acute care services
   c. The right to have all care paid for by the government
   d. The right to privacy when personal care is given.

3. When the resident is admitted to the long-term care facility, he should be:
   a. given a copy of the Resident's Bill of Rights.
   b. referred to by his room number.

   c. kept in his room alone until he has had time to adjust.
   d. undressed and kept in bed.

4. An example of a violation of the resident's right to confidentiality would be:
   a. discussing the resident's condition during a staff conference.
   b. reporting an observation to the nurse.
   c. discussing the resident's condition while in a crowded elevator.
   d. writing the resident's temperature on a scrap of paper.

5. What is your best response when a resident complains about the long-term care facility?
   a. Call the family and ask them to transfer the resident.
   b. Listen to the resident carefully and report the complaint to the nurse.
   c. Help the resident write a letter of complaint to the state.

d. Listen to the resident and then explain that some things cannot be changed.

6. When a resident feels that his rights have been violated, the resident has the right to:
   a. leave the facility without paying for the care.
   b. remain in the facility without paying any additional cost.
   c. call the police or sheriff.
   d. file a grievance.

7. When preparing the resident to take part in activities, it is important to:
   a. ask the resident which activities he or she would like to attend.
   b. take the resident to activities only after you have finished your other work.
   c. take the resident to the activity of your choice so that you may also attend.
   d. wait for the family to come and take the resident to the activity.

8. You see another nursing assistant hitting a confused resident. What is your best response?
   a. Call the resident's family immediately.
   b. Report this to your supervisor.
   c. Tell the other nursing assistant that you will not turn him in if he promises not to do this again.
   d. Do nothing, because it is not your responsibility to watch other employees.

9. You hear a housekeeper cursing at a resident because of a mess on the floor. You should:
   a. pretend that you did not hear.
   b. tell the other nursing assistants what happened and ask their advice.
   c. report this information to your supervisor.
   d. report this information to the housekeeper's supervisor.

10. You can assist residents in maintaining dignity and self-worth by:
    a. doing everything for each resident exactly the same.
    b. always calling residents endearing names, such as "honey" and "dear."
    c. doing things for the residents yourself so that you can get your work done quickly.
    d. allowing residents to make choices whenever possible.

11. Residents' possessions, such as photos and letters, should be:
    a. placed in the facility's safe.
    b. sent home with family members.
    c. handled with respect and care.
    d. put away where no one can see them.

12. The Resident's Bill of Rights:
    a. is a law for doctors to follow.
    b. must be respected by all employees of the health-care facility.

c. is a guideline for states to follow in providing services to residents.
d. is a guideline for residents to follow when interacting with facility staff.

13. What should you do when tidying a resident's room?
    a. Ask the resident before throwing anything away.
    b. Remove all plants and flowers from the room.
    c. Throw out any newspapers or old magazines.
    d. Clean the room without telling the resident.

14. When the resident exercises the right to refuse treatment,
    a. the resident must move out of the facility as soon as possible.
    b. the doctor and the family must be called immediately.
    c. the resident must inform the facility in writing.
    d. an explanation of the likely results of the refusal must be given to the resident.

15. The resident's right to privacy would be violated if you:
    a. opened the resident's mail without permission.
    b. closed the door after taking the resident into the bathroom.
    c. pulled the privacy curtains when the resident wanted to be alone.
    d. exposed only necessary body parts when bathing the resident.

16. A resident asks for help to go to the facility gift shop to buy a teddy bear for a new grandchild. Your best response is:
    a. "That teddy bear is expensive. How will you pay for it?"
    b. "It would be a waste of time. You don't have any money."
    c. "I'll try to take you after lunch or find someone who can."
    d. "Does your daughter know about this?"

17. Adaptive equipment is:
    a. surgically attached to the resident's body to replace a missing part.
    b. designed to help the resident be more independent.
    c. always used by the physician during an examination.
    d. used in emergencies only.

18. Restraints should:
    a. always be used to prevent wanderers from leaving the facility.
    b. be used to punish a resident for misbehaving.
    c. not be used if other measures will keep the resident safe.
    d. never be used.

19. Restraints:
    a. are a routine treatment for confused residents.
    b. must be used for all residents who are at risk of falls.
    c. may be applied if a resident becomes unruly.
    d. restrict freedom of movement and access to one's body.

20. Mr. and Mrs. Schneider have been married for 52 years. They reside in room 308 of your facility. You are about to enter the room to give bedtime care. You knock on the door and wait. No one answers, so you open the door. You find that Mr. and Mrs. Schneider are in the same bed. You should:
    a. apologize to the residents and leave the room at once.
    b. scold the residents for their childish behavior and assist them into their own beds.
    c. tell the other nursing assistants that you caught Mr. and Mrs. Schneider having sex.
    d. go about your duties in the room as if nothing is wrong.

21. You are assigned to care for Mrs. Sanchez, a 73-year-old resident who has heart problems. When you are bathing her, you notice that she has bruises on her upper arms. She tells you that Mary Atkins, another nursing assistant, held her down and forced her to eat. Mrs. Sanchez asks you not to tell anyone about the bruises. You should:
    a. say nothing, as this is what the resident wants.
    b. call the doctor and advise him of the bruises.
    c. ask Mary Atkins what happened.
    d. inform the nurse of the bruises.

22. You are assigned to care for Dr. Palmer, a retired physician who has had a stroke. Normally this resident is alert and able to visit with you when you help her with morning care. Today the resident seems confused and her speech is slurred. You should:
    a. inform the nurse of Dr. Palmer's condition right away.
    b. ask another nursing assistant what to do.
    c. do nothing, as mental confusion is a normal part of aging.
    d. assume that Dr. Palmer did not get enough sleep last night and allow her to rest.

23. You are working the 6:00 a.m. to 2:00 p.m. shift on C wing. Your unit is very busy this morning and Susan Birch, CNA, did not come to work. The nurse divides the residents in Susan's assignment and assigns a few of them to each of the other nursing assistants. You have three additional residents to care for from Susan's assignment. At 9:30 a.m., you enter Mrs. Mosier's room and find her sleeping with her side rails up. Her breakfast tray is uneaten on the overbed table. You should:
    a. remove the tray so that no one knows that you forgot to feed the resident.
    b. find the nursing assistant who passed the trays and advise her to feed Mrs. Mosier immediately.
    c. get another tray from dietary or warm the food in the microwave and feed Mrs. Mosier.
    d. tell the nurse that someone neglected the resident.

24. Mr. Springer likes to attend an activity called Current Events. You notice that this activity is scheduled for 9:00 a.m. Mr. Springer is scheduled to have a shower on the day shift. If the resident attends the activity, he will miss his shower time. What is the best way of handling the situation?
    a. Do not tell Mr. Springer about the activity.
    b. Ask Mr. Springer if he would like his shower at another time during the shift.
    c. Tell Mr. Springer that the activity is scheduled, but that he must take a shower before he can attend.
    d. Tell the activities director to schedule Current Events at a different time of day.

25. State surveyors are in the facility for their annual review. Mr. Connolly asks you to tell the surveyors that he wants to speak with them. You should:
    a. inform the nurse of Mr. Connolly's request so that he can tell the surveyors.
    b. tell the social worker to visit with Mr. Connolly immediately before he complains to the state.
    c. pretend that you did not hear Mr. Connolly and leave the room quickly.
    d. tell the resident that the surveyors are too busy reviewing care to speak with him.

26. Mr. James keeps the volume on his television loud. He likes to watch television late at night. The other residents complain that the noise from the television keeps them awake. Your best response would be to:
    a. tell the other residents that it is Mr. James's right to watch television if he wants to.
    b. go to Mr. James's room and turn the television off.
    c. close the doors of the residents who are still awake.
    d. tell Mr. James that the television is bothering others and ask him to turn the volume down.

CHAPTER 3
CROSSWORD PUZZLE

Directions: Complete the puzzle using these words found in Chapter 3.

abuse	exercise	protect
activities	explain	refuse
adaptive	grievance	reprisal
choices	law	restraints
communication	name	rights
confidentiality	neglect	self
councils	ombudsman	survey
dignity	privacy	vote

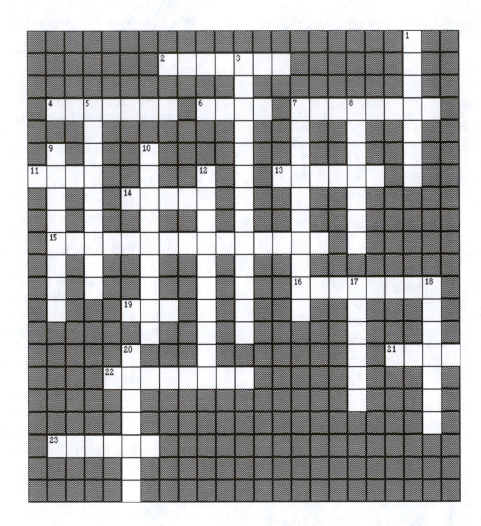

CHAPTER 3
PUZZLE CLUES

ACROSS

2. Offer the resident _____ whenever possible.
4. Treating residents with respect, honor, or esteem is treating them with _____ .
6. Call the resident by his preferred _____ .
7. A device that makes it easier for a resident to do something is called _____ equipment.
11. Residents have the right to _____ in elections.
13. Resident's Bill of _____
14. Intentional harm
15. Keeping facts or information private
16. The nursing assistant must help residents to _____ their rights.
19. The Resident's Bill of Rights is a _____ .
21. Making choices is good for the resident's _____ -esteem.
22. An act of revenge or retaliation
23. Residents may review state _____ findings.

DOWN

1. The resident has a right to _____ during procedures during which his body is exposed.
3. Writing letters and talking on the phone are forms of confidential _____ .
5. A complaint
7. Recreational and social programs
8. The nursing assistant must _____ the resident's rights.
9. Residents may organize and participate in resident and family _____ .
10. A resident advocate
12. Any equipment or devices that restrict freedom of movement and limit access to one's body
17. A resident has the right to _____ treatment.
18. If a resident refuses a procedure, health care workers must _____ the consequences of the refusal.
20. Deliberately or carelessly not taking care of a resident.

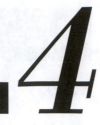

Mental Health and Social Needs

OBJECTIVES

In this chapter you will learn how you can help residents meet their mental health and social needs. After reading this chapter, you will be able to:

- Spell and define key terms.
- Identify characteristics of residents with mental health needs.
- Describe considerations to be given to the resident who has mental impairment.
- State the purpose of validation therapy.
- Describe techniques of behavior management.
- List guidelines for interacting with residents who have mental impairments.
- Describe ways to modify your behavior in response to resident behavior.

KEY TERMS

Alzheimer's disease: a disease of unknown cause that results in gradual loss of mental abilities. This irreversible disease may take from a few months to years to progress to the stage of complete helplessness

catastrophic reaction: unpredictable behavior that may become violent

confusion: behavior that is different from the usual and accepted; mixed up

dementia: impairment of mental abilities involving thinking, memory, and judgment

disorientation: loss of or confusion about one's identity, the place, or time

empathy: compassionately understanding how a resident feels, without feeling sorry for him or her

lethargy: abnormal drowsiness

mental illness: a disorder of the mind

mental retardation: lower-than-average intellectual development; can range from mild to severe

validation therapy: a program that helps confused residents feel good about themselves by helping them explore their thoughts and feelings

CHARACTERISTICS OF RESIDENTS WITH MENTAL HEALTH NEEDS

Many residents in long-term care facilities need some help in meeting their psychosocial needs. Individuals with some illnesses and conditions have special mental health needs. You will be caring for some residents who have mental disease. These residents may need physical care, but they will also need extra help related to their mental health problems. Knowing about mental impairments will help you care for these residents. Residents with **mental illness, mental retardation, Alzheimer's disease,** and other mental disorders will need special help from you. Individuals who have mental problems also have accompanying physical problems.

Mental Orientation

Residents who have mental impairments often experience **disorientation.** That is, they feel **confusion** about where they are and the current situation. It is a frightening experience to feel disoriented. Understanding this feeling in yourself will help you relate to the disoriented resident. Orientation is knowing:

- who you are.
- where you are.
- who other persons around you are.
- the time (year, month, date, day of week, and time of day).

POPULATION OF THE LONG-TERM CARE FACILITY

Many residents in the long-term care facility fit into broad categories of mental health needs. Residents with different health needs have different characteristics.

Residents with Mental Retardation

Residents with mental retardation often have the following characteristics:

- varying levels of ability
- difficulty adjusting to new situations
- poor judgment and inability to see the consequences of behavior
- socially inappropriate sexual behavior
- ability to learn appropriate and necessary ADL skills with proper training, support, and guidance from a knowledgeable, patient, and caring staff

Residents with Mental Illness

Residents with mental illness often reflect the following characteristics:

- changes in personality that vary between residents and type of mental illness
- tendency to benefit from medication, psychotherapy, and a supportive staff who know and understand behavior techniques

Residents with mental illness often display the following common behaviors:

- Inappropriate social behavior
  - varies from not sleeping to talking excessively
  - poor hygiene and grooming
  - alcoholism
  - sexual addiction
  - eating disorders

- Unusual level of activity
  - overactivity (pacing)
  - underactivity (refusing to move)

- Sleep disturbances
  - excessive sleeping
  - difficulty getting to sleep or awakening extremely early

- Delusions
  - having false beliefs

- Hallucinations
  - seeing, hearing, or smelling things that are not present

- Compulsive behaviors
  - performing a behavior repeatedly

- Other behavior
  - anxiety
  - confusion
  - angry outbursts (Figure 4-1)
  - weeping for no reason
  - laughing without cause
  - fear
  - withdrawal
  - suicidal thoughts and behavior
  - mood swings
  - depression
  - restless, agitated behavior
  - wandering and pacing

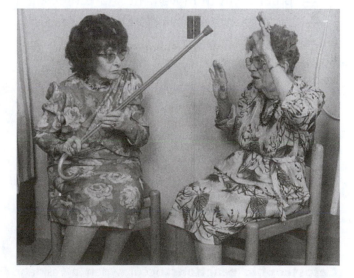

Figure 4-1 Residents with mental illness and dementia may have angry outbursts.

Residents with Alzheimer's Disease and Other Related Disorders

Alzheimer's disease is a form of dementia or mental illness of unknown cause. It creates changes in the brain tissue that cause a gradual loss of mental abilities. **Dementia** is a deterioration or decline of the brain that impairs mental capabilities. Dementia can be caused by acute (short-term) or chronic (long-term) disease. Characteristics of Alzheimer's and other dementias include:

- Sleep disturbances
  - difficulty sleeping
  - **lethargy,** depression, or restlessness

- Problems with wandering
  - wandering and confusion that worsen in the evening

- Memory and orientation
  - poor memory of recent events (short-term memory loss)
  - good long-term memory
  - lack of orientation to time and place
  - misidentification of people and common objects
  - lack of safety awareness

- Behavior problems
  - easily agitated and cannot be calmed readily
  - careless behavior
  - repetitive speech or behavior

- Neurological problems
  - problems with movement and coordination
  - incontinence of bowel or bladder
  - short attention span
  - poor judgment

- Other problems
  - creating new words
  - repetitive speech or verbally unresponsive
  - messy appearance

These symptoms may increase in severity over time until the resident needs help with all activities of daily living.

Catastrophic Reactions

Catastrophic reactions occur when a resident with Alzheimer's disease becomes overwhelmed by stimuli or is startled. Be careful when approaching a resident with Alzheimer's from behind. Speak quietly and gently so that you do not surprise the resident. Catastrophic reactions may be recognized by an increase in activity or talking. In a severe reaction, the resident becomes violent. Avoid catastrophic reactions by making sure that the resident is not stimulated by too much noise and activity. Make sure that the resident's basic physical needs, such as hunger, thirst, and elimination needs, are met. If a catastrophic reaction occurs, do not try to reason with the resident. Be calm and gentle in your approach. Touch may cause the resident to become more violent. Avoid restraining the resident, if possible.

If a resident has a catastrophic reaction or other behavior problem, do not take it personally. Understand that the problem is caused by the resident's disease.

CONSIDERATIONS FOR RESIDENTS WHO HAVE MENTAL IMPAIRMENTS

The resident with mental impairment needs the same physical care as any other resident. Remember, all people have the same basic physical and psychosocial needs. Be aware of these basic human needs as you care for residents who have Alzheimer's disease, dementia, or another mental impairment. Consider the following in caring for residents who have mental impairments:

- Environment
  - Provide a structured, safe environment.
  - Avoid change in routines.
  - Avoid excessive stimulation. Too much activity and noise often add to confusion and anxiety.
  - Avoid isolating the resident. Isolation leads to further confusion.
  - Supervise wandering residents adequately.

- Verbal communication
  - Call residents by their preferred names. All staff members should be consistent.
  - Maintain eye contact with the resident.
  - Use a calm voice and speak softly.
  - Keep communication simple. Give short, simple instructions.
  - Avoid arguing with the resident. A resident with dementia may have many false beliefs that you cannot change. Arguing will cause the resident to become very agitated. The resident has lost the ability to reason.
  - Allow time for the resident to respond.

— Mention the resident's emotions that are evident, such as fear or sadness.

- Body language

  — Approach residents from the front. Some residents with Alzheimer's disease have decreased ability to see side views.

  — Face the resident and make eye contact.

  — Bend down to the same level as the resident instead of standing over the resident when talking.

  — Use slow, deliberate hand movements to enhance understanding.

  — Remain calm and reassuring.

  — Use calm body language. Avoid jerky, rapid movements.

  — Use touch to reassure the resident, if he or she is not combative.

- Knowledge of residents' past

  — Listen to the resident's family. They can probably give suggestions or ideas to help you in the resident's care. Many families cared for residents for a long time at home.

  — Ask the nurse or social worker for information.

  — Remember that information about the resident is to be held in confidence.

VALIDATION THERAPY

Validation therapy is a behavior management technique that helps to maintain the resident's dignity and self-esteem by acknowledging how the resident feels. Validation therapy also acknowledges the resident's memories. It recognizes that all behavior has a purpose, even if we do not understand the reasons for the behavior. Sometimes the purpose of the behavior is a memory that the resident has. The nursing assistant should recognize that even confused residents are human beings and that they can feel pleasure by expressing their feelings and memories.

BEHAVIOR MANAGEMENT

All behavior has a purpose. It may mean one thing to the resident and something completely different to the staff. Understanding the resident's behavior may be very difficult. The behavior has meaning to the resident, however. Many behaviors that we consider problems are actually caused by fears, unmet needs, and lack of coping mechanisms. If an alert resident displays a behavior problem, it is usually because of an unmet psychosocial need.

Many residents have lost some control over their lives due to their disabilities. When they come to the long-term care facility, they feel that they have also lost control over their environment. They have given up many things that are important to them, including homes, possessions, and pets. This combination of losses often causes inappropriate behavior. Giving the resident control over routines and the environment will often reduce frustration and eliminate behavior problems. **Empathy** is compassionate understanding. Be empathetic. Understand how frustrated the resident is feeling.

When a resident who is mentally confused exhibits a behavior problem, it is often because of an unmet physical need, such as hunger, thirst, pain, need to use the bathroom, or need to change position. Sometimes the behavior is caused by too much noise and stimulation in the environment. Often the resident is unable to express the need in other ways. What we think is a behavior problem really is a method for the resident to tell us something. If the cause of the behavior can be discovered and eliminated, the behavior will stop.

Remembering that all behavior has meaning is important for the nursing assistant. Do not take the behavior personally (Figure 4-2). Treat each resident with patience, respect, and dignity.

Techniques to Reinforce Appropriate Behavior

Assist residents by reinforcing appropriate behavior in the following ways:

- Refer to the care plan regarding special methods, techniques, or strategies.

- Respond to appropriate behavior with genuine compliments and sincere praise.

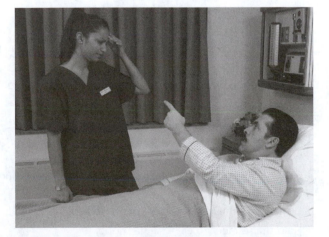

Figure 4-2 Do not take angry outbursts personally. Most of the time the resident is not mad at you. He is angry with his situation.

- Show pleasant responses to appropriate behavior by nonverbal communication such as a smile or soft touch.
- Never laugh at or ridicule a resident's behavior.
- Remember that all behavior has a meaning, even if you do not understand what the meaning is.

INTERACTING WITH RESIDENTS WHO HAVE MENTAL IMPAIRMENTS

This section lists some general techniques to follow when interacting with residents who have mental impairments. Because each resident is an individual, certain residents may have special instructions or restrictions. Being empathetic is important for the nursing assistant. Try to understand how the resident feels.

The need for individualized care is essential. Be sure to follow special instructions listed on the care plan for the resident. Consistency is important when caring for mentally impaired residents.

How to Respond to the Resident's Behavior

Become aware of your own responses and reactions to the resident's behavior, and modify your own behavior if necessary. Monitor your body language for hidden messages. Even mentally confused residents are sensitive to body language. Develop caring attitudes by demonstrating:

- patience
- kindness
- pleasantness
- gentleness
- caring
- understanding
- empathy

✔ **GUIDELINES for Interacting with and Caring for Residents Who Have Mental Impairments**

Keep in mind the following when caring for residents who have mental impairments:

☐ Reinforce feelings of belonging and safety by saying things such as, "You are safe here."

☐ Call the resident by her preferred name.

☐ Treat the resident with dignity and respect.

☐ Do not talk down to the resident or treat her like a child.

☐ Never call the resident degrading names or use degrading terms to refer to the resident.

☐ Always be calm in both verbal and nonverbal communications.

☐ Avoid changes in the resident's environment or routines.

☐ Dress and groom the resident appropriately.

☐ Make sure that the resident's physical needs are met.

☐ To be consistent, report all successes and failures at attempts to modify resident behaviors.

☐ Note when excessive behaviors occur. The resident may have a pattern that will give you important information about the cause of the behavior.

☐ Acknowledge the resident's feelings by saying things such as, "I can see that you are afraid," or "I can see you are feeling sad."

☐ Make the resident feel good about herself. Positive self-esteem decreases behavior problems.

☐ Allow the resident to be as independent as possible. Feeling independent helps increase the resident's feelings of self-worth.

☐ Support the resident's family and listen to their suggestions. Tell them about activities in which family involvement is encouraged.

☐ Understand the resident. Think how you would like to be treated if you or your parent were the resident.

☐ Help the resident to exercise her rights.

☐ Monitor the environment and eliminate safety hazards.

BEHAVIOR MODIFICATIONS FOR NURSING ASSISTANTS

This section describes specific ways in which you can change your behavior in response to the resident. These techniques can help you when working with residents who have mental impairments. With all techniques, remember to treat the resident with respect and dignity. Never assume that a particular behavior is "normal for the resident." If you can change a resident's behavior by eliminating the cause, be sure to share this information with the nurse and other members of the health care team.

Use of Body Language

Body language is an important tool for helping residents.

- Use body language that expresses a listening approach toward the resident (Figure 4-3).
- Place yourself near the resident, but do not get too close. This shows respect for the resident's personal space.
- Position yourself at the resident's level. Sit if the resident is sitting. Stand if the resident is standing.
- Face the resident and maintain eye contact.
- Assume an open posture by avoiding crossed arms and legs.

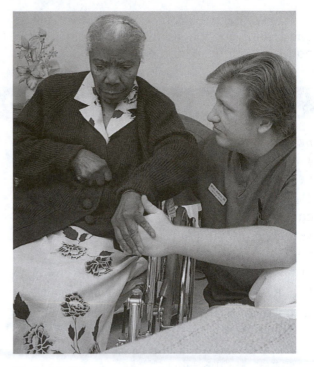

Figure 4-3 Show the resident that you care with your body language, calm demeanor, and gentle touch.

- Lean toward the resident.
- Appear relaxed and focus on the resident. Avoid looking around.

✔ GUIDELINES for Management of Agitated or Aggressive Behavior

The following guidelines will help you with behavior management:

- ☐ Base your actions on the principle that anger is a secondary emotional response to a primary feeling of fear, frustration, grief, or loss of self-esteem.
- ☐ If no risk to yourself or others exists, ignore the resident's behavior.
- ☐ Approach the resident from the front. Do not make the resident feel cornered.
- ☐ Move slowly and deliberately.
- ☐ Maintain eye contact.
- ☐ Your speech should be calm and firm. Speak with a low-pitched voice.
- ☐ Speak in short, simple phrases.
- ☐ Acknowledge feelings that are evident by saying, "I can see you are angry," or "I can see you are frightened."
- ☐ Be sure to tell the resident that she is safe.
- ☐ Allow the resident to talk about her anger.
- ☐ Listen to what the resident says.
- ☐ Monitor the resident's body language.
- ☐ If possible, use the resident's anger constructively by getting her to do things such as wiping a table, tearing rags, squeezing a ball, or rolling a ball of yarn.
- ☐ Use therapeutic isolation and physical restraints only when necessary and as indicated on the care plan.
- ☐ Report or record the resident's behavior and responses to your behavior.

- Use nonverbal behavior to show that you are interested in what the resident is saying by smiling, nodding your head, and so on.

- Report or record the resident's behavior and responses to your behavior.

KEY POINTS IN THIS CHAPTER

▲ Residents who have mental impairments need special assistance in meeting their psychosocial needs.

▲ The symptoms of mental impairment vary according to the disease.

▲ Special consideration must be given to the resident who has a mental impairment.

▲ Alzheimer's disease is a form of dementia resulting in gradual loss of mental and physical abilities.

▲ All behavior has meaning, even if the meaning is not clear to others.

▲ Attempt to determine the cause of the behavior and eliminate the cause.

▲ Report successes and failures in modifying resident behavior to the nurse.

▲ Inappropriate behavior often is caused by feelings of loss of control over life or by other unmet needs.

▲ Offering choices and allowing residents to do as much as possible gives them some sense of control and promotes feelings of self-esteem.

▲ Consistency in care is extremely important for residents who have mental impairment.

▲ The nursing assistant should modify his or her own behavior in response to the resident's behavior.

▲ Do not take resident behavior outbursts personally.

REVIEW QUIZ

1. A resident who is disoriented is:
   a. usually retarded.
   b. confused as to time and place.
   c. not allowed to eat.
   d. also destructive.

2. Changes in a resident's personality may be a sign of:
   a. mental illness.
   b. too much socializing.
   c. lack of exercise.
   d. manipulation.

3. Alzheimer's disease creates changes in the:
   a. brain.
   b. heart.
   c. lungs.
   d. spine.

4. A resident who has dementia needs:
   a. increased activity to stay alert.
   b. to be isolated from others.
   c. a structured, safe environment.
   d. freedom from rules.

5. All behavior has meaning to the:
   a. facility psychologist.
   b. person doing the behavior.
   c. person observing the behavior.
   d. person who is talking.

6. Inappropriate behavior is commonly caused by:
   a. abnormal vital signs.
   b. anger at the family or staff.

   c. a negative attitude.
   d. unmet needs.

7. When speaking with residents, the nursing assistant should call them:
   a. granny or gramps.
   b. the name preferred by the resident.
   c. "honey" or "dear."
   d. a friendly nickname.

8. When residents have feelings of positive self-esteem, behavior problems:
   a. decrease.
   b. increase.
   c. stay the same.
   d. get started.

9. When caring for residents who have mental impairments, you should keep the daily routine:
   a. full of recreational activities.
   b. varied to maintain interest.
   c. structured.
   d. free from any exercise.

10. To build feelings of self-esteem in residents who have mental illness,
    a. do things for them quickly so they do not have to wait.
    b. always feed them so they don't spill food.
    c. tell them what clothing to wear.
    d. allow them to do as much as possible for themselves.

11. When you empathize with residents, you are:
    a. understanding how the resident feels.
    b. feeling very sorry for them.
    c. feeling very happy for them.
    d. sympathizing with the situation.

12. A good listening approach to use when communicating with residents who have mental impairment is to:
    a. tell the resident to stop talking.
    b. stay at least six feet away from the resident.
    c. sit by a resident who is in a chair.
    d. avoid making eye contact.

13. When a resident is angry or agitated, the underlying feeling may be:
    a. fear.   c. hate.
    b. depression.   d. happiness.

14. A resident seems very angry and announces, "No one is going to tell me what to do." Your best response is to:
    a. apply a restraint.
    b. tell the resident to settle down.
    c. allow the resident to talk about the anger.
    d. confine the resident to her room.

15. A good example of providing choices to a resident would be to:
    a. tell the resident to go for a walk outside.
    b. allow the resident to choose a dessert if all of the dinner is eaten first.
    c. explain that if the resident chooses to be angry there will be no bingo games.
    d. allow the resident to pick out clothes to wear today.

16. Mr. Rimer is a 67-year-old resident with dementia. He is not able to express his needs verbally. He sits quietly much of the time, but you notice that he wanders quickly around the nursing facility about four times on your shift. Mr. Rimer usually urinates in his clothing when he wanders. What might be the purpose of Mr. Rimer's wandering behavior?
    a. The resident is bored.
    b. He is looking for the bathroom.
    c. He dislikes the noise in the environment.
    d. The resident is upset with you.

17. Mrs. Lee is an alert, demanding resident who uses the call signal frequently. If you do not answer it immediately, she yells, "Help! Help!" When you answer the call signal, her requests are never urgent. She speaks sharply to you when you are in the room. What would be your best response?
    a. Tell the nurse that Mrs. Lee doesn't like you and ask not to be assigned to her again.
    b. Take Mrs. Lee's call signal away.
    c. Tell Mrs. Lee that you have sick people to take care of and not to use the call signal unless it is an emergency.
    d. Give Mrs. Lee choices and control over her routines and environment.

18. Mr. Green is a 75-year-old resident who has a long history of mental illness. Mr. Green often smiles and talks when no one else is around. You are assigned to care for Mr. Green. He does not want to bathe and change his clothes. He says that God commanded him to wear the same clothes every day. Your best response would be to:
    a. check with the nurse or care plan for further directions.
    b. tell the resident that you are God and that he should change his clothes.
    c. attempt to remove Mr. Green's clothing anyway.
    d. leave and care for the next resident on your assignment.

19. You are caring for Mrs. Clark, a 69-year-old resident with Alzheimer's disease. It is time for lunch and you go to find the resident to take her to the dining room. Mrs. Clark is very upset when you enter her room. She is throwing things on the floor and yelling. You ask her what is wrong, but her response makes no sense. Your best response would be to:
    a. apply a restraint so that Mrs. Clark does not injure herself.
    b. acknowledge Mrs. Clark's feelings by saying, "I see that you are angry."
    c. tell Mrs. Clark to stop acting childishly.
    d. advise the resident that she will not be given lunch because of her temper tantrum.

20. Mr. Hassan is a confused resident who seems to get more confused late in the day. You are working the 2:00 p.m. to 10:00 p.m. shift on C station. There is quite a bit of activity on the unit after supper. Visitors are coming in and out, and staff members are busily trying to get residents ready for bed. Mr. Hassan is sitting in the chair by the nurse's station. You notice that he is becoming restless and agitated. You take him to the lounge, which is quiet, and put some music on the radio. You sit next to Mr. Hassan and talk to him. The resident calms down right away. Based on Mr. Hassan's response to your intervention, you should:
    a. always isolate the resident from others.
    b. put Mr. Hassan to bed immediately after supper.
    c. inform the nurse and other members of the health care team of Mr. Hassan's response.
    d. say nothing about Mr. Hassan's behavior, because it is just a coincidence.

CHAPTER 4
CROSSWORD PUZZLE

Directions: Complete the puzzle using these words found in Chapter 4.

Alzheimer's	disorientation	psychosocial
catastrophic	empathy	reality
confusion	lethargy	retardation
dementia	mental	validation

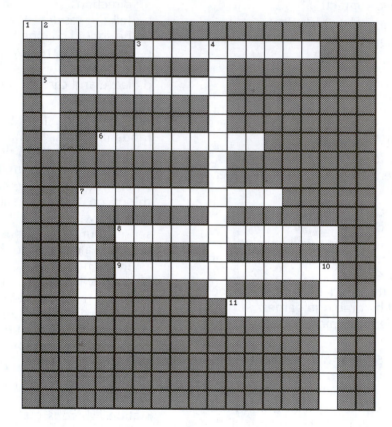

CHAPTER 4
PUZZLE CLUES

ACROSS

1. _____ illness is a disorder of the mind.

3. A program that helps confused residents explore their feelings and makes them feel good about themselves is _____ therapy.

5. _____ disease results in gradual loss of mental ability.

6. Behavior that is different from the usual; mixed up

7. Lower-than-average intellectual development is mental _____ .

8. Unpredictable behavior that may become violent is a _____ reaction.

9. _____ needs relate to mental and emotional activity.

11. Impaired thinking, memory, or judgment

DOWN

2. Understanding how a resident feels.

4. Confusion about identity, place, and time

7. A program to help the resident relearn dates, time, place, and identity is called _____ orientation.

10. Abnormal drowsiness or sleepiness

Communication

OBJECTIVES

In this chapter you will learn the importance of good communication with residents and other members of the health care team. After reading this chapter, you will be able to:

- Spell and define key terms.
- Explain why observation is an important part of effective communication.
- Demonstrate effective communication.
- Identify types of communication.
- List characteristics of therapeutic communication.
- Describe barriers to communication.
- Describe how to communicate with residents who have physical disabilities, vision loss, or hearing impairments, residents who are mentally confused, and residents who are unable to speak.
- Describe the importance of communication with staff.
- Give examples of observations to be reported.
- Describe the nursing assistant's role in recordkeeping.
- Identify common medical abbreviations and state their meaning.

KEY TERMS

abnormal: unusual, not normal

aphasia: the inability to speak or understand communication because of an injury, illness, or other medical condition

barrier: a barricade; something that interferes with, hinders, or separates

communication: the exchange of thoughts, feelings, and information by verbal or nonverbal messages

Health Insurance Portability and Accountability Act (HIPAA): a law that applies to resident privacy, confidentiality, and medical records. The HIPAA regulations protect all information by which a resident could be identified. The rules apply to paper, verbal, and electronic documentation, billing records, and clinical records. Staff are provided only the information needed to carry out their duties.

legible: plain, clear, easily read handwriting

medical record: the resident's chart. The medical record is a written legal record of the history, progress, and care plan of the resident.

nonverbal: sending a message without the use of words. Silence, appearance, room decor, and body language are methods of nonverbal communication.

objective: observations made by the senses of the observer; things you can see, feel, hear, and smell

observation: noticing a fact or occurrence

pain: a state of discomfort that is unpleasant for the resident. It is always a warning that something is wrong. It interferes with residents' function, well-being, and self-care.

prioritize: organizing your assignment so that the most important tasks are done first

sign: indication of illness, injury, or disease that can be seen by others

subjective: problems experienced by the resident that are not seen by others

symptom: indication of illness, injury, or disease felt by the resident, but not seen by others

verbal: sending a message by using words, tone of voice, and pitch of voice

EFFECTIVE COMMUNICATION

Effective **communication** is essential in your role as a nursing assistant. To do your job well in the long-term care facility, you must develop good communication skills for relating to residents, family members, visitors, and other staff (Figure 5-1). Communication includes three things:

- a sender
- a message
- a receiver

Effective communication occurs when the receiver understands the message in the same way that the sender meant the message. Communicating well takes time, practice, and skill. Because you will be spending much of your working day with individual residents, you have a responsibility to encourage residents to talk about their needs. Using the techniques listed will help encourage residents to talk about their needs.

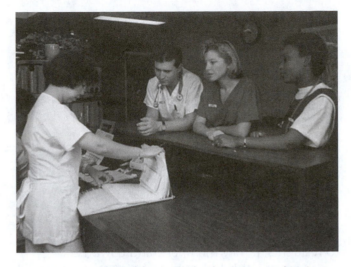

Figure 5-1 Good communication with other team members is essential for nursing assistants.

TYPES OF COMMUNICATION

Communication occurs in two ways: **verbal** and **nonverbal.** You will use both forms of communication as you work with residents. Verbal communication consists of:

- choice of words
- tone of voice
- speed of voice
- volume and pitch of voice

Monitor the resident's ability to understand the words you use. To achieve effective verbal communication, do the following:

- Get the message across by voice or words that the resident understands.
- Use verbal communication to give and receive information, report facts, and share experiences.

Nonverbal communication conveys a message without using words. Examples of nonverbal communication include:

- facial expression
- posture
- hand gestures
- touch
- dress
- movement
- raising of eyebrows
- smiles
- frowns
- silence
- resident's room decor

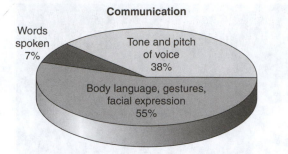

Communication

Words spoken 7%

Tone and pitch of voice 38%

Body language, gestures, facial expression 55%

Figure 5-2 Your body language and tone of voice are more important to the interpretation of a message than the words you use.

Remember that actions speak louder than words. Be aware of your nonverbal behavior when relating to residents, family members, and coworkers.

Over one-third of a message is communicated through the tone and pitch of your voice. If these things conflict with your spoken words, the tone and pitch will overshadow the message. Be aware of how the tone, pitch, and quality of your voice affect the way your message is interpreted. When speaking with others, always remember the impact of nonverbal communication. Your words represent only 7 percent of your message. The rest of the message is interpreted from facial expressions, gestures, and body language. Your tone of voice represents 38 percent of the meaning. Gestures, facial expressions, and other body language constitute 55 percent of your total communication (Figure 5-2).

THERAPEUTIC COMMUNICATION

The words *therapy* and *therapeutic* refer to healing or improving a resident's condition. Therapeutic communication can be either verbal or nonverbal. You have probably used therapeutic communication quite often. You have done this if you have discussed a problem with a friend, or helped someone through a sad situation by just being there. As a nursing assistant, you can provide therapeutic communication for residents (Figure 5-3). Successful therapeutic communication is possible only if you understand what the resident is really trying to tell you. Important points to remember in therapeutic communication are:

- Listen carefully to what the resident says.
- Observe the resident's body language, facial expression, movements, and actions.
- Be sensitive to the resident's feelings. Notice any difference between his words and his actions.
- Focus on what the resident is saying.
- Comment on the resident's feelings by giving appropriate responses.
- Respond to what is being said so both you and the resident understand what was communicated.

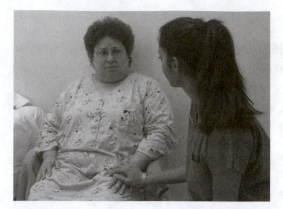

Figure 5-3 Whenever possible, take the time to sit and talk to residents, particularly if they are feeling stressed or upset.

- Report the resident's responses, actions, and behaviors to the nurse.
- Understand that people sometimes say what they think you want to hear.

COMMUNICATION BARRIERS

Anything that interferes with the communication process can be considered a **barrier**, something that makes communication difficult. The barrier can be from either the sender or the receiver and can interfere during any part of communication. Also, both verbal and nonverbal barriers can occur.

Barriers to Effective Communication

The following behaviors and conditions can pose barriers to communication:

- your physical position, if you are standing above the resident
- not listening
- background noise
- belittling a person
- talking to a resident as you would a child
- your body language
- your attitude or the resident's attitude, such as when you feel angry, anxious, or pressured
- a resident who is mentally confused
- when the resident's primary language is different from that of the nursing assistant
- taking over the conversation
- avoiding eye contact
- appearing too busy or in a hurry
- making judgments
- not acknowledging what the resident has said
- giving false or inappropriate answers

✔ GUIDELINES for Effective Communication

To communicate effectively, you must:

- ☐ Prepare the resident in advance if your time is limited, by stating how much time you have and when you will need to leave.
- ☐ Reduce background noise, such as music or television.
- ☐ Position yourself at the resident's level.
- ☐ Make good eye contact.
- ☐ Be polite.
- ☐ Make sure your body language says you are listening.
- ☐ Speak at a pace the resident understands.
- ☐ Use terms that are familiar to the resident; avoid slang and sound-alike words, such as "hall" and "haul."
- ☐ Give the resident time to talk.
- ☐ Express an interest in what the resident says.
- ☐ Ask questions or make comments to show that you are interested in what the resident says.
- ☐ Match body language with what is said.
- ☐ Speak clearly and at an appropriate loudness level so the resident can hear you.
- ☐ Do not chew gum when talking.
- ☐ Do not cover your mouth with your hands.
- ☐ Refer to the resident by the name he prefers.
- ☐ Use touch to communicate caring, if appropriate.

- using words the resident does not understand
- sensory impairments, such as impaired vision and hearing
- residents with glasses not wearing them, or glasses dirty
- residents with hearing aids not using them; hearing aid batteries dead, or hearing aid in poor repair
- physical disability related to injury or disease, such as **aphasia,** which is the inability to speak or understand
- being insensitive to the needs of a resident from a different culture
- preconceived ideas or beliefs

Communicating with Residents Who Have Vision Impairment

Because some vision loss is part of the normal aging process, you will be working with vision-impaired residents. Vision impairment often is a barrier to communication. The care plan identifies specific methods for helping residents who have visual impairments. Helpful techniques for communicating with residents who have visual impairments are:

- Identify yourself when approaching the resident.
- Knock before entering the room.
- Call the resident by the name the resident wants to be called.
- Remember that glare from a window behind you can interfere with the resident's ability to see clearly.
- Encourage the use of eyeglasses and help the resident as needed. The nursing assistant is responsible for keeping the glasses clean.
- Offer your arm to guide the resident. Walk slightly ahead of the resident.
- Speak clearly and slowly, using a moderate tone of voice.
- Do not talk to the resident as if he were a child.
- Provide adequate light in the room. Changes in vision due to aging make seeing in the dark more difficult.
- Make sure the light source is behind the resident, and not behind you (in the resident's eyes).
- Use touch to communicate, if appropriate, but do so slowly and gently so the resident is not startled.
- Tell the resident what you are doing when working in the room.
- Tell the resident when you are finished.
- Replace everything in its original location. Tell the resident where items are.

- You may discuss new things you see, interesting changes, and what others are doing. This is not offensive. You are the resident's eyes!

- Always ask the resident what he would like to wear. Describe the color and style of the clothes.

- When seating the resident, place the resident's hand on the back or arm of the chair.

- Do not leave a resident who is visually impaired or blind in an open area. Lead him to the side of a room, chair, or landmark from which he can obtain a direction for travel.

- Tell the resident when you are leaving the room. Make sure he is comfortable and safe, with the call signal and needed personal items within reach.

Communicating with Residents Who Have Hearing Impairment

Some hearing loss occurs in the normal aging process. Hearing loss can be a severe barrier to communication. Specific suggestions will be listed on the resident's care plan. Helpful techniques for communicating with residents who have hearing impairments are:

- Identify yourself to the resident.

- Gently touch the resident to get his attention.

- Make sure that the light source is behind the resident, not you, so that the resident can see your mouth clearly.

- Eliminate outside distractions and noise from the radio, television, or other sources.

- Face the resident when speaking. Use hand gestures and facial expressions to help the resident understand you.

- Speak clearly and slowly. Be aware of your own speech patterns and practice so you can speak in a way the resident will understand.

- Keep sentences short.

- Keep your hands away from your face when speaking.

- Stand or sit near the resident.

- Do not eat or chew gum when talking to the resident.

- If the resident does not understand you, choose new words to say the same thing. Do not repeat what you said in a louder tone of voice.

- Write and use other assistive devices to communicate with the resident.

- If the resident uses a hearing aid, help insert it.

Care of the hearing aid. Caring for the resident's hearing aid is the responsibility of the nursing assistant. A hearing aid is expensive and difficult to replace. Be sure that is not accidentally dropped in the linen when the bed is changed. Check the resident's ears daily for buildup of wax or other **abnormal** conditions. Follow the manufacturer's instructions or the care plan for cleaning and inserting the hearing aid.

Several different types of hearing aids are available. Some are very small and are worn completely within the ear. Others are larger and have an ear mold. Some are contained within the arm of the resident's eyeglasses. Rules for hearing aid care are as follows:

- Handle the hearing aid with care. Be sure that it is not dropped.

- Do not allow the hearing aid to get wet. If the hearing aid has an outside ear mold, the earpiece can be washed only with mild soap and water. The part of the hearing aid containing the batteries should never get wet. Always remove the hearing aid when bathing the resident, washing the hair, or using a hair dryer.

- Turn the hearing aid off when the resident is not using it.

- If the hearing aid has a cord, check it daily for cracks or breaks.

- Be sure that the ear mold is clean. If the hearing aid is the cannula type, it may be cleaned with a small pipe cleaner or special appliance cleaner. If excess wax is present, notify the nurse.

- Allow the resident to assist as much as possible.

- Organize your work so that male residents who are shaved with an electric razor can be shaved before the hearing aid is applied. If this is not possible, turn the aid off or remove it before using the electric razor. The buzzing of the razor is very loud and annoying with a hearing aid in place.

- Insert the hearing aid properly. If the resident complains that it hurts, advise the nurse. Sometimes the shape of the ear changes with aging, and the hearing aid may have to be refitted.

- If the resident has difficulty with letters or numbers, say, "M as in Mary, 2 as in twins, B as in boy." Say numbers separately, such as "six seven," instead of 67.

- Follow the same guidelines that you use when communicating with a resident who has hearing impairment.

- Remove the hearing aid and allow the ear to "cool" before taking a tympanic temperature.

✓ **GUIDELINES for Troubleshooting Hearing Aid Problems**

Never try to repair a hearing aid yourself. If the resident has problems with the hearing aid, you can perform a few simple activities that may resolve the problem:

☐ Make sure the aid is turned on. Some aids have settings marked on them. These are "M" for microphone, "T" for telephone, and "O" for off. Set the switch to the "M" setting.

☐ Check the volume of the aid; make sure it is turned up loud enough.

☐ Hold the aid in the palm of your hand. Turn the volume up all the way. Cup the aid between your hands. You should hear a loud whistle. If the sound is weak or absent, the battery is low.

☐ Before changing the battery, check the position of the old battery. Put the new one in the same way. Insert a new battery gently. Avoid forcing it.

☐ Check the ear mold and remove wax buildup.

☐ Ask the nurse to check the resident's ears with an otoscope.

☐ If the hearing aid makes a whistling sound when it is in the resident's ear, check the position. Make sure it is securely in the ear. Hair, ear wax, and clothing should not interfere with the position. Check the tubing for cracks. Whistling may indicate an air leak.

☐ Check for dirt under and around the battery if the aid works intermittently or makes a scratchy sound. Check the volume control and connections. Make sure the connecting wire is plugged in tightly and is not cracked or bent.

☐ Notify the nurse if the hearing aid does not work properly.

COMMUNICATING WITH RESIDENTS WHO HAVE DISABILITIES AND OTHER SENSORY IMPAIRMENTS

Many residents in the long-term care facility have disabilities and sensory impairments. Some of these problems interfere with communication. You may be unsure of what to say to residents who have disabilities, without being offensive. People with disabilities are like you. They have the same problems, wants, and needs. They can do many of the same things you can. However, they may need to adapt or change the environment to be able to do them. People with disabilities may perform the task differently, but the end result will be the same. Their bodies just work differently! As a rule, people with disabilities do not want to be treated differently from anyone else. Many are self-sufficient. Most have led productive lives. People with disabilities are valuable and equal members of society. You must treat them as such. Although they are physically challenged, most have developed other abilities using nonphysical skills.

You must emphasize the uniqueness and worth of all persons. Treat residents who have disabilities the way you like to be treated.

Communicating with Residents Who Have Problems with Language and Understanding

Some residents have illnesses or injuries that affect their ability to speak and understand what is spoken to them. They may understand some things, but not others. Assume that they understand you. Communicate with them as you would other residents. Speak when you are caring for them. If you are silent, the resident may interpret this as a negative message. Some residents may be able to speak, but what they say does not make sense. Certain words or phrases may have meaning to the resident, but not to you. Try to understand what the resident is saying. Avoid frustration. Be empathetic. If you learn what the resident is saying, share this information with others. This will help all team members to meet the resident's needs. Some residents understand what is spoken to them, even if they cannot speak.

Do not assume that residents with speech problems are mentally confused. Test the resident's ability. If he can answer yes-or-no questions, or follow simple directions, he understands you.

Communicating with Residents Who Have Problems Speaking

Residents with some diseases and injuries are unable to speak. Although they can make sounds, they cannot form words. Residents with this problem usually understand what you are saying. Do not make the mistake of thinking that the resident is mentally confused. Some residents will regain their speech with speech therapy. Some develop other methods of communication. They often make their needs known by using gestures, writing, or other adaptive communication devices.

✔ **GUIDELINES for Communicating with Residents Who Have Disabilities**

- ☐ Avoid referring to the resident as a condition, such as "the paraplegic in 525." Say instead, "Mrs. Smith in 525." Avoid identifying the resident by condition. Always emphasize the person over the condition.
- ☐ Use common sense when speaking. Talk to the person the same way you would anyone else. People with disabilities do not want to be treated differently.
- ☐ Do not assume that someone is *not* disabled because you cannot see the disability. Some conditions are severely disabling, but not visible.
- ☐ You may shake hands gently with residents who have upper extremity disabilities or prostheses.
- ☐ Before helping someone who has a disability, ask if you can help. Do not assume that the person needs help without asking.
- ☐ It is all right to ask residents about their disabilities. Many residents are comfortable and will talk about them. However, it is also all right if they do not want to talk about it. A resident who is newly disabled may not have accepted the disability, and may be uncomfortable talking about it.
- ☐ Do not assume that the resident can or cannot do something. Assuming is offensive. Always ask.
- ☐ Stress the resident's ability and not the disability.
- ☐ Avoid assuming that residents who use wheelchairs, canes, walkers, and crutches are sick. Avoid making assumptions.
- ☐ Do not treat residents who use wheelchairs as if they are mentally impaired! Most have no mental problem. Speak with the person in the wheelchair, not the person's companion.
- ☐ Position yourself at the resident's eye level when speaking with a resident in a wheelchair.
- ☐ Be polite. Use good manners.
- ☐ Excuse yourself if you walk in front of a resident in a wheelchair.
- ☐ If you are in a crowded area, avoid standing in front of a person in a wheelchair. Standing in front of the resident blocks his view.
- ☐ The wheelchair is an extension of the resident's body. Leaning or hanging on the chair is an invasion of the resident's personal space.
- ☐ It is all right to use words such as "see," "hear," "run," and "walk" when speaking with residents who have disabilities.
- ☐ Select words that are positive and nonjudgmental. Avoid using demeaning words like "cripple," "gimp," "spastic," and "retard." Using words like these promotes negative perceptions of people who are physically challenged. Tables 5-1 and 5-2 give examples of acceptable and unacceptable words to use. Always emphasize the person first. Emphasizing the disease is demeaning. Table 5-2 lists phrases to use when speaking about persons who have disabilities.
- ☐ People with disabilities like to laugh and have fun. Do not leave them out!
- ☐ Seeing-eye dogs, hearing-ear dogs, and other canine companions are on duty. Do not feed or pet them without permission. This prevents them from doing their job.
- ☐ Do not park in spaces reserved for persons who are disabled. They need them more than you do. Often someone will pull into a disabled parking spot while a companion runs into a store. The driver remains in the car so it can be moved if the police come. When a driver with a disability pulls in, he has no place to park!

TABLE 5-1

Words to Avoid When Speaking with or About Persons Who Have Disabilities

abnormal	cripple	deformity	maimed	stricken with
afflicted	crippled	diseased	moron	sufferer
burden	deaf and dumb	epileptic	normal	suffers with
cerebral palsied	deaf mute	gimp	palsied	suffering
confined to a wheelchair	defect	invalid	poor	unfortunate
courageous	defective	imbecile	spastic	victim

TABLE 5-2

Offensive and Unacceptable—Do Not Use in Conversation	Acceptable—Use This Instead
Disabled person	A person with a disability (or who has a disability)
Blind person	A person who is vision-impaired
Deaf person	A person who is hearing-impaired
A hunchback	A person who has curvature of the spine
The disabled	People who are disabled; the disabled community
He is a cripple	He has a disability
Dumb (or deaf and dumb)	A person who has a speech or hearing impairment
She is nuts, crazy	She has an emotional disability or mental illness
Retard	A person who is mentally retarded
Birth defect	A person who is disabled from birth
Fit (or has fits)	Seizure (has a seizure disorder)
Normal person as compared with a person who has a disability	A person who is not disabled as compared with a person who is
Confined to a wheelchair	A person who uses a wheelchair

✓ GUIDELINES for Communicating with Residents Who Have Problems with Language and Understanding

☐ Knock on the door and identify yourself by name and title before entering the room. Call the resident by the preferred name.
☐ Be courteous and friendly when approaching the resident.
☐ Assist the resident with glasses and hearing aids, if used.
☐ Explain what will be done.
☐ Use short, simple words. Speak clearly and slowly.
☐ Focus on one topic.
☐ Use short sentences.
☐ Show that you care with gentle touch.
☐ Keep conversations short but frequent.
☐ Use gestures and facial expressions to communicate.
☐ Allow time for the resident to respond.
☐ Do not finish a sentence for the resident.
☐ Listen carefully. Pay attention.
☐ If you think you understand what the resident is saying, paraphrase the words to give the resident feedback.
☐ Do not cut the resident off when he is speaking.
☐ Avoid communicating frustration through your body language.
☐ If you cannot get a response, assume that the resident understands.
☐ Help the resident point to things and use gestures.
☐ Use adaptive devices, such as picture boards, if available. The speech-language pathologist will often provide these devices and teach the resident to use them.
☐ Tell the resident when you leave the room. Make sure that he is comfortable and safe, with the call signal and needed personal items within reach.

✔ **GUIDELINES for Communicating with Residents Who Have Problems Speaking**

☐ Knock on the door and identify yourself by name and title before entering the room. Call the resident by the preferred name.

☐ Be courteous and friendly when approaching the resident.

☐ Assist the resident with glasses and hearing aids, if used.

☐ Explain what will be done.

☐ Keep conversations short but frequent.

☐ Ask the resident questions that can be answered yes or no. Instruct the resident to nod his head in response. If the resident cannot nod the head, tell him to blink the eyes once for yes and twice for no.

☐ Allow time for the resident to respond.

☐ See if the resident can write, or use assistive communication devices, such as picture or word boards.

☐ Listen carefully to the response.

☐ If you think you understand what the resident is saying, repeat it.

☐ Do not pretend to understand if you do not.

☐ Emphasize words and gestures that you do understand.

☐ Allow time to complete the conversation.

☐ Avoid showing impatience.

☐ Avoid communicating frustration through your body language.

☐ If you cannot get a response, assume that the resident understands.

☐ Help the resident point to things and use gestures.

☐ Tell the resident when you leave the room. Make sure that he is comfortable and safe, with the call signal and needed personal items within reach.

Communicating with People Who Are Mentally Retarded

Three percent of the population in the United States has mental retardation. A person who is mentally retarded has learning problems. The condition was caused by conditions before birth or in early childhood. The resident did not cause the problem. There are many levels of retardation, ranging from profound to mild. Residents with profound retardation function at the level of a newborn. People with mild retardation function at about the fourth-grade level. Most people with mental retardation are mildly retarded. People who are mentally retarded have the same needs as you do. They learn more slowly. Their learning may be limited. Most live productive lives. Mental retardation is like any other disability.

Residents who are mentally retarded need acceptance and attention. Treat them with dignity and respect. Allow them to express themselves and relieve stress. They may become overwhelmed if they are frustrated. They can make simple choices. Limit the options to avoid frustrating the resident. Consistency is important in their routines. Use the care

plan to ensure consistent care. Most are happy and loving. They like to help and feel like they are contributing. Make the resident feel worthwhile.

Avoid pressuring residents with mental retardation to learn or perform new tasks. They can learn new things, but you must be patient and teach them gradually. They may not function well in high-pressure situations, or large, loud, confusing groups. Support a resident who is in this situation. Residents with mental retardation know if others are making fun of them, and feel hurt and rejection.

COMMUNICATING WITH RESIDENTS' FAMILIES, FRIENDS, AND VISITORS

You represent the long-term care facility to visitors. Speak and smile when you see visitors in the hallway. Ask if you can be of assistance. Be friendly and supportive. Show them where the lounges, vending machines, cafeteria, restrooms, and smoking areas are. Answer questions about policies and procedures. You must protect resident confidentiality, even with family members. If they ask you questions about the resident's condition, refer them to the nurse. You may tell them something about the resident's activities,

✔ GUIDELINES for Communicating with People Who Are Mentally Retarded

☐ Use short, simple words and sentences.

☐ Give simple, clear, concise instructions.

☐ Avoid talking down to the resident.

☐ Avoid treating the residents like children. They are adults. Avoid dressing them in childish clothing.

☐ Listen carefully when the resident speaks. He may know more than you think.

☐ People who are mentally retarded are sensitive to the moods of others. If you are upset, the resident will be too. Happiness is contagious.

☐ Limit choices to two if making decisions upsets the resident.

☐ If the resident becomes frustrated, slow down. Do not push.

☐ Praise and compliment the resident frequently.

☐ Treat the resident with respect.

such as, "He ate a good lunch." Avoid giving them information about other residents.

Families may show anxiety or anger in reaction to a resident's problems. Be patient and understanding. Avoid arguing. Listen carefully and be empathetic. If you believe that family members are upsetting the resident, inform the nurse. Relay all complaints to the nurse.

If visitors are in the room and you must perform a procedure, ask them to step out. Show them where they can wait. When you are done with the procedure, inform them that they can return to the room. If the procedure is not urgent, wait until the visitors are gone.

ANSWERING THE TELEPHONE

If answering the telephone is your responsibility, answer the phone by stating the name of your facility or unit. State your name and title. Be courteous and polite. A nurse must take the call if a physician is on the line to give orders. If the caller is not a physician, obtain the information, or transfer the caller to the proper person. You may answer the caller's questions. However, avoid giving out personal information about residents. Take a clear message if the person being called cannot come to the telephone. Write down the date, time of the call, name of the caller, and a brief message. Sign your name and title to the message. Inform the caller that you will deliver the message. Thank the person for calling.

COMMUNICATION WITH STAFF

Nursing assistants have frequent and close contact with residents and therefore have the opportunity to observe residents more closely than the supervising nurse. Communicating with the nurse about residents is absolutely necessary for continuity of care.

The care plan is an essential tool for staff communication regarding each resident's care. The care plan is a written plan that clearly identifies a resident's needs. Your responsibilities for the resident's care are listed on the care plan. Your supervising nurse will help you develop your assignment based on information in the care plan. Ask the nurse any questions you have when you receive your assignment. Your supervising nurse will help you decide how to **prioritize**, or arrange, your assignment. Setting priorities means that the most important tasks are completed first, and all essential care is done in a timely manner. Remember, the Resident's Bill of Rights gives the resident the right to privacy of medical records and information. Be sure you discuss the resident's condition with the nurse in a private setting.

Report

The facility will have a change-of-shift report at the beginning of every shift. Usually, the offgoing nurse gives a verbal report to the oncoming nurse. Some facilities use a tape-recorded report. The report provides information about the residents' conditions during the previous shift. Resident illness, pain, hospitalization, and other notable changes will be discussed. In some facilities, all nursing staff listen to this report. In other facilities, only the nurses receive the report. They in turn will have a report for the nursing assistants after the offgoing shift leaves. Although the procedure varies from one facility to the next, it is safe to say that you will receive some type of report at the beginning of every shift.

Having a report at the beginning of the shift helps to ensure continuity of care. The report will provide information you will need to set priorities and plan the care you will give the residents during your shift. It will alert you to things you should be monitoring. Baseline information is provided, such as "Mrs. Romcevich's temperature was 97.8°F. She complained of feeling cold, so we gave her extra blankets." From hearing this, you will know that you should monitor this resident for feeling cold during your shift. The nurse may also ask you to check her temperature. If you find it is significantly different from the previous shift, notify the nurse immediately. Likewise, if the resident complains of feeling hot, or the skin feels hot to the touch for no obvious reason, inform the nurse promptly.

You will report information to the nurse throughout your shift. At the end of the shift, you will report off on all your residents. You will describe your observations, care, and other information. The nurse will use this as a basis for reporting to the oncoming shift and completing his assessments and documentation. As you can see, your shift begins with communication. You communicate with others throughout the shift, then end the shift with more communication. Recording information on the residents' records is also a form of communication. Making observations, communicating with residents and other staff, reporting, and recording are important skills to master.

REPORTING OBSERVATIONS

Because of your close contact with residents, you must know what should be reported to the nurse. Certain **observations** must be reported immediately. If you have any doubts, err on the side of caution and report the change to the nurse right away (Figure 5-4). Report the following observations:

- changes in the resident's physical or mental status, or general mood
- residents' reactions and behaviors
- what the resident says about his health (e.g., pain, numbness, dizziness)
- what you observe using your senses of hearing, sight, touch, and smell
- care that seems to work best for the resident
- care that does not seem to work well

If you report your observations to the nurse and the resident's condition seems to worsen, report to the nurse again. If you make an observation and report it, and you are not sure whether the nurse has responded, ask the nurse for his opinion on what you observed. This will serve as a gentle reminder to the nurse to check the resident if he has not already done so.

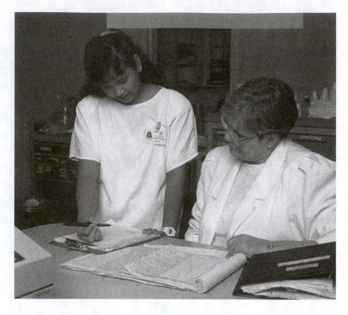

Figure 5-4 Accurately monitoring of residents' conditions and reporting of observations to the nurse are essential for residents' well-being.

How to Recognize and Report Abnormal Signs and Symptoms

A **sign** is an indication of disease. Signs are **objective** findings that can be detected by others. They are things you can see, feel, hear, and smell. Examples of signs are bruises or reddened areas on the skin. A **symptom** is a **subjective** finding. Symptoms cannot be seen by others. They are felt by the resident, who usually tells you about them. An example of a symptom is pain.

The following signs and symptoms tell you something is abnormal. They may indicate disease or illness in the resident and must be brought to the nurse's attention.

- Evidence of pain
  - in the chest
  - when moving
  - while urinating
  - while having a bowel movement
- Skin changes
  - redness that does not go away quickly when pressure is relieved
  - unusual color, such as blue or gray, of the skin, lips, nailbeds, lining or roof of mouth, or mucous membranes
  - breaks or tears in the skin
  - bruises
  - lumps
  - rashes

— abnormal sweating

— swelling of feet, ankles, or hands

— skin that is very warm or cool to the touch

- Respiratory changes

— coughing

— slow, rapid, or irregular breathing

— shortness of breath or difficulty breathing

— gasping for breath

— noisy breathing

- Digestive changes

— sores or ulcers inside the mouth or gums

— nausea

— vomiting

— choking

— frequent belching

— appetite changes

— excessive thirst

— difficulty in chewing or swallowing

— dark or bloody stool

— loose, watery stool

— hard stool or difficulty passing stool

— unusual color of stool

- Urinary changes

— difficulty urinating

— dark color

— strong odor

— blood, mucus, or sediment in urine

— urinating frequently in small amounts

— burning or pain while urinating

— suddenly cannot control the passage of urine

- Musculoskeletal changes

— cannot move arms or legs

— shaky or jerky motions

— obvious deformities

— changes in ability to sit, stand, walk, or move

— pain on movement

- Change in mental status

— drowsiness

— sleepiness for no apparent reason

— restlessness

— suddenly more confused

— problems with coordination

— changes mood quickly

- Other changes

— fever or chills

— any unusual body discharge, such as pus or mucus

PAIN

Pain is a state of discomfort that is unpleasant for the resident. It is always a warning that something is wrong. It interferes with the resident's function, well-being, and self-care. Unrelieved pain contributes to complications of immobility, increasing the risk of pneumonia, skin breakdown, and other problems. Pain may cause acting out, crying, and other strange, belligerent, or combative behavior. It is a major preventable public health problem that slows recovery in individuals with acute illness, complicates chronic illness, and increases health care costs. Relieving pain has always been an important nursing responsibility. Nursing staff must identify residents who are having pain, and those who are at risk of pain, then take the appropriate action(s) to make residents as comfortable as possible.

Residents' Responses to Pain

Residents' responses to pain vary widely. Some individuals do not feel pain as acutely as others. Some try to ignore pain. Other residents may try to deny pain because they are afraid of what it means. Ignoring or denying pain increases the risk of injury, because the normal warning that pain provides goes unrecognized or unheeded. Confused residents may display behavior problems when they are having pain. Some moan, sigh, or yell during movement. Never ignore body language or other signs of pain in residents. Always report signs and symptoms of pain to the nurse. Your observations are a valuable contribution to the nursing assessment and residents' comfort.

Identifying Residents Who Are in Pain

Pain is a serious condition that affects well-being and quality of life. Residents have the right to timely pain assessment and management. Many factors affect residents' reactions to pain. The reactions may be different from one moment to the next, and from one resident to the next. Pain is usually categorized into four types:

- Acute pain—Occurs suddenly and without warning; usually the result of tissue damage, caused by conditions such as injury or surgery. Typically decreases over time, as healing takes place.

- Persistent (chronic) pain—Pain that lasts longer than six months. (Another, older term for this type of pain is *chronic pain*). It may be intermittent or constant.

- Phantom pain—Occurs as a result of an amputation. A body part, such as a leg, has been removed, but the residents complains of pain in the toes of the missing leg. The pain is real, not imaginary.
- Radiating pain—Moves from the site of origin to other areas. For example, when a resident is having a heart attack, the pain may radiate from the chest to the jaw or arm.

Observing and Reporting Signs and Symptoms of Pain

Body language is often the first clue that a resident is having pain. This may be the only clue in some cognitively impaired residents, those from other cultures, and residents who are comatose. Look for pain on movement, facial expressions, crying, moaning, rigid posture, and guarded positioning. Some residents will yell out, grimace, or cry during transfers or movement. This may be interpreted as confusion instead of pain. The resident may withdraw when he is touched or repositioned. Watch for restlessness, irregular or erratic respirations, periodic breath holding, dilated pupils, and sweating. The resident may favor one extremity. He may become irritable, fatigued, or withdrawn. The resident may refuse to eat for no apparent reason. He may act the opposite of normal. Always suspect pain if the resident's behavior changes. Report your observations to the nurse and compare with the normal behavior for the resident.

The resident's self-report of pain is the most accurate indicator of the existence and intensity of pain, and should be respected and believed. Avoid making assumptions about a resident's pain. Although many residents with pain display outward signs through their body language and behavior, avoid making assumptions about the presence or absence of pain if the resident is laughing, talking, or sleeping. For example, some health care workers assume that residents who are smiling or laughing cannot be in pain. Vital signs may be normal. These workers believe that residents who are having pain should be grimacing, frowning, or crying. This is untrue. Some residents may appear comfortable while having severe pain. Once again, avoid judging the resident. His self-report of pain is the most accurate and reliable indicator of pain. Notify the nurse without passing judgment.

When asking about pain, make sure the resident can see and hear you. Allow enough time for the resident to process your questions and respond. Be patient. Use language that is appropriate for the resident's age and mental status. Remember that residents may use different words for pain, such as *hurt, sore,* or *tender.* Residents who are mentally confused may surprise you. Some can describe their pain accurately. Always ask residents who are crying, have body language suggesting pain, and those whose behavior suggests pain if they are having pain or discomfort.

Response to Pain

Pain always requires further intervention. It should never be ignored. Always report verbal complaints of pain, describing the pain in the resident's exact words. Be aware of signs and symptoms of pain in residents who have difficulty communicating, such as residents who cannot speak and residents who are cognitively impaired. Pain is always an observation that must be reported immediately. A nursing assessment of pain involves many different factors. Your observations contribute to this assessment and the resident's well-being.

Using a pain rating scale. Your facility will have policies and procedures for pain management. Most facilities have adopted several different pain rating scales to evaluate the level of residents' pain. In fact, many facilities now consider pain the "fifth vital sign." In these facilities, pain is regularly and frequently evaluated.

Because pain is personal and subjective, consistent pain evaluation between health care workers is a concern. Using a pain rating (assessment) scale helps nurses assess the resident and keeps caregivers from forming their own opinions about the level of a resident's pain. Using a pain scale prevents subjective opinions, eliminates some barriers to pain management, and gives the resident a means of describing the pain accurately. Pain scales are important tools for communication. The resident selects the scale that helps *best describe* his pain. Pain rating scales can be used to evaluate pain in residents of all ages and cultures.

Although you will not directly assess residents' pain, you must understand the purpose of the scales used in your facility and how they are interpreted. Many facilities use a 0 to 10 scale, with 0 meaning no pain and 10 meaning intolerable pain. If the resident tells you that he is having pain at "level 5," for example, you must know what this means and report the problem to the nurse. Likewise, if the resident complains of pain at "level 9" an hour after receiving pain medication, this suggests a potentially serious problem and must be reported immediately.

Many different pain scales are used in health care (Figure 5-5). These scales are for example only. Your facility may use similar or different tools for evaluating pain. Pain scales use pictures, words, or numbers to help the resident describe pain intensity. Most scales range from no pain to very severe pain. Picture scales use smiling faces, neutral faces, frowns, and tears.

Managing Pain

Unrelieved pain has a negative effect on the resident's health and functional status. Notify the nurse

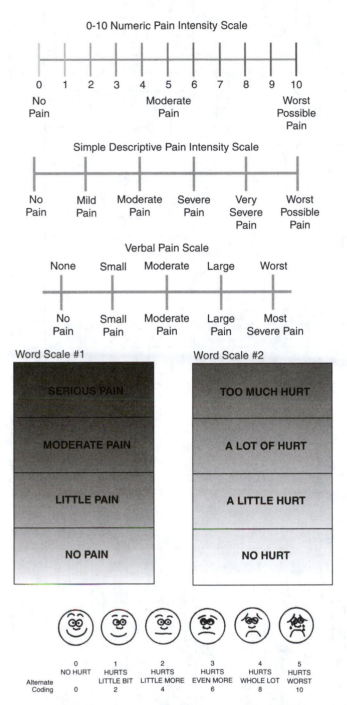

0-10 Numeric Pain Intensity Scale

| 0 | 1 | 2 | 3 | 4 | 5 | 6 | 7 | 8 | 9 | 10 |

No Pain   Moderate Pain   Worst Possible Pain

Simple Descriptive Pain Intensity Scale

No Pain   Mild Pain   Moderate Pain   Severe Pain   Very Severe Pain   Worst Possible Pain

Verbal Pain Scale

None   Small   Moderate   Large   Worst

No Pain   Small Pain   Moderate Pain   Large Pain   Most Severe Pain

Word Scale #1

SERIOUS PAIN

MODERATE PAIN

LITTLE PAIN

NO PAIN

Word Scale #2

TOO MUCH HURT

A LOT OF HURT

A LITTLE HURT

NO HURT

	0 NO HURT	1 HURTS LITTLE BIT	2 HURTS LITTLE MORE	3 HURTS EVEN MORE	4 HURTS WHOLE LOT	5 HURTS WORST
Alternate Coding	0	2	4	6	8	10

Figure 5-5 The resident will select the pain scale that best helps him communicate the level and intensity of his pain. (FACES pain scale from Wong, D. L., Hockenberry-Eaton, M., Wilson, D., Winkelstein, M. L., & Schwartz, P. (2005). *Wong's essentials of pediatric nursing,* 7th ed. St. Louis, MO: Mosby, p. 1259. Copyrighted by Mosby, Inc. Used with permission)

as soon as the resident complains, before pain becomes severe or out of control. Report your observations objectively. Observe the resident carefully after pain medication has been given, and report your observations to the nurse.

Sometimes the physician orders several different medications for a resident's pain. The nurse will select which drug to use based on an assessment of the resident. Your observations, the resident's self-report of pain intensity, and physical assessment findings are all considered when determining which medication to administer, when more than one is ordered. If the first drug does not relieve the pain, the nurse may have the option of administering another, so always report unrelieved pain.

Pain management is an important part of resident care. Take complaints of pain very seriously. Respect and support residents' right to pain assessment and management without judgment or disbelief. Although nursing assistants are not directly responsible for pain management, your observations and nursing care are very important, because you work so closely and intimately with residents. Understanding the responsibilities that health care providers have for pain relief will help you provide nursing comfort measures, monitor for signs and symptoms of pain, and report your observations to the nurse. The quality of pain control is influenced by the education, experience, and attitude of the workers who care for the resident.

RECORDKEEPING

The resident's **medical record** is often called the resident's *chart*. This is a legal document that contains the history and progress of the resident's care in the facility. It is a true, accurate, and complete record of the resident's care. Recordkeeping policies, or charting, are not the same at all facilities. In many facilities, the nursing assistant is responsible for some important recordkeeping. Patterns or changes in the resident's behavior are noticed and treated because of the nursing assistant's reporting and recording. Most facilities require nursing assistants to do checklist charting (Figure 5-6). Examples of forms that you would use for checklist charting are:

- activities of daily living (ADL) sheets (Figure 5-7)
- bowel sheets

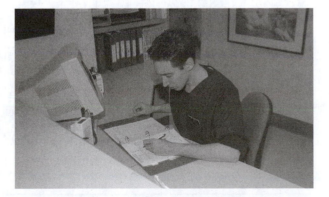

Figure 5-6 Medical records are an objective legal record. They are an important part of resident care. In fact, they validate that care was given, as stated on the care plan. Accurate and complete documentation helps others determine what has been done. Team members use this information to plan additional clinical approaches for residents' care.

NURSE ASSISTANT CARE RECORD—A.M. SHIFT

(Reference tags: F309, F310, F312, F315-F318, F327; Cross reference tags: F221, F222, F241, F246-F247)

INSTRUCTIONS: Identify the appropriate code for each item listed under the correct date column. Unless otherwise indicated refer to the following response key: **Y** = Yes; **N** = No; **I** = Independent; **A** = Assist; **D** = Dependent; **— —** = Not Applicable. Initial each day's documentation and identify your initials by signing (one time) on the reverse where indicated. Additional notes and comments should also be documented on the reverse.

Month		Year	Code	1	2	3	4	5	6	7	8	9	10	11	12	13	14	15	16	17	18	19	20	21	22	23	24	25	26	27	28	29	30	31
FEEDING	Breakfast		% Eaten																																
	Lunch		% Eaten																																
	Self/Assisted/Fed		S-A-F																																
	Ate in-Bed/Room/Dining Room/Chair		B-R-D-C																																
	Nourishment-Taken/Refused		T-R																																
BODY CARE	Bath-Bed/Shower/Tub/Partial/Whrpl/Shampoo		B-S-T-P-W-SH																																
	Nail Care-Fingers/Toes		F-T																																
	Skin-Clear/Other (Report "O" to Nurse)		C-O																																
	Positioned qh		¼-½-1-2 / I-A-D																																
	Pads-Air/Water/Foam/Synthetic		A-W-F-S																																
BLADDER	Continent-Bedpan/Urinal/BRP/Commode		P-U-B-C																																
	Incontinent		# Times																																
	Catheter		C-N																																
	Intake		cc's																																
	Output		cc's																																
BOWEL	Continent-Bedpan/BRP/Commode		P-B-C																																
	Incontinent		# Times																																
	Enema-Tap Water/Soap/Fleets		T-S-F																																
	Loose Stool		# Times																																
BEHAVIOR	Cooperative-Accepts Assist		C-N																																
	Resistant-Refuses Assist		R-N																																
	Alert-Oriented to Reality		Y-N																																
	Confused/Noisy/Agitated (if ✓'d note reason on reverse)																																	
	Behavior Monitored (specify)		# Times																																
	Feeding Program		Y-N																																
	Oral Hygiene		I-A-D																																
	Hair Care		I-A-D																																
	Shave		I-A-D																																
	Dressing/Undressing with ROM		I-A-D																																
RESTORATIVE CARE	Range of Motion-Passive/Active		P-A																																
	Transfers		I-A-D																																
	Bowel & Bladder Program		Y-N																																
	Up in Chair		I-A-D																																
	Restraints-Bed/Wheelchair		B-W																																
	Ambulation-Walker/Cane/Assist/Self		W-C-A-S																																
	Scheduled Activities-Attended/Refused		A-R																																
SAFETY DEVICES	Side Rails Up/Down/Release		U-D-R																																
	Geri Chair/Vest/Wrist/Waist/Pelvic		G-V-W-WA-P																																
	Safety Device/Restraint-Released qh		2-1-1½																																
	Checked q 30 minutes		✓																																
	Positioned qh		½-1																																
OTHER																																			
	CHARGE NURSE NOTIFIED (record reason on back)		Y-N																																
	OUT OF FACILITY		Y-N																																
AIDE INITIALS																																				

NAME—Last   First   Middle   Attending Physician   Chart No.

CFS 6-3AHH   © 1992 Briggs Corporation, Des Moines, IA 50306 (800) 247-2343   Printed in U.S.A.

NURSE ASSISTANT CARE RECORD
A.M. SHIFT

Figure 5-7 Most long-term care facilities use flow sheets to record daily care. (Compliments of Briggs Corporation, Des Moines, IA (800) 247-2343)

- intake and output (I&O) sheets
- meal acceptance sheets
- temperature, pulse, and respiration (TPR) and blood pressure (BP) sheets.

Charting is always done after you have given care. Never document a procedure before you actually do it. Charting must be accurate, clearly stated, **legible,** confidential, dated, and signed. Charting is done in chronological order according to the time. Things that happen or are observed first are charted first. Sign your charting with your name (or first initial and last name) and title.

Confidentiality and privacy. The medical record is a private, confidential document. Protect medical records from access by unauthorized persons. Likewise, you should not read resident charts out of curiosity. Medical records should be accessed only by those with a need to know the information. In 1996, Congress passed the **Health Insurance Portability and Accountability Act (HIPAA).** This law has many provisions. One portion applies to resident privacy, confidentiality, and medical records. The HIPAA rules:

- Increase residents' control over their medical records.
- Restrict the use and disclosure of resident information.
- Make facilities responsible for protecting resident data.
- Require the facility to implement and monitor their information release policies and procedures.

The HIPAA regulations protect all health information that can identify an individual. The rules apply to paper, verbal, and electronic documentation, billing records, and clinical records. Staff should be provided only with the information needed to carry out their duties. Because of this, resident information is disclosed on a "need to know" basis. For example, the dietary department would need to know if the resident had an order for a diabetic diet. They would not need to know that the resident has an infected area on the face. The nursing assistant needs to know about both the diabetes and the infection.

Facilities must monitor how and where resident information is used. Policies must protect resident charts, places where residents are discussed, faxing and electronic transmission of information, and disclosure of other personal information. Each facility writes policies and procedures to meet its needs according to the HIPAA guidelines.

MEDICAL ABBREVIATIONS

Many different abbreviations are used for written communication in health care facilities. Your facility will have a list of abbreviations that may be used. Use only abbreviations that are on the list. In 2004, some regulatory agencies started requiring facilities to eliminate abbreviations that are confusing or may be misinterpreted because of illegible handwriting. The following list includes common abbreviations that are often used in long-term care. However, it is possible that some of these are not used in your facility. Know and follow your facility policies.

ī, īī	_____	one, two, etc.
ʒ	_____	ounces
ʒī, ʒīī	_____	one ounce, two ounces, etc.
↓	_____	down
↑	_____	up
Abd.	_____	abdomen
āc	_____	before meals
ad lib	_____	as desired
ADL	_____	activities of daily living
adm	_____	admission
AIDS	_____	acquired immune deficiency syndrome
Amb.	_____	ambulate; to walk
AROM	_____	active range of motion
ax	_____	under the arm
B & B	_____	bowel and bladder program
b.i.d.	_____	twice a day
BM	_____	bowel movement
B/P	_____	blood pressure
BR	_____	bed rest; bathroom
BS	_____	blood sugar
BSC	_____	bedside commode
c̄	_____	with
Ca	_____	cancer
CC	_____	chief complaint
CHF	_____	congestive heart failure
c/o	_____	complains of
COLD	_____	chronic obstructive lung disease
COPD	_____	chronic obstructive pulmonary disease
C & S	_____	culture and sensitivity
CVA	_____	cerebrovascular accident, stroke, brain attack
DNR	_____	do not resuscitate
DOB	_____	date of birth
dx	_____	diagnosis
e	_____	enema

et	_____	and	rehab	_____	rehabilitation
ext	_____	extremities	res, Res	_____	resident
fx	_____	fracture	resp	_____	respirations
I&O	_____	intake and output	R/O	_____	rule out
MI	_____	myocardial infarction, heart attack	ROM	_____	range of motion
			Rx	_____	treatment
mL	_____	milliliter	s̄	_____	without
mm	_____	millimeter	S.O.B.	_____	shortness of breath
MRSA	_____	methicillin-resistant *Staphylococcus aureus*	S/S, SS, S & S	_____	signs and symptoms
Na	_____	sodium	Stat	_____	immediately, at once
n/c	_____	no complaints	STD	_____	sexually transmitted disease
NG	_____	nasogastric			
NPO	_____	nothing by mouth	Std. prec.	_____	standard precautions
N&V	_____	nausea and vomiting	Sx	_____	symptoms
O, PO	_____	oral	T, temp	_____	temperature
O₂	_____	oxygen	t.i.d.	_____	three times a day
OBS	_____	organic brain syndrome	TPR	_____	temperature, pulse, respiration
p̄c	_____	after meals			
PRN, prn	_____	whenever necessary	Tx	_____	traction, treatment
PROM	_____	passive range of motion	UA, U/A	_____	urinalysis
PT	_____	physical therapy	URI	_____	upper respiratory infection
q̄	_____	every, each	UTI	_____	urinary tract infection
q.i.d.	_____	four times a day	VRE	_____	vancomycin-resistant *Enterococcus*
q̄h	_____	every hour			
q̄2h, q̄3h, q̄4h, etc.	_____	every two hours, every three hours, every four hours, etc.	VS	_____	vital signs
			WA, W/A	_____	while awake
			w/c	_____	wheelchair
			WNL	_____	within normal limits
q̄s	_____	sufficient quantity	wt	_____	weight
R	_____	rectal, respirations	XR, X/R	_____	X-ray
reg	_____	regular			

KEY POINTS IN THIS CHAPTER

▲ Effective communication occurs when the message received is the same as the one sent.

▲ Communication can be either verbal or non-verbal.

▲ A barrier to communication is anything that blocks or interferes with communication.

▲ Common barriers to effective communication with elderly residents are vision, hearing, speech, and mental impairments.

▲ People with disabilities should be treated the way you like to be treated. Some people with disabilities have special communication needs.

▲ Courtesy is important when answering the telephone in the health care facility.

▲ The nursing assistant has the most opportunities in the long-term care facility to observe residents. Reporting these observations to the nurse is an important role of the nursing assistant.

▲ Recordkeeping must be accurate, legible, and confidential. Documentation must be signed and dated by the person doing the recording.

▲ Medical abbreviations are used in the health care setting to help you communicate well.

REVIEW QUIZ

1. Communication is effective when the message is:
   a. sent correctly.
   b. received as the sender wants it to be received.
   c. received as the receiver wants to receive the message.
   d. sent as the sender intends but is received differently.

2. Which of the following is a good communication technique?
   a. Finishing sentences for a resident who has a speech problem
   b. Teasing and kidding the resident
   c. Standing over the resident with the light behind you
   d. Listening carefully to what the resident says

3. Verbal communication is:
   a. sending a message using words.
   b. using touch to send a message.
   c. the same as nonverbal communication.
   d. sending a message without the use of words.

4. What is an example of a communication barrier?
   a. listening attentively
   b. observing facial expressions
   c. maintaining eye contact
   d. talking down to a person

5. When communicating with a resident who has a vision impairment, it is important to:
   a. speak louder than usual.
   b. encourage the resident to wear his glasses.
   c. give the resident written instructions.
   d. keep the room as dark as possible to avoid eyestrain.

6. Communication with a resident who has a hearing impairment may be improved by:
   a. yelling in the resident's good ear.
   b. standing with the light behind you.
   c. using sign language.
   d. keeping sentences short.

7. What member of the nursing staff has the most frequent contact with the resident?
   a. the medication nurse
   b. the director of nursing
   c. the nursing assistant
   d. the charge nurse

8. The essential tool in staff communication regarding resident care is the:
   a. care plan.
   b. interdisciplinary progress note.
   c. flow sheet.
   d. nurses' notes.

9. Which of the following is important for you to report to the nurse?
   a. gifts brought to the resident
   b. the television programs the resident watches
   c. any change in the resident's health
   d. personal information the resident tells you

10. When observing skin changes in the resident, you should notice and report:
    a. shortness of breath.
    b. redness or swelling.
    c. digestive disturbances.
    d. drowsiness or restlessness.

11. The legal document that contains the resident's medical history and progress is the:
    a. care plan.
    b. assignment sheet.
    c. medical chart.
    d. Medicare report.

12. All of the following are true about charting in the medical record *except:*
    a. Charting must be accurate.
    b. Charting must be clearly written.
    c. No signature is required on any charting.
    d. The information is confidential.

13. Medical terms and abbreviations are used in the health care setting to:
    a. encourage staff to learn new words.
    b. discourage residents from understanding medical findings.
    c. keep information in code in case it is overheard by visitors.
    d. assist in making staff communication clear and concise.

14. What does "BP b.i.d." mean?
    a. Take blood pressure twice a day.
    b. Give the resident the bedpan when in bed.
    c. Take blood pressure at the bedside.
    d. Give the resident the bedpan every 2 hours.

15. Abnormal changes that you should recognize and report are:
    a. the resident needs a shave and shower.
    b. the resident is wearing clothes that do not match.
    c. the resident's clothing is soiled.
    d. the resident's lips and nailbeds are blue.

16. The abbreviation for three times a day is:
    a. 3xid.
    b. t.i.d.
    c. 3 i.d.
    d. t.o.d.

17. When communicating with a resident who uses a wheelchair, you should avoid using the word:
    a. see.
    b. run.
    c. walk.
    d. cripple.

18. When caring for residents who have vision or hearing loss, you should:
    a. be as quiet as possible when you are in the room so the resident is not disturbed.
    b. make as much noise as possible when you are in the room so the resident knows what you are doing.
    c. announce yourself by name and title when you enter the room.
    d. always approach the resident from behind.

19. When caring for residents who have problems with speech or understanding, you should:
    a. explain the care you will be giving in medical terms.
    b. choose short, simple words and use short sentences.
    c. use sign language that the resident understands.
    d. not explain procedures, because the resident will not understand.

20. When caring for a person who is mentally retarded, you should:
    a. treat the resident with courtesy and respect.
    b. not explain procedures.
    c. never smile, because this is upsetting to the resident.
    d. treat the resident like a child.

21. You answer the telephone on your unit. The caller identifies herself as Dr. Gonzales and states that she wants to give orders for Mrs. Keene. You should:
    a. ask the doctor to hold while you get the nurse.
    b. write down the orders the doctor gives you.
    c. tell the doctor to call back later.
    d. ask a more experienced assistant to take the call.

22. An abnormal change in the digestive system that you should report is:
    a. dark, hard stools.
    b. pain while urinating.
    c. shortness of breath.
    d. dry, red skin.

23. Mr. King is an 83-year-old resident with a diagnosis of congestive heart failure. He is alert and able to do most of his care by himself. He is usually up, dressed, and in the dining room before breakfast. He remains up and is active in the facility during the day. When you make your first round on the day shift, you enter Mr. King's room and discover that he is still in bed. His ankles are swollen, his breathing is rapid, and he complains of a headache. You should:
    a. tell Mr. King to get up and get ready for breakfast.
    b. notify the nurse immediately of your observations.
    c. help Mr. King get dressed, as he does not feel well.
    d. call the kitchen and order a room tray for the resident.

24. You are assigned to help in the facility dining room at lunchtime. Mrs. Hazeldon is an 84-year-old mentally confused resident who wears thick glasses. You observe that she has eaten everything on her plate. However, the resident has not eaten any of her fruit or dessert. She has not taken a drink of milk or water. You should:
    a. return the resident to her room because she has finished eating.
    b. leave the resident alone.
    c. make sure that Mrs. Hazeldon can see her fruit, dessert, and beverages.
    d. report the resident to the nurse.

25. Mr. Ardlean is an 87-year-old resident who is very hard of hearing. He wears a hearing aid when he is up and about in the facility. You are assigned to care for Mr. Ardlean on Wednesday. You are assigned to give him a shower, wash his hair, shave him, and make his bed. You should:
    a. leave the hearing aid in during the shower.
    b. check the bed linen before removing it to make sure that the hearing aid was not accidentally dropped in the bed.
    c. tell Mr. Ardlean to insert the hearing aid by himself.
    d. put the hearing aid in before using the electric razor.

26. You are assigned to work the 2:00 p.m. to 10:00 p.m. shift on third floor. When you come on duty, Mr. Allen, the charge nurse, gives you report and posts the assignment sheet. After you get report, you should:
    a. complete your charting for the shift.
    b. ask another nursing assistant what you should do first.
    c. review the assignment sheet and set your priorities for the shift.
    d. begin bringing residents to the dining room for supper.

27. You have been off work for the past two days. You are scheduled to work the 2:00 p.m. to 10:00 p.m. shift when you return. You are assigned to care for Mrs. Fulmer, a 71-year-old resident who is mentally confused and does not speak. You are helping Mrs. Fulmer undress and

get ready for bed. She is wearing a cardigan sweater and a short-sleeved blouse. When you remove her sweater, you notice a large bruise on Mrs. Fulmer's arm. Because you did not work yesterday, you do not know how or when she got the bruise. You should:

a. report the bruise to the nurse.

b. say nothing about the bruise, as this is not your responsibility.

c. do nothing about the bruise, as you know that it did not happen on your shift.

d. apply a hot pack to the bruise.

28. You are assigned to care for Mr. Stine, a 77-year-old resident who is normally mentally alert. Mr. Stine speaks with you normally at the beginning of your shift, but as the shift progresses, the resident becomes more confused. You should:

a. do nothing, as this is normal in the elderly.

b. notify the nurse of the resident's confusion.

c. call Mr. Stine's daughter and inform her of the confusion.

d. say nothing, but record your findings in the medical record.

29. You are assigned to care for Miss Williams, a 32-year-old resident who has cerebral palsy. The resident has multiple physical deformities and requires total care. Miss Williams is unable to speak, but she understands what others say to her. She is able to nod her head to answer yes-or-no questions. When Miss Williams is using the toilet, you must stay in the bathroom with her because she is not able to balance herself on the toilet seat. You notice that she makes a face when she is urinating. Her urine has a very strong odor. You should:

a. report your observations to the nurse.

b. notify Miss Williams's doctor of your observations.

c. call Miss Williams's brother and advise him of the problem.

d. say nothing, because this is normal in cerebral palsy.

CHAPTER 5
CROSSWORD PUZZLE

Directions: Complete the puzzle using these words found in Chapter 5.

abbreviation
abnormal
aphasia
barrier
communication
hearing

impaired
legible
medical
nonverbal
objective
observation

sign
subjective
symptom
therapeutic
verbal

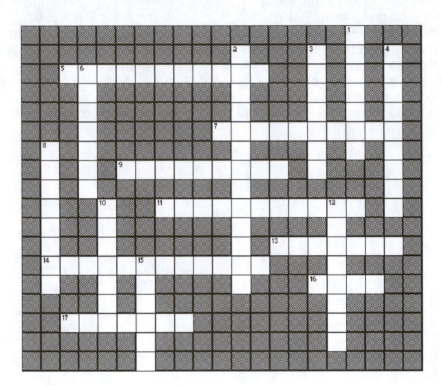

CHAPTER 5
CROSSWORD CLUES

ACROSS

5. Noticing a fact
7. A problem experienced by a resident that cannot be seen by others
9. Indication of illness, disease, or injury that can be detected by using the senses of the observer
11. Care designed to cure, heal, or preserve health
13. A subjective change in the body that may indicate illness, injury, or disease
14. Shortened form of words, used for communication
16. An objective indication of disease, illness, or injury
17. Plain, clear, easily read

DOWN

1. Inability to speak or understand
2. Exchanging thoughts, ideas, and information
3. Document your observations in the _____ record.
4. Sending a message without the use of words
6. A barricade
8. Unusual
10. A device that some residents use so that they can hear what you are saying is a _____ aid.
12. A resident who cannot see well is vision _____ .
15. Speaking is _____ communication.

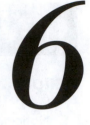

Infection Control

OBJECTIVES

In this chapter, you will learn the principles of infection control. You must understand these principles to prevent the spread of disease in the health care setting. After reading this chapter, you will be able to:

- Spell and define key terms.
- List principles of medical asepsis.
- Define *infection*.
- Describe the common methods by which infections are spread.
- List the times when you should wash your hands.
- Describe standard precautions.
- Demonstrate proper handwashing.
- Describe when to use gloves, protective eyewear, and surgical masks.
- Perform isolation procedures.
- List the types of isolation and describe personal protective equipment worn in each.

KEY TERMS

airborne precautions: a category of transmission-based precautions that health care workers use to prevent the spread of airborne pathogens

airborne transmission: the spread of disease by very small microbes carried or suspended in the air

aseptic: the absence of any disease-causing microbes

bacteria: one-celled microorganisms, some of which cause disease

biohazardous waste: waste products contaminated by contact with blood or body fluid that require special handling

blood and body fluid transmission: a method of transmitting disease that occurs when blood or any body fluid except sweat contacts nonintact skin or mucous membranes

chain of infection: a description of the factors necessary for an infection to spread

communicable: diseases that are easily transmitted to other persons

contact precautions: a category of transmission-based precautions used when caring for patients who have infections that are spread by skin and wound drainage, secretions, excretions, blood, body fluids, or contact with mucous membranes

contact transmission: the spread of pathogens by direct or indirect contact, such as touching an infectious object or person

contaminated: unclean, soiled articles or equipment

disinfection: the process that destroys or slows the growth of disease-causing microorganisms

droplet precautions: a category of transmission-based precautions used to prevent the spread of infection from patients whose infection is spread by respiratory droplets in the air

droplet transmission: the spread of disease in the air. Droplets usually remain within three feet of the resident. Droplet transmission occurs by inhaling droplets of secretions that contain pathogens

droplets: moist secretions produced by sneezing, coughing, laughing, talking, and singing that are spread into the air

drug-resistant pathogens: pathogens that cannot be destroyed by most antibiotics

germs: a common name for disease-causing microbes

high-efficiency particulate air (HEPA) filter respirator: respirator that prevents transmission of tuberculosis and other tiny pathogens that are spread by the airborne method of transmission

HBV (hepatitis B virus): the virus that causes hepatitis B, a disease of the liver

HCV (hepatitis C virus): a serious infection of the liver caused by the hepatitis C virus; can be spread through contact with blood or body fluids

HIV (human immunodeficiency virus): the virus that causes HIV disease and AIDS

infection: a disease state caused by germs invading the body

isolation: protective techniques used when caring for a resident who has a communicable disease

medical asepsis: the practices and techniques used in the health care setting to prevent the spread of microorganisms from one person or place to another

microbe: a microorganism

microorganisms: living plants and animals that are so small they can be seen only with a microscope

mite: microscopic parasite that lives on the skin of animals and humans, causing rashes and irritation

MRSA (methicillin-resistant *Staphylococcus aureus*): a pathogen that is very difficult to eradicate because it is resistant to most antibiotics

N95 respirator: a respirator used when caring for a resident in airborne precautions

necrotizing fasciitis: an invasive skin and tissue infection that is commonly caused by group A Streptococcus, the same bacterium that causes strep throat. (It may be caused by other bacteria, or a combination of bacteria.) This microbe also may be called "flesh-eating strep." The bacterium enters the body through a break in the skin, such as a paper cut or pressure ulcer. Toxins quickly multiply in the tissue and the disease becomes widespread in the body, causing shock, tissue decay, and death

pathogen: a microbe that is harmful and causes disease; disease-causing microbe

personal protective equipment: common medical equipment, such as gloves, gowns, masks, and other items, that prevents the spread of infection by contact with blood or any other body fluids, secretions, excretions, mucous membranes, or nonintact skin

PFR95 respirator: a respirator used when caring for a resident in airborne precautions

pseudomembranous colitis: a very serious condition in which diarrhea is caused by a bacterium called *Clostridium difficile (C. difficile)*. Some health care workers refer to this condition and microorganism by its nickname, "C. diff"

scabies: a mite that cannot be seen with the eye that causes severe itching and skin rash, and is highly contagious

shingles (herpes zoster): a condition that occurs only in people who have had chickenpox. The resident develops blister-like lesions on the torso that follow the nerve pathways, and are extremely painful. The condition is infectious through the airborne and contact routes until all lesions crust over

standard precautions: special protective procedures and practices used in the care of all residents; standard precautions protect both the nursing assistant and the residents

sterile: free from all microbes

sterilization: a process that destroys all microbes

TB (tuberculosis): a serious disease that is spread by airborne transmission

transmission-based precautions: The Centers for Disease Control (CDC) recommendations for preventing the spread of infection in residents known or suspected to have certain diseases

virus: extremely small microbes that grow in living plants and animals; viruses cause infections that cannot be eliminated by antibiotics

VRE (vancomycin-resistant *Enterococcus*): a pathogen found in health care facilities that is resistant to most antibiotics

MEDICAL ASEPSIS

Medical asepsis means practices and techniques used in the health care facility to prevent the spread of disease. **Germs** are also called **microorganisms** or **microbes.** Some of these microorganisms cause disease. **Aseptic** means free from disease-causing microorganisms. The staff in a health care facility must use the principles of medical asepsis to prevent the spread of diseases. An understanding of microorganisms will help you to realize the importance of medical asepsis. Practicing medical asepsis protects both the nursing assistant and the resident (Figure 6-1).

Microorganisms

Microorganisms are small, living plants and animals that cannot be seen without a microscope. Microorganisms, also called microbes, are found everywhere. They are in the air, in soil, in water, on food, on clothing, and on our bodies. Microbes need food, warmth, and moisture to grow and thrive. They grow best in warm, dark, damp areas. Microorganisms do not grow as well in light and dry areas. Disease-causing microbes are called **pathogens.** Some pathogens can be destroyed by **disinfection.** When something is **sterile,** it is free from all microorganisms. **Sterilization** is required to kill all

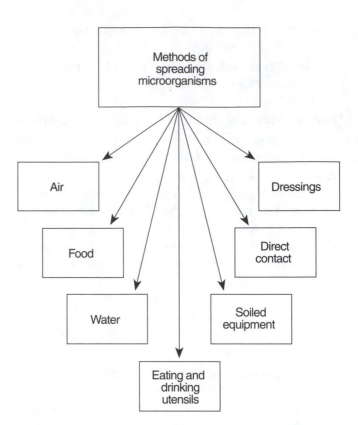

Figure 6-2 Microorganisms can be spread by many different methods.

microorganisms. Sterilization can be done by using heat, gas, or chemicals.

In the long-term care facility, all persons are exposed to many microorganisms. Practicing the principles of medical asepsis is important to protect both nursing assistants and residents. Many residents do not have strong resistance to disease, because of age and illness. In the health care facility, you must prevent the spread of disease from resident to resident, resident to staff, or staff to resident (Figure 6-2). Sometimes visitors are ill when they come to the long-term care facility. If you believe that a visitor is ill, inform the nurse.

Principles of Medical Asepsis

Principles of medical asepsis include the following:

* Handwashing

  — This is the single most important measure in preventing the spread of infection (Figure 6-3).

* Proper handling of food
* Separation of clean and dirty

  — Follow facility policy for separation of clean and dirty items. For example, the food cart (clean) should be kept at least one room away from the housekeeping cart (dirty) or soiled linen hamper (dirty). Some facilities require

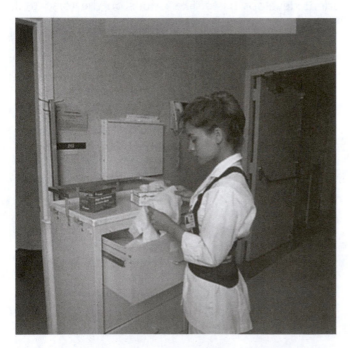

Figure 6-1 Medical asepsis prevents the spread of infection.

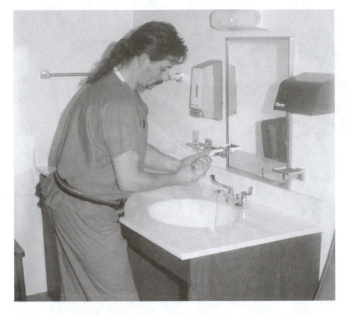

Figure 6-3 Handwashing is the most important method of preventing the spread of infection.

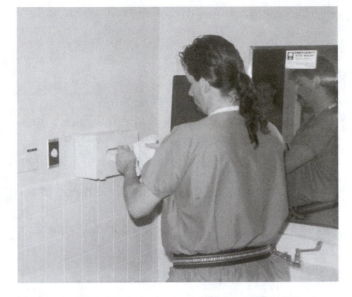

Figure 6-4 Wear gloves when contact is likely with blood, body fluids (except sweat), secretions, excretions, mucous membranes, or nonintact skin.

that dirty items be completely removed from the hall during food service.

- Disinfection of supplies and equipment

    — As a nursing assistant, you will be responsible for disinfecting reusable resident care items. Take this responsibility very seriously, and disinfect equipment according to facility policy.

- Proper handling of linens

    — Wear gloves when handling linen **contaminated** with blood or any moist body fluid except sweat. The term *contaminated* means the same as dirty.

    — Do not let clean or dirty linens touch your uniform. Carry them away from your body.

    — Do not take more linen into a room than you need. If linen is stacked in the room, it can only be used there. It is considered contaminated if it is removed.

    — Do not place soiled linen on the floor.

    — Avoid shaking linens.

    — If clean linen falls on the floor, place it in the soiled linen hamper.

    — Know and follow facility policy for placing clean and soiled linen while you are making a bed and performing resident care in the room.

- Proper disposal of liquids

    — Dispose of soiled liquids directly into sinks, toilets, or according to facility policy.

    — Avoid splashing.

- Facility policy for wearing gloves

    — Wear nonsterile gloves when contact with blood, body fluids, and contaminated items is anticipated (Figure 6-4).

    — Some facilities allow one glove to be worn in the hallway to hold a soiled item. The ungloved hand is used to open doors, turn on faucets, and so on. Some facilities prohibit the wearing of gloves in the hallway. An alternative is to hold a paper towel in the palm of your hand. Use the paper towel to contact soiled items and the ungloved hand to contact environmental surfaces.

    — Always avoid touching environmental surfaces with used gloves, even if the gloves do not look soiled.

    — Know and follow facility policy for disposing of used gloves.

- Proper handling of body waste

    — Wear gloves when contact is likely with blood, body fluids (except sweat), secretions, excretions, mucous membranes, or nonintact skin. If you are already wearing gloves, change them immediately before contacting nonintact skin or mucous membranes.

    — Dispose of body waste properly.

    — Follow the infectious waste policy of your facility.

- Maintain good health
  - Eat properly.
  - Get enough sleep.
  - Get adequate exercise.
  - Maintain good mental health.
  - Be sure that your own immunizations (hepatitis B, tetanus, and others) are current.
- Personal illness
  - Staff and visitors should avoid coming to the facility when they are ill.
  - Follow your facility policy for notifying your supervisor of illness.
- Personal protective equipment
  - Select the proper type of **personal protective equipment** for the task you are performing.
- Handwashing
  - Remember that handwashing is the single most effective way to prevent the spread of disease.

INFECTION

An **infection** is a disease state that results from the invasion and growth of pathogens in the body. The infection may be localized, or confined to a certain body part. The infection may also be generalized, involving the whole body.

Development of Infection

The **chain of infection** (Figure 6-5) is a set of factors necessary for an infection to spread. If any of the factors is missing, an infection will not spread. These factors are the:

- *source:* a carrier of the germ that causes the disease. The source can be human or environmental
- *reservoir* or *host:* a place where the source or germ can grow
- *carrier:* a reservoir or host, usually a person, who has an infection; the person may not know that she is carrying the disease
- *causative agent:* the germ that causes the disease
- *transmission:* the way in which a pathogen is spreads from one person to another
- *portal of exit:* the method by which the pathogen leaves the host. This is commonly in excretions,

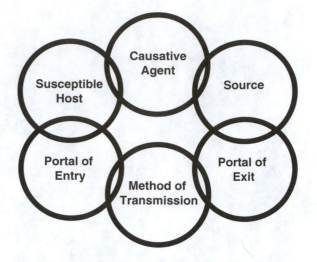

Figure 6-5 The chain of infection. If one link in the chain is broken, the infection cannot spread.

secretions, or body fluids such as urine, saliva, mucus, or drainage from open wounds

- *portal of entry:* a place where the germ can get into the susceptible host's body
- *susceptibility:* the ability or inability of the susceptible host's body to resist the disease-causing germ

Disease Resistance

It is important to know how infection develops because you will be working with people who can become ill very easily. A person's ability to resist infection and illness is related to:

- age
- general health and nutritional state
- medications taken by the person
- presence of other illnesses and underlying diseases

Spread of Infection

Infections can be spread in many ways. The most common methods are airborne, contact, droplet, and blood and body fluid transmission.

Airborne transmission. In **airborne transmission,** very small pathogens are suspended in the air or in dust particles and may travel for long distances. They are inhaled by the susceptible host.

Contact transmission. In **contact transmission,** pathogens are spread by two different types of contact. Pathogens spread by *direct contact* are spread when the susceptible host actually touches the source. Touching an infected area or secretions is a form of direct contact. Pathogens that are

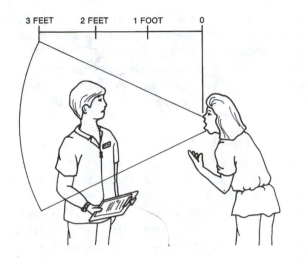

Figure 6-6 Colds can be spread by droplet transmission of pathogens. The droplets are respiratory secretions that are large and heavy. They usually remain within three feet of the host.

spread by *indirect contact* are spread when the susceptible host contacts a contaminated item, such as soiled linen.

Droplet transmission.   Droplets are moist particles created when coughing or sneezing. Pathogens are spread into the air with the droplets. This is called **droplet transmission.** The pathogens usually do not travel beyond three feet from the source (Figure 6-6). The susceptible host usually inhales them.

Blood and body fluid transmission.   Blood and body fluid transmission of microbes is a form of contact transmission. Diseases can occur when the susceptible host comes into direct or indirect contact with blood, body fluid, mucous membranes, nonintact skin, or any moist body substance except sweat.

COMMON DISEASES

Health care workers must learn to protect themselves and others from many diseases present in health care facilities. Some diseases are very serious. Practicing medical asepsis, applying standard precautions, and using **isolation** precautions help protect both the nursing assistant and residents from contracting diseases.

Since the discovery of antibiotics, many lives have been saved. Antibiotics kill **bacteria,** some of which cause disease. Over the years, however, common pathogens have developed resistance to antibiotics so that antibiotics no longer eliminate those pathogens. Sometimes this occurs because people took antibiotics until they felt better but did

not finish taking the prescription. The pathogen was still present in the person's body and developed resistance to the antibiotic used. Over time, these pathogens have become quite powerful and now resist most antibiotics. These are called **drug-resistant pathogens.** Although some antibiotics can kill resistant germs, these drugs often are very expensive and may have toxic side effects, particularly in the elderly.

Some diseases are caused by a very tiny organism called a **virus.** Antibiotics do not kill viruses.

Several diseases in health care facilities are referred to using abbreviations. Some common diseases are:

- **HBV,** or **hepatitis B virus.** This virus causes permanent damage to the liver and is spread by contact with blood and body fluid.

- **HCV** or **hepatitis C virus.** The hepatitis C virus causes a serious infection of the liver. It can be spread through contact with blood or body fluids. The infected person may not know of the infection, but the virus is slowly destroying the liver. The hepatitis C virus is the leading cause of the need for liver transplants in the United States.

- **HIV,** or **human immunodeficiency virus.** This virus causes HIV disease and AIDS, a progressively fatal disease that weakens the immune system. It is spread by contact with blood and body fluid. Not everyone who has contact with the virus develops AIDS.

- **MRSA,** or **methicillin-resistant *Staphylococcus aureus.*** This drug-resistant pathogen can be spread by either the droplet method of transmission or contact transmission, depending on the location of the germ in the carrier's body. It usually causes skin infections, but can cause other illnesses in the lungs and urinary tract. This microbe is resistant to most forms of antibiotic therapy. Some people are *colonized* with MRSA. This means that the microbe is in their body, but they do not have an active infection. The pathogen can only be spread to others if the person has an infection.

- **VRE,** or **vancomycin-resistant *Enterococcus.*** This dangerous drug-resistant germ emerged in the 1990s. The pathogen originates in the intestine, but can cause infection in any part of the body. It is commonly spread by the contact method of transmission.

Tuberculosis, or **TB,** is a disease spread by airborne transmission. TB is like MRSA in that some people have the TB pathogen in their body but are not infectious. If a tuberculosis skin test is done on such a person, it is interpreted as positive. This form of TB is a *latent* infection. Although the microbe is present, the immune system contains it so that it cannot be spread to others. If the individual is treated with drugs, the TB will be eliminated. If the person is not treated, the TB may become active in the future. Some forms of TB also are drug-resistant.

We think of TB as a disease of the lungs, but it can also be found in other parts of the body. All, however, are caused by the susceptible host inhaling the TB microbe. This microbe is very tiny and can spread over long distances in the air on dust and moisture. For this reason, special ventilation systems are used, and all caregivers who enter the room wear **high-efficiency particulate air (HEPA) filter respirators** (Figure 6-7). Alternatives to the HEPA mask are the **N95 respirator** or **PFR95 respirator.** Any mask worn in an airborne precautions room must be approved by the National Institute of Occupational Safety and Health (NIOSH). The pathogen that causes TB is very small and may fit through the air holes of a regular surgical mask. The respirator mask has extremely tiny pores, and the pathogen cannot fit through them. Not everyone can wear a respirator mask. Before you use one of these masks, you must be fit-tested by a qualified professional. You must also have a medical examination. The physician must state that use of the respirator mask will not harm you. You will learn how to check the fit on the respirator mask yourself. Every time you put a respirator mask on, you must check to be sure that there are no air leaks around your face. The mask must seal tightly to be effective. All respirator masks have two elastic straps that fit around the head. This maintains a tight seal around

the face. Men with facial hair cannot wear the respirator mask because the hair prevents a tight seal. Special hoods are available. Some respirator masks are disposable. Disposable masks are used once and thrown away. Other respirator masks are reusable. Many masks are color-coded according to fit size.

Other Problematic Infections

Scabies.   Another disease commonly seen in health care facilities is **scabies.** This disease is spread by contact transmission. Scabies is caused by a **mite,** a tiny parasite that can be seen only under a microscope. It lives on the skin and causes severe itching, skin conditions, and rashes. Special lotions and creams are used to kill the mite. More than one application may be necessary. The environment, furniture, and resident's clothing must also be cleaned to eliminate the mite. Products containing the chemical lindane are not recommended. These can cause toxicity in susceptible individuals. The scabies mite may also be resistant to treatment.

Pseudomembranous colitis.   Many bacteria live in the bowel of healthy people. Most of them are harmless, and some friendly bacteria help with digestion. A few of these have the potential to be troublemakers if they get out of control. Most of the time, the bad bacteria are outnumbered by the good bacteria, and no harm comes to the person. Taking antibiotics can upset the balance in the colon. Many people develop a brief bout of diarrhea because the balance is upset, but the condition resolves quickly on its own.

Pseudomembranous colitis is a very serious condition in which diarrhea is caused by a bacterium called *Clostridium difficile (C. difficile)*. It is often called by its nickname, "C. diff." This condition develops in residents who have been on antibiotic therapy. The friendly (good) bacteria die as a result of the antibiotic, and the harmful (bad) bacteria grow out of control. Pseudomembranous colitis occurs because the antibiotics destroy the friendly bacteria in the bowel, but leave *C. difficile.* Without the other friendly bacteria to keep it in check, *C. difficile* breeds rapidly, producing toxins that cause serious illness. The toxins cause inflammation of the intestine. This results in sudden, severe, foul-smelling, watery diarrhea. Stopping the antibiotic will not stop the diarrhea. The resident may become dehydrated rapidly and develop other serious imbalances within the body. If the condition is not promptly identified and treated, it can cause ruptured bowel and a condition in which the bowel becomes severely distended and retains stool.

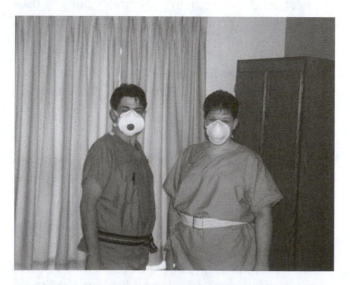

Figure 6-7 A HEPA respirator filter (left) and N95 respirator (right). Both are NIOSH-approved for working in airborne precautions rooms.

C. difficile is very common in health care facilities. It is picked up on the hands on the bedpans, bedside commodes, toilets, sinks, countertops, bed rails, doorknobs, and other surfaces that have been contaminated by stool. It spreads into the body (most commonly the mouth) by unwashed hands. A resident who has been diagnosed with this condition will be placed in isolation. Use good handwashing with antibacterial soap and water. *Do not use alcohol-based hand cleaners* when caring for residents who have this condition. The disease is spread by spores, and alcohol will not eliminate them. The friction and running water will remove them from your hands during handwashing.

Shingles. **Shingles** (herpes zoster) is a condition that occurs only in people who have had chickenpox. Although the person recovers from the chickenpox, the virus that caused the condition remains hidden in the body. The virus resides in the nervous system. The immune system keeps it in an inactive state. However, the immune system weakens with age. In some people, it weakens to the point that it is no longer able to contain the virus. The resident develops painful, blister-like lesions on the torso that may be mistaken for a rash. The lesions follow the nerve pathways. Workers who have not had chickenpox should not enter the room, if possible. Inhaling airborne viruses will cause chickenpox in workers who are not immune. The lesions are infectious in the blister state. Airborne precautions may be used for residents with a widespread outbreak, and those who have conditions that weaken the immune system. Contact precautions are also used, at least until all blisters have burst and crusted over. For a minor, localized outbreak, standard precautions may be used.

Necrotizing fasciitis. **Necrotizing fasciitis** is a very serious skin and tissue infection that is commonly caused by group A Streptococcus, the same bacterium that causes "strep throat." (It may be caused by other bacteria, or a combination of bacteria.) This microbe also may be called "flesh-eating strep." The bacterium enters the body through a minor injury or break in the skin, such as a paper cut or pressure ulcer. Toxins quickly multiply in the tissue and the disease becomes widespread, causing shock, tissue destruction, and death. Amputation of an infected body part may be necessary.

Fifteen to 30 percent of the population carries Strep A at any given time. The carrier usually has no symptoms. You may be a carrier, so always cover your mouth when sneezing or coughing. Throw away used tissues, then wash your hands immediately. Frequent handwashing is the best method of prevention. Avoid contact with persons who have sore throats. Wash and care for even small cuts. Keep them covered with a plastic bandage strip, if possible.

Early in this condition, signs and symptoms may be mistaken for the flu. However, the pain in the broken area of skin may be out of proportion to the injury. As the condition progresses, the resident becomes seriously ill very quickly. The condition cannot be treated in the long-term care facility. The resident will be transferred to the hospital.

STANDARD PRECAUTIONS

Standard precautions are measures that health care workers use to prevent the spread of infection to themselves and others (Figure 6-8). Standard precautions require that all health care workers routinely use appropriate techniques when contact is anticipated with blood or any other moist body fluid (except sweat), secretions, or excretions. They are also used for contact with mucous membranes and nonintact skin. These precautions are used for all residents, regardless of their disease or diagnosis. A health care facility may develop specific policies, but most generally include the following:

- Wear gloves when in contact with any blood, body fluid or body discharge (except sweat), secretion, or excretion. Wear gloves for contact with mucous membranes and nonintact skin. If you are already wearing gloves, change them *immediately before* touching mucous membranes and nonintact skin, even if the gloves do not appear to be soiled. Wearing gloves does not replace the need for handwashing, because the gloves may have small defects that you cannot see, or may get torn during use. Your hands may also accidentally become contaminated when you remove the gloves.
- Wash your hands before applying gloves and after removing gloves.
- Change gloves after contact with each resident.
- Dispose of gloves according to facility policy.
- Always carry gloves with you.
- Wear gloves, gown, mask, cap, face shield, or goggles when indicated to protect against direct contact with body fluids or accidental splashing of secretions. When you wear goggles or a face shield, you must always wear a face mask as well. A good rule to follow is that you can wear a mask without eye protection, but you cannot wear eye

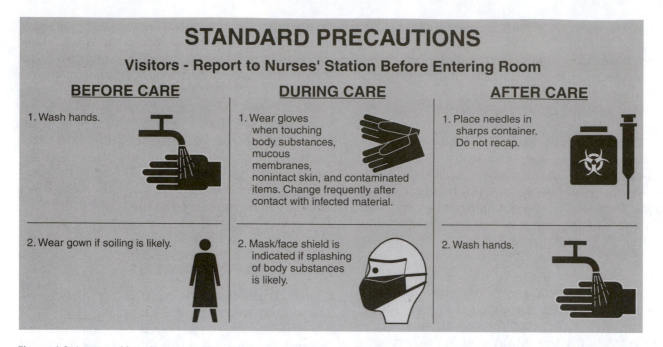

STANDARD PRECAUTIONS

Visitors - Report to Nurses' Station Before Entering Room

BEFORE CARE

1. Wash hands.

2. Wear gown if soiling is likely.

DURING CARE

1. Wear gloves when touching body substances, mucous membranes, nonintact skin, and contaminated items. Change frequently after contact with infected material.

2. Mask/face shield is indicated if splashing of body substances is likely.

AFTER CARE

1. Place needles in sharps container. Do not recap.

2. Wash hands.

Figure 6-8 Agent and host factors are difficult to control. Because of this, infection control practices are used to interrupt the transfer of microbes from one person (or object) to another person. Most suggestions for preventing the spread of infection are based on this concept. Residents can spread infection even though they do not appear ill. Likewise, the nursing assistant can spread pathogens to a resident, or pick up pathogens and move them from one resident to another. To reduce the risk of infection, standard precautions are used in the care of all residents, regardless of disease or diagnosis. (Courtesy of Briggs Corporation, Des Moines, IA (800) 247-2343)

protection without a mask. You must choose the proper protective equipment for the task you are doing. Isolation procedures are discussed later in this chapter.

- Dispose of trash and linen properly (Figure 6-9). Place in a sturdy plastic bag. Do not allow soiled material to touch the outside of the bag.

- Laundry and trash bags should be labeled as contaminated or as indicated by facility policy. Some facilities require these items to be double-bagged. The Centers for Disease Control (CDC) state that double-bagging is not necessary unless the outside of the bag becomes contaminated or torn.

- Trash that has contacted blood or body fluid requires special labeling and handling. Follow your facility policy for handling this **biohazardous waste** (Figure 6-10). The biohazard symbol should have a red or orange background with a contrasting color emblem. It means that the contents of the container are potentially contaminated with blood or body fluid. Biohazardous waste requires special storage, handling, and removal. It is not thrown into the regular trash can. Most facilities require staff to dispose of used

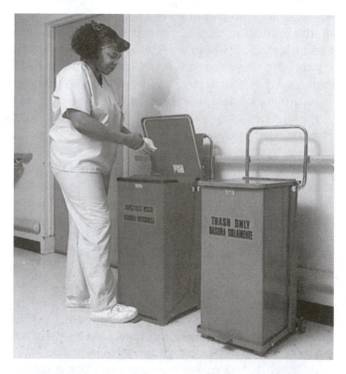

Figure 6-9 Discard trash in the proper container. Items contaminated with blood, body fluid, secretions, or excretions should be placed in the biohazardous trash. Other items may be discarded in regular trash containers.

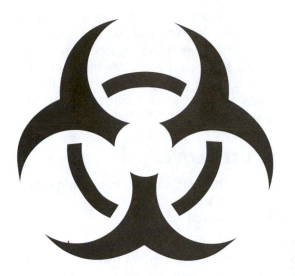

Figure 6-10 The biohazard emblem is black with a red or orange background. The emblem is used for trash, linen, and other items contaminated with blood, body fluids, secretions, or excretions.

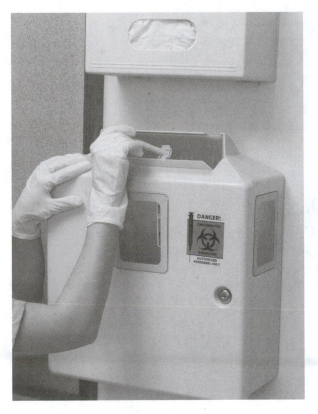

Figure 6-11 Discard needles, razors, and other sharps in a puncture-resistant container.

disposable gloves in a covered trash can. Contaminated disposable gloves and biohazardous waste are discarded in designated covered trash cans. A red bag may be used to line the can, but is not required. The outside of the container should be labeled with the biohazard emblem.

- Know and follow facility policy and procedure regarding special situations.
- Needles, razors, and other sharps must be disposed of in puncture-resistant containers (Figure 6-11). Never recap, cut, or bend needles.
- Clean up broken glass with a broom and dustpan. Never use your hands.

HANDWASHING

As you have learned, handwashing is the single most effective way to prevent the spread of infection. Handwashing should be done:

- when beginning work.
- before and after caring for each resident.
- before and after using gloves.
- before handling food.
- after personal use of the bathroom.
- after combing your hair, using a tissue, eating, drinking, or smoking.
- after handling a resident's belongings.
- after working with anything soiled.
- before using lip balm.
- before and after any oral contact.

- before and after manipulating contact lenses.
- before adjusting your eyeglasses.
- after contact with blood, nonintact skin, mucous membranes, moist body fluids (except sweat), secretions, excretions, or equipment or articles contaminated by them.
- before leaving work at the end of the day.

Waterless Hand Cleaners

Many facilities provide dispensers containing waterless hand cleaners (Figure 6-12) in various locations in the facility. The hand cleaners contain an alcohol-based gel, lotion, or foam that is dispensed in small dime- to quarter-sized portions. Alcohol-based products are often less irritating to the hands than washing repeatedly with soap. Most alcohol solutions contain moisturizers that prevent drying of the skin. In addition, paper towels are not necessary when alcohol products are used. Paper towels contain wood fibers that can be very irritating to sensitive skin.

Each facility has directions for using such products and policies and procedures for when waterless hand cleaners may be used. Waterless hand cleaners may be safely used instead of handwashing during

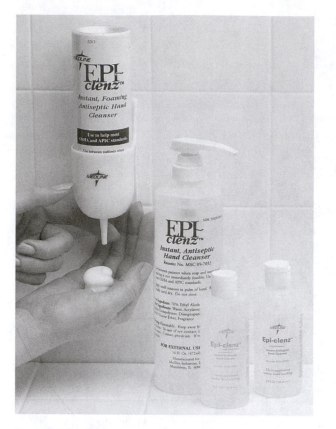

Figure 6-12 Alcohol-based hand cleaners may be safely used instead of washing at the sink unless your hands are contaminated with a protein substance, or the patient has an infectious condition that is spread by spores. (Courtesy of Medline Industries, Inc. 1-800-MEDLINE)

hand. Rub the product into the hands until it dries, making sure to rub all areas and surfaces, including the nailbeds and between the fingers. This should take at least 15 seconds. Become familiar with the products used by your facility and their application. They are very effective in reducing infection and eliminating pathogens from the hands.

WHEN TO USE GLOVES

Residents need to be touched. Avoid wearing gloves for routine contact and care.
Gloves should always be used:

- when touching excretions, secretions, blood, body fluids, mucous membranes, or nonintact skin. If gloves become contaminated with body substances, remove them, wash your hands, and put on a clean pair of gloves before continuing the procedure or care.

- when your hands have cuts, are chapped or scraped, or you have a rash or other skin condition.

- when cleaning spills of any body fluid.

- when cleaning any equipment or environmental surface that may be contaminated.

- when washing or caring for a resident's eyes, nasal discharges, or discharges from the mouth.

- when providing mouth or oral care, or assisting with a dental procedure.

- when shaving residents.

- any time you perform a procedure in an area where the resident's skin is cut, scraped, torn, or otherwise not intact.

routine resident care. However, washing at the sink should be done any time the hands are visibly soiled. To use the waterless cleaning product, dispense the proper amount into the palm of your

---

✓ GUIDELINES for Handwashing

Follow these guidelines each time you wash your hands.

☐ Use warm, running water.

☐ Do not lean against the sink when washing. The sink is contaminated.

☐ Always keep your fingertips pointed down when washing your hands.

☐ Wash hands for a minimum of 15 seconds.

☐ Avoid shaking water from your hands. Shaking water may spread microbes.

☐ *Friction* is required in handwashing. Friction is created by rubbing the hands together briskly. Friction is important to remove germs from the hands.

☐ Dry your hands thoroughly.

☐ Always turn the faucet off by using a clean paper towel.

☐ Put lotion on your hands frequently. Frequent washing dries your hands. Dry skin on hands may crack, creating a place for pathogens to enter.

☐ Follow facility policy for use of soap or other hand-cleaning agents. Some facilities use waterless hand-cleaning products for most routine care.

- when changing colostomy or ileostomy bags.
- when collecting specimens.
- when performing perineal care or when cleaning episodes of incontinence.
- during any procedure when you are not sure if an area is contaminated.

Change your gloves:

- before each resident contact.
- after each resident contact.
- *immediately before* touching mucous membranes.
- *immediately before* touching nonintact skin.

PERFORMANCE PROCEDURE

2   Handwashing

1 Stand away from the sink. Your uniform and hands must not touch the sink. Roll up long sleeves and push your watch up above your wrist.

2 Turn on warm water. Adjust water to a comfortable temperature.

3 Wet hands, keeping your fingertips pointed down.

4 Apply soap over hands and wrists, working it into a lather.

5 Rub your hands together vigorously to create a lather. Rub the hands together in a circular motion for at least 15 seconds. Rub all surfaces of the hands. Pay particular attention to the area between your fingers. Wash your thumbs well. Keep your fingertips pointed down (Figure 6-13).

6 Rub the fingernails against the palm of the opposite hand. Clean the nails with a brush or an orange stick if they are soiled.

7 Rinse your hands from the wrist to the fingertips. Make sure that all soap residue is removed. Keep the fingers pointed down.

8 Do not shake water from hands.

9 Dry hands with a clean paper towel. Discard paper towel properly.

10 Use a clean, dry paper towel to turn off the faucet. Do not touch the faucet handle with your hand.

11 Discard the paper towel in the wastebasket.

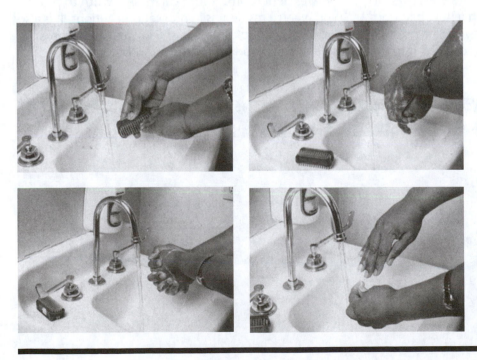

Figure 6-13 Scrub your hands with soap for at least 15 seconds. Keep your fingertips pointed down.

- after you touch a resident's secretions or excretions, before moving to care for another part of the body.
- after touching blood or body fluids, before moving to care for another part of the body.
- after touching contaminated environmental surfaces or equipment.
- any time your gloves become visibly soiled.
- if your gloves become torn.
- before caring for another resident.

Avoid:

- double- or triple-gloving, unless you are specifically instructed to do so by the nurse.
- washing your gloved hands.
- touching an environmental surface with used gloves, even if the gloves are not visibly soiled. Gloves are contaminated after resident contact.
- contaminating clean supplies, linen, equipment, or environmental surfaces with gloved hands. Remove one glove and use your ungloved hand, or place a clean paper towel under one glove and contact environmental surfaces with the towel.
- wearing the same gloves to care for more than one resident.

Discarding Used Gloves

Dispose of used gloves according to facility policy. Generally, they are not discarded in an open wastebasket in the resident's room. Some facilities place extra plastic bags in the bottom of the wastebasket. Replace the one currently in use with a new bag from the bottom of the wastebasket. If you must throw soiled gloves and other contaminated items into the wastebasket, remove the bag, tie it, and take it with you when you leave the room. Discard the bag in the biohazardous waste or other designated location.

USE OF PROTECTIVE EYEWEAR

Eye protection should be used any time you anticipate splashes of blood or body fluids. This could occur during a resident care procedure, when cleaning equipment and supplies, or while rinsing linen. Protective goggles that fit tightly offer protection to the mucous membranes of the eyes. The goggles do not protect the mucous membranes of your nose and mouth. You must wear a surgical mask in addition to the goggles. Face shields are also available. These cover the entire face, from the forehead to the chin. It is possible for secretions to splash under the shield. Additional protection is provided by wearing a surgical mask.

Select eyewear that allows you to see clearly. Protective eyewear that fits over regular eyeglasses is available. Some eyewear is disposable. It is used once and discarded. Other eyewear is reusable. It is disinfected after each use. Become familiar with the eyewear used by your facility before you need it.

USE OF A SURGICAL MASK

The surgical mask is worn to protect the mucous membranes in your nose and mouth. Some facilities buy masks that have an eye shield attached (Figure 6-14). Masks are disposable. They are worn once, then discarded. They should not be used in more than one resident room. A surgical mask is worn to protect you when a resident is in droplet precautions. It is also worn with goggles or face shield to protect you from splashes of blood and other moist body fluids.

✔ GUIDELINES for Wearing a Mask

To ensure full protection, follow these guidelines for wearing a mask:

- ☐ Wash your hands before putting on the mask.
- ☐ The mask should cover your nose and mouth. Bend the nosepiece of the mask so that it fits securely.
- ☐ If your face becomes wet, change the mask. It is not effective when moist.
- ☐ Do not let the mask hang around your neck.
- ☐ Do not remove the mask when you are performing resident care. Wait until you finish the procedure.
- ☐ The mask is used only for the care of one resident, then discarded.
- ☐ Handle the mask only by the ties or elastic straps.
- ☐ Never touch the front of the mask when you are wearing it.
- ☐ Wash your hands before removing the mask.

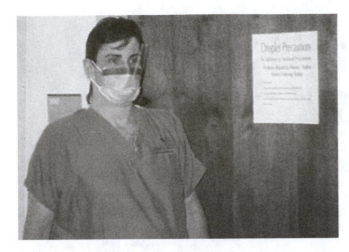

Figure 6-14 An alternate type of surgical mask has an eye shield attached. This mask protects the eyes, as well as the mucous membranes of the nose and mouth.

ISOLATION PROCEDURES

Isolation is a method or technique of caring for residents who have **communicable** or contagious diseases. The purpose of isolation is to prevent the spread of the disease. Knowing isolation procedures will help you stay healthy and prevent the spread of disease.

The procedures for isolation vary with the disease and how it is transmitted from one person to another. Most facilities use a system that lists which procedures to follow. Some isolation procedures include wearing a mask, gown, and gloves (Figure 6-15). *Standard precautions are always used in addition to isolation procedures.*

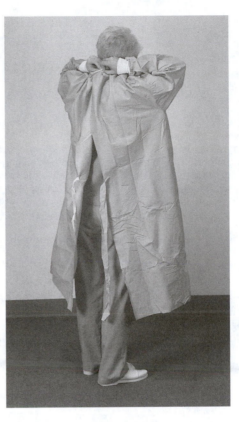

Figure 6-15 Follow facility policies and procedures for preventing the spread of infection.

Transmission-Based Precautions

In 1996, the Centers for Disease Control (CDC) issued guidelines that included **transmission-based precautions.** These precautions were designed to replace the isolation categories used previously. The CDC recommends three types of transmission-based precautions. Standard precautions are used

✔ GUIDELINES for Putting on Protective Eyewear and a Mask

- ☐ Wash your hands.
- ☐ Apply the surgical mask.
- ☐ Apply the face shield or goggles.

✔ GUIDELINES for Removing Protective Eyewear and a Mask

- ☐ Wash your hands.
- ☐ Remove the face shield or goggles.
- ☐ Remove the surgical mask.
- ☐ Wash your hands.

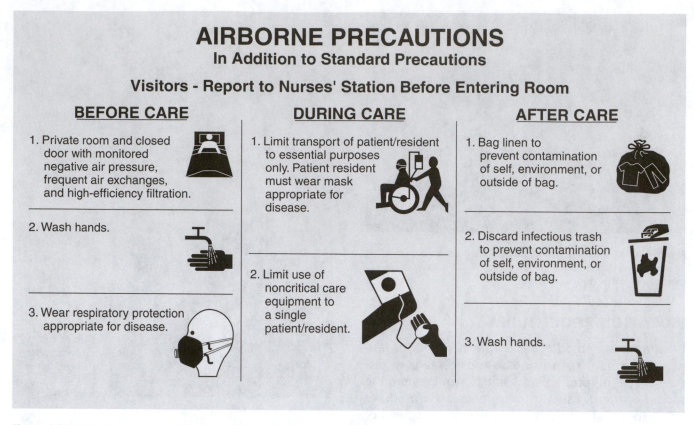

Figure 6-16 Airborne precautions. (Courtesy of Briggs Corporation, Des Moines, IA (800) 247-2343)

with transmission-based precautions. The type of precautions used is selected by the nurse manager and physician according to the mode of transmission of the infection. Transmission-based precautions are used because normal cleanliness and standard precautions are not adequate to prevent the spread of infection with certain pathogens. A private room is used. This confines the pathogen to a single unit. In some situations, residents with the same pathogen will share a unit.

Airborne precautions. **Airborne precautions** are used for diseases that are spread a long distance in the air, ventilation system, or by airborne dust and moisture particles (Figure 6-16). An example of a disease requiring use of airborne precautions is tuberculosis. Residents in airborne precautions must have a special ventilation system in their room. Care givers must wear NIOSH-approved respirators when giving care. The HEPA respirator filter, N95, and PFR95 respirators are all approved for use in the airborne precautions room. Standard precautions are also used. Figure 6-17 describes how to apply a respirator and check the fit.

Droplet precautions. **Droplet precautions** protect you when a resident has a disease in which the causative agent is spread into the air by large droplets (Figure 6-18). The droplets can be spread by sneezing, coughing, talking, singing, or laughing. An example of a disease requiring use of droplet precautions is influenza. The droplets usually do not travel more than three feet. A surgical mask is worn when caring for a resident in this type of isolation. Standard precautions are also used.

Contact precautions. **Contact precautions** are used for conditions in which a disease is spread by either direct or indirect contact (Figure 6-19). An example of a disease requiring use of contact precautions is scabies. Many skin and urinary tract infections also require the use of contact precautions. Contact occurs by touching the contaminated area on the skin. In the case of a urinary tract infection, contact occurs by touching the urine. Indirect contact can also occur in this type of infection by touching an item, such as linen, that has come in contact with the infectious material. Gloves are put on before you enter the room. Gloves should be changed if they contact highly contaminated matter. After you remove the soiled gloves, wash your hands, then apply clean gloves. Remove the gloves and wash your hands immediately before you leave the room. Use a paper towel to turn the door handle.

A gown is worn when you enter the room if you think that your clothing may contact the resident or items in the room. The gown is removed before you

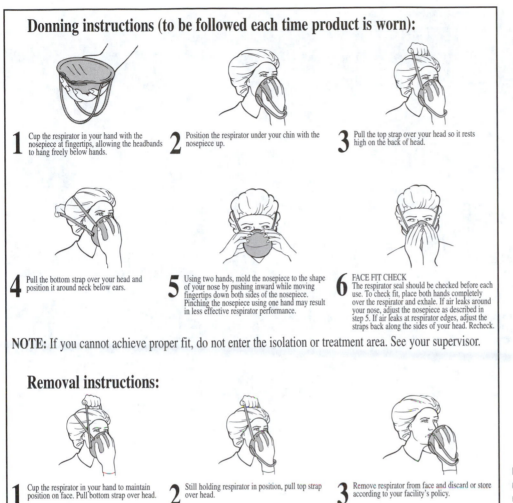

Donning instructions (to be followed each time product is worn):

1 Cup the respirator in your hand with the nosepiece at fingertips, allowing the headbands to hang freely below hands.

2 Position the respirator under your chin with the nosepiece up.

3 Pull the top strap over your head so it rests high on the back of head.

4 Pull the bottom strap over your head and position it around neck below ears.

5 Using two hands, mold the nosepiece to the shape of your nose by pushing inward while moving fingertips down both sides of the nosepiece. Pinching the nosepiece using one hand may result in less effective respirator performance.

6 FACE FIT CHECK
The respirator seal should be checked before each use. To check fit, place both hands completely over the respirator and exhale. If air leaks around your nose, adjust the nosepiece as described in step 5. If air leaks at respirator edges, adjust the straps back along the sides of your head. Recheck.

NOTE: If you cannot achieve proper fit, do not enter the isolation or treatment area. See your supervisor.

Removal instructions:

1 Cup the respirator in your hand to maintain position on face. Pull bottom strap over head.

2 Still holding respirator in position, pull top strap over head.

3 Remove respirator from face and discard or store according to your facility's policy.

Figure 6-17 Check the fit of the respirator each time it is worn. It must fit securely, with no air leaks. (Courtesy of 3M Health Care)

DROPLET PRECAUTIONS
In Addition to Standard Precautions

Visitors - Report to Nurses' Station Before Entering Room

BEFORE CARE	DURING CARE	AFTER CARE

BEFORE CARE

1. Private room. Maintain 3 feet of spacing between patient/resident and visitors.

2. Mask/face shield for staff and visitors within 3 feet of patient/resident.
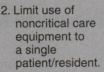

DURING CARE

1. Limit transport of patient/resident to essential purposes only. Patient/resident must wear mask appropriate for disease.

2. Limit use of noncritical care equipment to a single patient/resident.
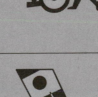

AFTER CARE

1. Bag linen to prevent contamination of self, environment, or outside of bag.

2. Discard infectious trash to prevent contamination of self, environment, or outside of bag.

3. Wash hands.

Figure 6-18 Droplet precautions. (Courtesy of Briggs Corporation, Des Moines, IA (800) 247-2343)

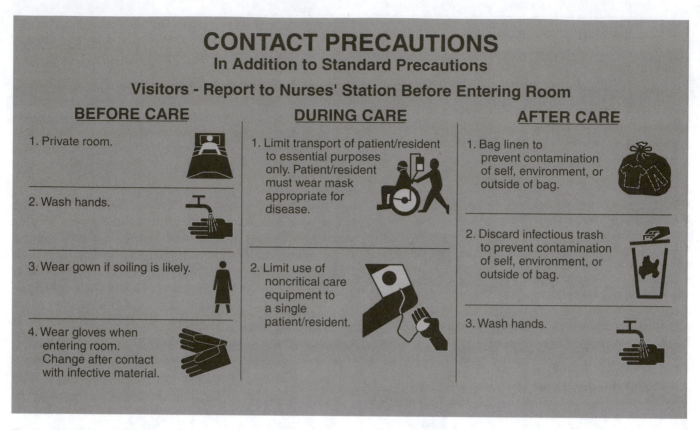

Figure 6-19 Contact precautions. (Courtesy of Briggs Corporation, Des Moines, IA (800) 247-2343)

leave the room. After removing the gown, make sure your uniform does not contact the resident or items in the environment. For example, if you are entering the room to leave a food tray on the overbed table, you would wear gloves only. If you will be making the bed or touching the sheets with your uniform, wear both a gown and gloves. Standard precautions are also used.

PERFORMANCE PROCEDURE

3   Isolation Procedures

Putting on disposable gown, gloves, goggles, and mask (Figure 6-20A)

1 Remove your watch and place it on a clean paper towel. You will carry your watch with you into the isolation room on the paper towel.

2 Wash your hands and dry them thoroughly.

3 Put on a gown. Tie the neck ties.

4 Tie the waist ties of the gown, making certain the gown is overlapping and covering your uniform.

5 Put a mask on, and adjust it over your nose and mouth. Tie the mask securely at the back of your head, or slip the elastic straps over your ears.

6 Position goggles over eyes and adjust to fit.

7 Put on gloves, covering the cuffs of the gown with the top edge of the gloves.

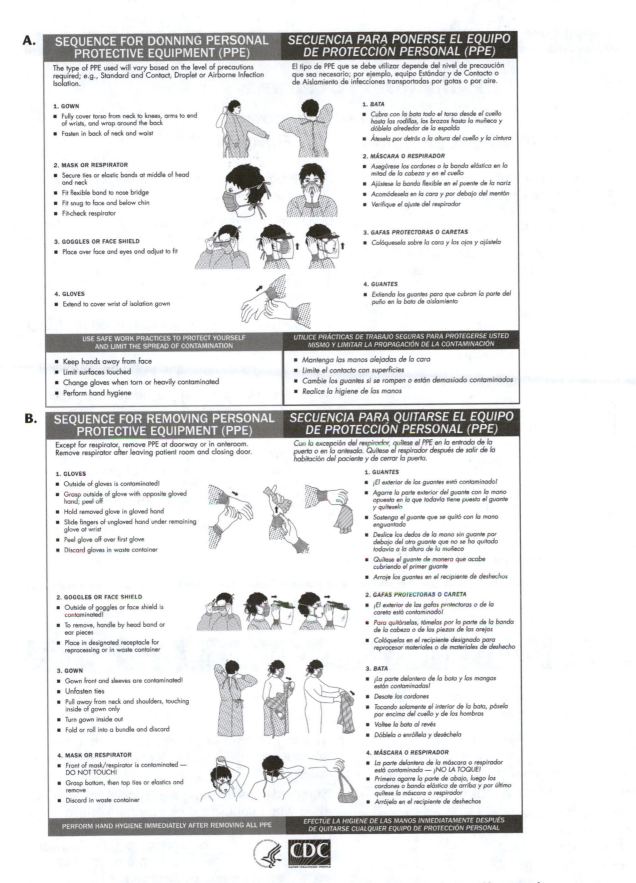

Figure 6-20 Follow these guidelines for applying and removing personal protective equipment. (Courtesy of Centers for Disease Control and Prevention)

PERFORMANCE PROCEDURE

4 Isolation Procedures

Removing disposable gown, gloves, goggles, and mask (Figure 6-20B)

1 Make sure that all jobs in the isolation unit are complete and that the resident is comfortable and safe. Place needed personal items and the call signal within the resident's reach.

2 Remove gloves by turning them inside out, and dispose of them in the biohazardous waste receptacle.

3 Remove goggles or face shield, handling only by the elastic.

4 Untie the waist ties of the gown.

5 Untie the neck ties of the gown and loosen the gown at the shoulders.

6 Slip the fingers of one hand under the cuff of the gown on the opposite arm. Do not touch the outside of the gown. Pull it down over your hand.

7 With your hand inside the gown, pull the gown off the other arm.

8 Fold and roll the gown away from your body, with the contaminated side facing in.

9 Dispose of the gown in the covered biohazardous waste container.

10 Remove the mask by grasping only the ties. Untie the bottom tie first, then the top tie, or slip the elastic over your ears.

11 Discard the mask in the covered trash container.

12 Wash and dry your hands. Turn off the faucet with a clean paper towel.

13 Pick up your watch and put it on your wrist.

14 Holding the clean upper side of the paper towel, pick up the towel and discard it in the trash.

15 Obtain a clean paper towel from the dispenser and use it to open the door of the room.

16 Discard the towel inside the room.

17 Repeat handwashing if this is your preference or facility policy.

KEY POINTS IN THIS CHAPTER

▲ Medical asepsis refers to practices performed to prevent the spread of disease.

▲ Microorganisms are found everywhere. Many are present on the body.

▲ Microorganisms thrive in warm, dark, damp areas.

▲ Pathogens are microbes that cause disease.

▲ Most residents in the long-term care facility have lower resistance to disease, which means that most are susceptible to illness.

▲ Proper handwashing is the single most effective way to prevent the spread of disease.

▲ Alcohol-based hand cleaners may be used for most routine care. Wash with soap and water if hands are soiled.

▲ Friction is required when washing hands.

▲ Infections can be localized or generalized.

▲ The most common routes by which infection spreads are airborne, droplet, and contact transmission.

▲ Standard precautions are special procedures used when contacting blood or any moist body fluid (except sweat), secretions, excretions, mucous membranes, or nonintact skin. Standard precautions are used in the care of all residents, regardless of disease or diagnosis.

▲ Isolation procedures may be necessary to prevent the spread of communicable disease.

REVIEW QUIZ

1. Practices used in health care facilities to prevent the spread of disease are called:
   a. sterilization.
   b. disinfection.
   c. medical asepsis.
   d. techniques.

2. Which of the following is *not* true regarding microorganisms?
   a. All microorganisms are harmful to humans.
   b. Microorganisms are small, living plants or animals.
   c. Microorganisms need food, warmth, and moisture to grow.
   d. Microorganisms are present in many places.

3. What is the *most* important measure nursing assistants can take to prevent the spread of infection?
   a. Sterilize all items.
   b. Wear isolation gowns.
   c. Wash hands.
   d. Wear gloves.

4. Proper handling of linens includes all of the following *except:*
   a. hold linens against your uniform.
   b. avoid shaking linen.
   c. wear gloves if linens have moist body fluid, secretions, or excretions on them.
   d. never place soiled linen on the floor.

5. Microorganisms can be spread by all of the following *except:*
   a. contaminated dressings.
   b. sterile items.
   c. food and water.
   d. secretions and excretions.

6. Scabies is spread by:
   a. droplets.
   b. the ventilation system.
   c. the airborne method.
   d. direct contact.

7. A germ that causes a disease is the:
   a. source.
   b. host.
   c. carrier.
   d. portal.

8. Principles of standard precautions include wearing gloves:
   a. at all times when giving care to residents.
   b. for residents in isolation only.
   c. for contact with all moist body fluids (except sweat), secretions, and excretions.
   d. for contact only with body fluids that contain visible blood.

9. When performing the handwashing procedure, you should:
   a. turn the faucet off with a clean paper towel.
   b. wash for a minimum of five seconds.
   c. shake the excess water off your hands.
   d. keep your fingertips pointed up.

10. Friction in handwashing is caused by:
    a. lotion applied to hands.
    b. rubbing the hands together.
    c. using a mild soap.
    d. using warm water.

11. A disease state caused by invasion of microorganisms into the body that can be either localized or generalized is:
    a. transmission.
    b. disability.
    c. infection.
    d. contamination.

12. Microorganisms live best in:
    a. cool, dry areas.
    b. warm, sunny areas.
    c. cold, bright, wet areas.
    d. dark, damp, warm areas.

13. Microorganisms that cause disease are called:
    a. toxins.
    b. pathogens.
    c. disinfections.
    d. aseptics.

14. Waterless hand cleaners may be used:
    a. when hands are visibly soiled.
    b. when caring for residents with *C. difficile*.
    c. only if no sink is available.
    d. before and after routine resident care.

15. When working with a resident who has tuberculosis, you should wear a:
    a. surgical mask.
    b. NIOSH-approved respirator.
    c. negative pressure filter.
    d. gown and goggles.

16. Pathogens that cannot be killed by most antibiotics are:
    a. sterile.
    b. parasites.
    c. drug-resistant.
    d. immune-deficient.

17. Shingles is caused by the virus that causes:
    a. HIV.
    b. measles.
    c. hepatitis.
    d. chickenpox.

18. Standard precautions are used when caring for:
    a. all residents.
    b. residents with HIV disease only.
    c. residents with MRSA only.
    d. residents in isolation only.

19. Wash your hands:
    a. after applying gloves.
    b. before removing gloves.
    c. after touching soiled linen with your gloves.
    d. for at least 15 seconds.

20. An example of indirect contact is:
    a. touching a resident.
    b. touching a tissue used by a resident.
    c. sneezing.
    d. giving a backrub.

21. Droplet secretions usually do not travel farther than:
    a. one foot.
    b. two feet.
    c. three feet.
    d. twenty feet.

22. When entering an isolation room, you should put on your protective equipment in this order:
    a. goggles, mask, gown, gloves.
    b. gown, mask, goggles, gloves.
    c. gloves, mask, gown, goggles.
    d. gloves, goggles, gown, mask.

23. When leaving an isolation room, your protective equipment should be removed in this order:
    a. mask, goggles, gloves, gown.
    b. goggles, gown, gloves, mask.
    c. gloves, goggles, gown, mask.
    d. mask, gown, gloves, goggles.

24. Most residents in the long-term care facility have:
    a. low resistance to disease.
    b. strong resistance to disease.
    c. immune deficiency syndrome.
    d. infectious diseases.

25. You should wear gloves for contact with the resident's:
    a. arms.
    b. perspiration.
    c. hair.
    d. saliva.

26. You are assigned to care for Debra Barber, a 43-year-old resident. Ms. Barber is in a coma and cannot speak to you. She does not have control over her bowels and bladder. You should wear gloves when:
    a. combing her hair.
    b. rubbing her back.
    c. washing her perineum.
    d. touching her exposed skin.

27. You are assigned to change the bed for James Tucker, a 77-year-old resident in contact precautions because of an MRSA infection in a wound on his foot. The wound is draining heavily through the bandage. When you go into the room, the resident is sitting in a chair next to the bed. You notice a large amount of drainage from his foot on the top sheet. Select the personal protective equipment that you will need to wear when changing the bed.
    a. gloves only
    b. gloves and gown
    c. gloves, gown, and mask
    d. gloves, gown, mask, and face shield

CHAPTER 6
CROSSWORD PUZZLE

Directions: Complete the puzzle using these words found in Chapter 6.

AIDS
airborne
aseptic
bacteria
biohazardous
carrier
communicable
contact
contaminated
disinfection
droplet
germs
gloves
gown

handwashing
HEPA
HIV
indirect
infection
isolation
mask
microbe
microorganism
mite
MRSA
pathogen
portal
protective

reservoir
resistant
scabies
source
standard
sterile
susceptibility
sweat
TB
transmission
virus
VRE

CHAPTER 6
PUZZLE CLUES

ACROSS

1. A special mask worn when working with a resident who is in airborne precautions
4. A skin condition that is highly infectious and is transmitted by a mite
5. Touching linen that is contaminated with pathogens is an example of _____ contact.
6. Touching a wound spreads pathogens by direct _____.
7. Extremely small microbe that grows in living plants and animals that cannot be killed by antibiotics
11. A living plant or animal that is so small it can be seen only through a microscope
14. Waste products contaminated with blood or body fluid are disposed of in the _____ waste.
15. Personal protective equipment that covers your uniform
16. Unclean
22. Some way for the germ to get from the reservoir or host to another host
23. Free from all microbes
24. The causative organism for AIDS
26. Process that slows growth of microorganisms
29. Personal protective equipment worn on your hands
30. Inhaling pathogens after a resident sneezes is an example of _____ spread of infection.
31. Diseases that are easily spread to others are _____.
34. Perspiration
35. The place where the germ enters the host's body is the _____ of entry.
36. The abbreviation for a drug-resistant germ that is commonly found in the intestine
37. A _____ of infection
38. A place where the source or germ grows

DOWN

2. Absence of disease-causing microbes
3. One-celled microorganisms
4. Routine measures the nursing assistant uses when contacting blood or any moist body fluid (except sweat), secretions, and excretions are _____ precautions.
8. Techniques used when caring for a resident who has a communicable disease
9. A microbe that causes disease
10. Personal _____ equipment
12. The ability of the host to resist the disease-causing germ
13. The single most important measure the nursing assistant uses to prevent the spread of infection
17. Progressively fatal disease caused by the human immunodeficiency virus
18. Personal protective equipment worn to cover the nose and mouth
19. The abbreviation for a drug-resistant germ that causes skin infections
20. Pathogens that cannot be killed by most antibiotics are said to be drug-_____.
21. The parasite that causes scabies
25. Disease state caused by pathogens invading the body
27. Common name for disease-causing microbes
28. The abbreviation for tuberculosis
31. A reservoir or host who may not have signs of disease
32. A microorganism
33. Tiny pathogens that travel long distances in the air are spread by the _____ method of transmission.

Safety and Emergency Measures

OBJECTIVES

In this chapter, you will learn the safety and emergency measures you need to know when working in a long-term care facility. After reading this chapter, you will be able to:

- Spell and define key terms.
- Describe common accident hazards in the health care facility.
- List appropriate safety and accident prevention measures for residents.
- List rules to follow when using restraints.
- Apply a vest and belt restraint.
- List beginning procedure actions and procedure completion actions.
- Explain why alternatives to restraints are necessary.
- Describe your role in fire safety measures.
- Identify situations that call for emergency action and perform emergency procedures.

KEY TERMS

cardiopulmonary resuscitation (CPR): an emergency procedure used to establish effective circulation and respiration in a victim whose heart has stopped beating

emergency: an event that calls for immediate action

gait belt: a strong and sturdy belt, usually made of canvas, that is used to move, lift, ambulate, or support residents by placing it securely around their waists

geriatric chair or **geri chair:** a chair with wheels and a tray attached to it

hazard: a potential source of danger

Heimlich maneuver: a procedure done to expel a foreign object from the airway of a person who is choking

immobile: unable to move

impairment: anything that hinders proper function

incident: an unusual occurrence or event

obstructed airway: a blockage of the air passages

oxygen: a tasteless, colorless, odorless gas that is essential for breathing

protective device: a type of restraint that keeps the resident from harm

transfer belt: same as gait belt

RESIDENT SAFETY

As a nursing assistant, you must always make sure that residents are safe. All staff must be concerned for the safety of residents. Many are frail or weak because of disease or old age.

Some residents have **impairments** in vision, hearing, or balance, as well as other disabilities. These, along with decreased strength, may increase the chance of accident or injury. Other residents may have a mental impairment or may be confused. Any of these conditions puts the resident at higher risk of injury or accident. Newly admitted residents who may not be familiar with the surroundings also are at high risk of injury. Some residents with mental impairments who are ambulatory or use wheelchairs are at high risk of wandering away from the facility.

Potential Hazards

Some common **hazards** found in many long-term care facilities are:

- Substances that the resident may swallow, such as disinfectants, cleaning supplies, medications, denture cleaning tablets, and nail polish remover. Some of these substances may also harm the resident if they contact the skin or get into the eyes (Figure 7-1).
- Lack of proper lighting. Glare is especially hazardous to the elderly person. As we age, our eyes need more light in the room to see properly.
- Lack of glasses, hearing aids, and other devices that help the resident stay in touch with the environment. It is the nursing assistant's responsibility to see that these devices are clean and that the residents who use these devices wear them.
- Unsafe equipment.
- Slippery floors (Figure 7-2).
- Unlocked wheelchairs, **geriatric chairs (geri chairs),** shower chairs, or beds.
- Errors such as giving the resident the wrong tray, treatment, or medication.

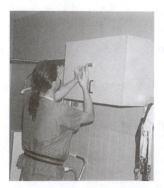

Figure 7-1 Keep hazardous chemicals locked in a secure location.

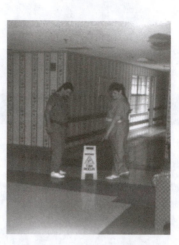

Figure 7-2 Place a "wet floor" sign to warn others of a slippery floor.

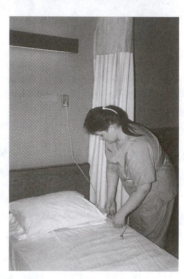

Figure 7-3 Check the call signal each day to be sure it works properly. Make sure it is within the resident's reach at all times.

- Improper use or application of restraints and safety devices.
- Improperly placed or nonworking call signal (Figure 7-3).
- Unsafe or improperly performed procedures.
- Unsupervised use of smoking materials.
- Cluttered hallways.

PREVENTION OF ACCIDENTS

Preventing accidents is the responsibility of everyone in the health care facility. By being aware of the hazards, an alert staff can prevent many accidents. Ways to prevent injuries or accidents are:

- Respond to emergency calls immediately.
- Follow the care plan at all times.
- Answer call signals as soon as possible.
- Check resident identification before giving care and performing procedures.
- Many injuries occur in the bathroom. Be alert when toileting residents.

- Use wheel locks on beds, lifts, shower chairs, geri chairs, and wheelchairs.
- Fasten safety belts when residents are in shower chairs and whirlpool lift chairs.
- Use side rails as indicated on the care plan.
- Use safety devices and restraints only when indicated on the care plan, and only according to manufacturers' directions.
- Clean up spills immediately.
- Be alert for sharp objects and remove them.
- Put all equipment and supplies on the same side of the hallway, leaving the opposite side free of clutter.
- Do not overload electrical outlets or use extension cords.
- Report unsafe equipment, and follow facility policy for removing it from service.
- Know procedures and do them properly. Avoid shortcuts.
  — Ask questions if you are unsure of how to do the task.
  — Do not perform tasks you have not been taught.
- Get help when necessary.
- Know the fire safety policy of the facility. Be alert to fire safety violations. Know smoking rules, oxygen safety, use of electrical equipment, unsafe wires, overuse of extension cords.
- Recognize that some residents cannot stay in the sunlight very long, because of medications or medical conditions. Follow the resident's care plan.
- Maintain your own health. Stay away from the facility if you are ill. Be sure to call the facility when illness prevents you from working.
- Use proper precautions when working with contaminated items.
- Monitor residents who wander. Know what clothing they are wearing and check their whereabouts frequently.
- Be alert for any safety hazard.
- Think safety each time you enter or leave a room.

Falls

Falls are a serious threat or hazard to residents. They are a common cause of accidents in the long-term care facility. If a resident starts to fall while you are walking with him, you should:

- Gently guide the resident to the floor while grasping the **transfer (gait) belt,** or wrap your arms around the resident's midsection.

- Lean the resident onto your leg as you go down to the floor.
- Protect the resident's head so it does not hit the floor.

Call for the nurse immediately. Use the call signal or follow your facility policy. Stay with the resident. Do not attempt to move the resident until the nurse has checked him. If you find a resident on the floor, stay with the resident and call for help.

Incidents

When an accident or injury occurs, an incident report must be filled out (Figure 7-4). An **incident** is any event that is not part of the routine care or routine operation of the facility. An incident may involve the resident, the staff, or visitors.

RESTRAINTS AND SAFETY DEVICES

Restraints are **protective devices** that limit a resident's freedom to move about and limit access to his own body. These safety devices are an infringement on the resident's rights and may be used only when ordered by a physician. The resident or legal guardian must also consent to the use of a restraint. Restraints must be used only when absolutely necessary and when other means of protecting the resident have been unsuccessful. They should be the last choice after other alternatives have been tried, such as behavior modification, physical therapy, and changing environmental factors that put the resident at risk of injury.

Reasons for Using Restraints

Restraints may be used to:

- enable a resident to function at the highest possible level by providing proper positioning and support.
- prevent injury, such as falling.
- prevent the resident from injuring others.
- prevent pulling on tubing or wound coverings.
- prevent residents from accidentally injuring themselves.

Types of Restraints

A variety of protective devices are available. If a resident does not have the physical or mental ability to remove a device, it may be considered a restraint. Common items are not always recognized as restraints. Examples of these items are sheets pulled tightly, trays that attach to the chair with velcro, and seat belts with plastic buckles that are difficult to release. Nursing personnel often cover the resident's

RESIDENT INCIDENT REPORT

IF INJURY SERIOUS, GIVE IMMEDIATE NOTICE TO THE ADMINISTRATOR AND DIRECTOR OF NURSING SERVICE   **NOTE: PLEASE COMPLETE IN DETAIL**

INSTRUCTIONS: Completed report to D.O.N. for review and filing in Administrator's Office. Make detailed report in Nurses Notes/Resident Records.

DATE OF OCCURRENCE 1/4/XX PLACE Room 304 TIME 4:30 AM (PM)

NAME Jane Walther TEMP 98⁴ BLOOD PRESSURE 134/88 PULSE 80 RESPIRATIONS 16

ASSISTANCE NEEDED (Partial or Total)	FUNCTIONING (Partial or Total)	MENTAL STATUS*** Yes No	BEHAVIOR PROBLEMS 1-Minimum 2-Moderate 3-Maximum
P T Ambulation	P T Bedfast	(Y) N Lucid	2 Confused
P T Amb. w/Cane, Crutch, Walker	P T Fecal Incontinent	Y (N) Labile	0 Withdrawn
(P) T Transferring	P T Urinary Incontinent	(Y) N Disoriented	0 Hyperactive
(P) T Wheelchair Mobility	(P) T Blindness	Y (N) Comatose	0 Wanders
P T Bedside Chair	P T Deafness	Y (N) Semi-Comatose	0 Suspicious
(P) T Bathing	P T Aphasia	(Y) N Forgetful	0 Combative
(P) T Dressing	P T Speech Problem	Y (N) Controlled with Medication	2 Supervised for Safety
P T Grooming			0 Causes Mgt. Problems

RESTRAINTS ORDERED: ☐ YES ☑ NO ☐ NOT APPLICABLE   ***Complete this section ONLY IF mental status contributed to incident/accident

IF NOT USED, WHY? _____

WAS PRN MEDICATION ADMINISTERED BEFORE INCIDENT? ☐ YES ☑ NO ☐ NOT APPLICABLE

NAME OF DRUG ADMINISTERED & TIME ADMINISTERED _____

DESCRIPTION OF INCIDENT (include circumstances under which incident occurred): Resident attempted to transfer self from bed to w/c unassisted. No witnesses to incident. Res. was found on floor. Brakes to w/c were not locked. Footrests to w/c were in down position. Res. had socks on feet, but no shoes. States "I slipped".

INDICATE ON FIGURES PART OF BODY AFFECTED AND DESCRIBE EXTENT OF INJURY:

Bruise (L) temple
Skin tear (R) forearm
Bruise (L) ankle

PHYSICIAN'S NAME John Dennis, D.O.

PHYSICIAN NOTIFIED: DATE 1/4/XX TIME 4:50 AM (PM)

PHYSICIAN'S ORDERS, TREATMENT OR STATEMENT: Cleanse skin tear + apply dry dressing.

HOSPITALIZED: ☐ YES ☑ NO NAME OF HOSPITAL _____

Figure 7-4 An incident report must be completed for any unusual occurrence involving a resident, visitor, or staff.

lap with a sheet, blanket, or lap robe when the resident is in a wheelchair. If the cover is tied around the back of the chair, it is a restraint. Many other pieces of equipment used in long-term care facilities can restrain residents whose physical or mental abilities are impaired.

Vest and belt restraints are the restraints most commonly used in long-term care. Some states have discussed eliminating vest restraints completely because they create a high risk of injury, including strangulation and death. Most states, however, still permit facilities to use the vest restraint.

Extremity restraints are used to hold the resident's arms and legs. They are usually used to prevent pulling at tubes or dressings, and to keep the resident still during medical procedures. Many different extremity restraints are available. The most common are mittens and cuffs. Most of these are padded

with sheepskin or foam, so additional padding is not necessary. If your facility uses unpadded restraints, wrap a washcloth or other padding around the extremity before applying the restraint, to prevent circulatory problems. Some facilities require the nursing assistant to place handrolls in the resident's hands when wrist restraints are used. Use commercial handrolls. Rolled washcloths should not be used as handrolls, because they promote squeezing and can cause deformities.

Side rails on beds are restraints. They can also be an enabler. Many residents pull on the rails to position and turn themselves in bed. Some residents feel more secure if the rails are up. The rails must be up if the resident is restrained in a vest, belt, or extremity restraint.

When side rails are used, it is important to check the space between the rail and the mattress.

Hospital beds are used for many years. Mattresses wear out and are replaced. There have been cases of injury and death in which residents became trapped between the mattress and side rails because the replacement mattress was not the same size as the original. Residents at high risk of entrapment include those with conditions such as confusion, restlessness, lack of muscle control, or a combination of these factors. *Make sure that the gap between the mattress and the side rail is not large enough to cause injury.* This is an important safety issue. Figures 7-5A and 7-5B show potential areas of entrapment. Padded foam barriers may be used to close the space between the mattress, side rails, and bed frame (Figure 7-5C). Limiting the space reduces the risk of choking, entrapment, and other injuries.

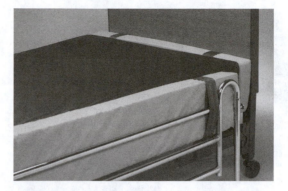

Figure 7-5C Various foam wedges and pads may be used to close the space between the side rails, bed frame, and mattress, reducing the risk of injury. (Courtesy of Skil-Care Corporation, Yonkers, NY; (800) 431-2972)

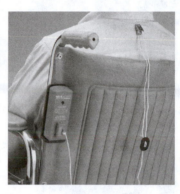

Figure 7-6 The personal alarm is a versatile restraint alternative that may be used in the bed or chair. (Courtesy of Skil-Care Corporation, Yonkers, NY; (800) 431-2972)

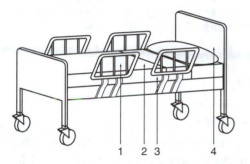

Figure 7-5A Entrapment between the mattress and side rails occurs in one of the following ways: (numbered 1 to 4 in the diagram):

1. through the bars of an individual side rail
2. through the space between split side rails
3. between the side rail and mattress
4. between the headboard or footboard, side rail, and mattress

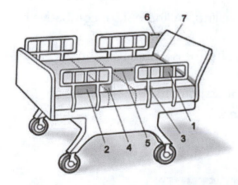

Figure 7-5B Potential areas of entrapment:

Zone 1—Within the rail
Zone 2—Between the top of the compressed mattress and the bottom of the rail, between rail supports
Zone 3—Between the rail and the mattress
Zone 4—Between the top of the compressed mattress and the bottom of the rail, at the end of the rail
Zone 5—Between the split bed rails
Zone 6—Between the end of the rail and the side edge of the headboard or footboard
Zone 7—Between the headboard or footboard and the end of the mattress

Studies have shown that serious injuries can occur if residents attempt to climb over side rails and fall. This is a common cause of hip fractures. Leaving the rails down is safer for some residents. Alarms that sound if the resident attempts to get up may be used to alert staff (Figure 7-6). Facilities and commercial manufacturers have developed many excellent alternatives to the use of side rails. Each resident's care plan will provide instructions regarding use of side rails or alternative devices. Before applying restraints or raising side rails, ask yourself if the risks of using them outweigh the benefits. If a less restrictive restraint is available, consider using it first. Other possible alternatives to the use of side rails are:

- Keeping the bed in the lowest possible position with the wheels locked
- Using beds that can be raised and lowered close to the floor
- Placing mats on the floor next to the bed (Figure 7-7) so that if a fall occurs, the resident falls on a padded surface instead of the hard floor
- Anticipating reasons why the resident might get up, including need to use the bathroom, hunger, thirst, restlessness, and pain. Meet these needs promptly.

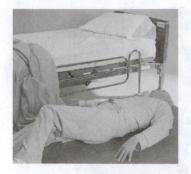

Figure 7-7 Placing foam mats on the floor reduces the risk of injury if the resident falls from the bed. (Courtesy of Skil-Care Corporation, Yonkers, NY; (800) 431-2972)

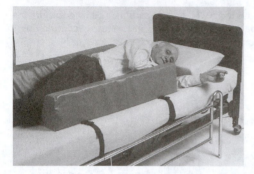

Figure 7-8 Bed control bolsters eliminate the need for side rails, and help prevent injuries. (Courtesy of Skil-Care Corporation, Yonkers, NY; (800) 431-2972)

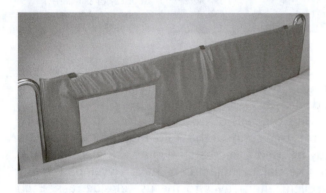

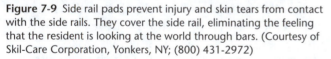

Figure 7-9 Side rail pads prevent injury and skin tears from contact with the side rails. They cover the side rail, eliminating the feeling that the resident is looking at the world through bars. (Courtesy of Skil-Care Corporation, Yonkers, NY; (800) 431-2972)

- Using side rail bolster cushions (Figure 7-8) and side rail pads (Figure 7-9).
- Pressure-sensitive alarms that sound when a resident attempts to get up (Figure 7-10).

Each health care facility has policies addressing when side rails may be used. Know and follow your facility policies.

Side Effects of Restraints

Restraints can have many negative side effects. These include:

- Swelling of the legs, ankles, and feet
- Decreased appetite and weight loss

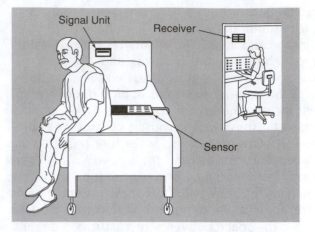

Figure 7-10 The pressure-sensitive pad is placed under the sheet. The sensor box is placed in the room. When the resident relieves pressure from the pad, a distinctive alarm sounds. The alarm may be set to sound only at the desk, at both the desk and the resident's room, or in the room only. (Courtesy of RN⁺ Systems, Boulder, CO; (800) 727-1868)

- Dehydration
- Confusion, frustration, and anxiety
- Lowered self-esteem
- Change in patterns of bowel and bladder elimination, leading to constipation, urinary tract infection, or incontinence
- Loss of self-care ability
- Weakness
- Decrease in mobility and loss of ability to walk
- Muscle wasting and contractures
- Depression
- Screaming, yelling, calling out, or combative behavior
- Pneumonia, shortness of breath, and accumulation of fluid in the lungs
- Bruising, redness, or cuts
- Pressure ulcers
- Falls

NOTE TO THE STUDENT

The direct care procedures begin in this chapter and continue through the remainder of the text. The beginning and ending steps of all procedures are the same. These steps have been printed inside the covers of your textbook for easy reference. Your text will instruct you to "Perform your beginning procedure actions." Turn to the front cover to refer to these steps. Refer to the back cover when the text instructs you to "Perform your procedure

✓ GUIDELINES for the Use of Restraints

Follow these guidelines when using restraints:

- ☐ Instructions for restraints must be written in the care plan with an order from the physician that specifies the type of restraint, when it is to be applied, the reason for the restraint, and when to release the restraint. The information required to be in the doctor's order varies from state to state.

- ☐ Information on the care plan also varies according to state. Check the date of the restraint order on the care plan to be sure it has not expired. Sometimes restraints are ordered for limited periods of time.

- ☐ Restraints are used only when other means of keeping the resident safe have not been effective.

- ☐ Use the least restrictive restraint that will keep the resident safe.

- ☐ Restraints must never be used for the convenience of the staff. For example, do not restrain a resident who wanders so that you do not have to watch him.

- ☐ Always explain to the resident the reason for the restraint.

- ☐ The restraint must be applied according to manufacturers' directions. Improperly applied restraints put the resident at high risk of injury. For example, vest restraints that cross over in the front should not be put on backwards.

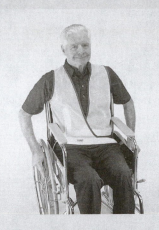

Figure 7-11 Always apply the vest restraint so the straps cross in front. Thread the straps between the seat and the armrest, not through the armrests. This keeps the resident's hips down, reducing the risk of injury. (Courtesy of the J.T. Posey Co., Arcadia, CA)

- ☐ Using the proper size restraint for the resident is very important. If the restraint does not fit the resident, there is a high risk of injury.

- ☐ When the resident is in a wheelchair, the straps to most belt and vest restraints should be placed across the resident's lap, then threaded *between* the seat and armrest of the chair. This keeps the resident's hips down and prevents standing and tipping the chair. The straps should not be threaded *through* the armrest (Figure 7-11). Follow the manufacturer's directions.

- ☐ Restraints must always be tied in a slipknot so that they can be removed quickly in case of an emergency (Figure 7-12).

- ☐ Apply the restraint securely, but do not cut off the resident's circulation. Always check the fit by slipping your fingers under the restraint to be sure that it is not too tight.

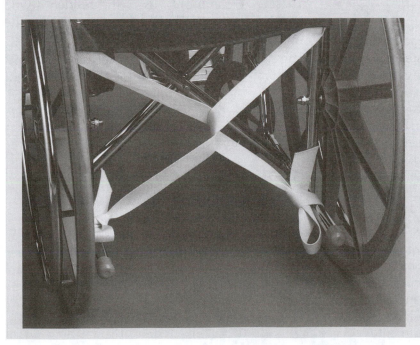

Figure 7-12 Position the straps at the bottom of the chair, instead of behind the seat where the resident can reach them. Tie the restraint in slipknots for quick release in an emergency. (Courtesy of the J.T. Posey Co., Arcadia, CA)

❑ When using restraints in bed, be sure that they are tied to the moveable part of the bed frame and not the stationary part.

❑ Check the skin under the restraint for signs of irritation.

❑ The call signal, water, and needed personal items should be within the resident's reach, even if the resident is mentally confused.

❑ The nursing assistant should visually check the resident who is in restraints every 15 to 30 minutes to be sure that he is safe.

❑ The resident must be completely released from the restraint every 2 hours or more often. The resident should be repositioned in the bed or chair, allowed to walk, use the bathroom, or be given range-of-motion exercises according to instructions on the care plan. Check pressure areas on the resident's skin for redness or irritation. The resident must be out of the restraint for a minimum of 10 minutes before it is reapplied.

❑ The use and release of the restraint must be recorded on the resident's medical record. Many facilities use a flow sheet for this purpose.

completion actions." Eventually, the steps will be committed to memory. Review them often, because they are very important. Table 7-1 and Table 7-2 summarize these important beginning and ending actions.

ALTERNATIVES TO RESTRAINTS

The OBRA legislation requires nursing facilities to provide alternatives to restraints and to promote a restraint-free environment. Care of residents in restraints is more time-consuming compared with caring for residents who are not restrained. Restraints may cause serious complications. Sometimes residents who are restrained attempt to remove the restraints by burning or cutting the straps and are seriously injured.

Restraints can be psychologically damaging and cause the resident to feel a loss of self-esteem, humiliation, abandonment, anger, and depression. Because of the serious side effects, we must seek other ways to keep residents safe. Examining the reason that the resident is in the restraint in the first place is also important. If we can detect the cause of the behavior that caused the resident to have to be restrained and eliminate that cause, we can probably eliminate the need for restraints.

Most facilities are equipped with the following alternatives to restraints:

- A wheelchair lap tray is a useful restraint alternative. Trays fasten to the back of the wheelchair with Velcro straps. They can be used for residents to lean on and as tables during meals and activities. They also are reminders for the resident not to leave the chair. *Trays are heavy*. If a mentally

confused resident pushes the tray off, it may land on her legs, causing injury. Use these trays only for residents who will not attempt to push them forward. Also note that *lap trays are considered to be restraints* if they are used for residents who do not have the physical or mental ability to remove them.

- Lateral body supports improve sitting posture for residents who lean to the side. They are commonly used for residents who are paralyzed on one side of the body. The foam support keeps the resident from leaning to the side, and the armrest supports the resident's arm.

- Lateral stabilizer armrest bolsters are also useful for residents who lean to the side (Figure 7-13). These are commonly used for residents who have no paralysis. They provide support for the resident's upper body.

- The slide guard wedge is also called a "pommel cushion." The wedge shifts the resident's weight

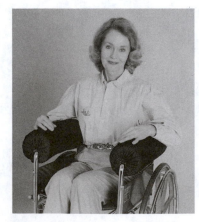

Figure 7-13 The armrest bolsters help keep the resident securely positioned and prevent leaning to the sides. (Courtesy of Skil-Care Corporation, Yonkers, NY; (800) 431-2972)

Table 7-1

Beginning Procedure Action	Rationale
1. Assemble equipment and take to the resident's room.	Improves efficiency of the procedure. Ensures that you do not have to leave the room.
2. Knock on the resident's door and identify yourself by name and title.	Respects the resident's right to privacy. Notifies the resident who is giving care.
3. Identify the resident by checking the identification bracelet.	Ensures that you are caring for the correct resident.
4. Ask visitors to leave the room and advise them where they may wait.	Respects the resident's right to privacy. Shows hospitality to visitors by advising them where to wait.
5. Explain what you are going to do and how the resident can assist. Answer questions about the procedure.	Informs the resident of what is going to be done and what to expect. Gives the resident an opportunity to get information about the procedure and the extent of resident participation.
6. Provide privacy by closing the door, privacy curtain, and window curtain.	Respects the resident's right to privacy. All three should be closed even if the resident is alone in the room.
7. Wash your hands, or use an alcohol-based hand cleaner.	Applies the principles of standard precautions. Prevents the spread of microorganisms.
8. Position the resident for the procedure. Ask an assistant to help, if necessary, or support the resident with pillows and props. Make sure the resident is comfortable and can maintain the position throughout the procedure. Drape the resident for modesty.	Ensures that the resident is in the correct position for the procedure. Ensures that the resident is supported and can maintain the position without discomfort. Respects the resident's modesty and dignity.
9. Set up the equipment for the procedure at the bedside. Open trays and packages. Position items within easy reach. Avoid positioning a container for soiled items in a manner that requires crossing over clean items to access it.	Prepares for the procedure. Ensures that the equipment and supplies are conveniently positioned and readily available. Reduces the risk of cross-contamination.
10. Apply gloves if contact is likely with blood, moist body fluids (except sweat), secretions, excretions, or nonintact skin.	Applies the principles of standard precautions. Protects the nursing assistant and the resident from transmission of pathogens.
11. Apply a gown if your uniform will have substantial contact with linen or other articles contaminated with blood, moist body fluid (except sweat), secretions, or excretions.	Applies the principles of standard precautions. Protects your uniform from contamination with bloodborne pathogens.
12. Apply a gown, mask, and eye protection if splashing of blood or moist body fluids is likely.	Applies the principles of standard precautions. Protects the nursing assistant's mucous membranes, uniform, and skin from accidental splashing of bloodborne pathogens.
13. Raise the bed to a comfortable working height.	Prevents back strain and injury caused by bending at the waist.
14. Lower the side rail on the side where you are working.	Provides an obstacle-free area in which to work.

Table 7-2

Procedure Completion Actions	Rationale
1. Remove gloves.	Prevents contamination of environmental surfaces from the gloves.
2. Check to make sure the resident is in good alignment.	All body systems function better when the body is correctly aligned. The resident is more comfortable when the body is in good alignment.
3. Replace the bed covers, then remove any drapes used.	Provides warmth and security.
4. Elevate the side rails, if used, before leaving the bedside.	Prevents contamination of the side rail from gloves. Promotes the resident's right to a safe environment. Prevents accidents and injuries.
5. Remove other personal protective equipment, if worn, and discard according to facility policy.	Prevents unnecessary environmental contamination from used gloves and protective equipment.
6. Wash your hands or use an alcohol-based hand cleaner.	Applies the principles of standard precautions. Prevents the spread of microorganisms.
7. Return the bed to the lowest horizontal position.	Promotes the resident's right to a safe environment. Prevents accidents and injuries.
8. Open the privacy and window curtains.	Privacy is no longer necessary unless preferred by the resident.
9. Leave the resident in a comfortable and safe position, with the call signal and needed personal items within reach.	Prevents accidents and injuries. Ensures that help is available. Eliminates the need to call or reach for needed personal items.
10. Wash your hands, or use an alcohol-based hand cleaner.	Although the hands were washed previously, they have contacted the resident and other items in the room. Wash them again before leaving to prevent potential transfer of microorganisms to areas outside the resident's unit.
11. Remove procedural trash and contaminated linen when you leave the room. Discard in appropriate container or location, according to facility policy.	Applies the principles of standard precautions. Prevents the spread of microbes and reduces the risk of cross-contamination.
12. Inform visitors that they may return to the room.	Demonstrates courtesy to visitors and resident.
13. Report completion of the procedure and any abnormalities or other observations.	Informs the supervisor that your assigned task has been completed, so that further resident care can be planned and you can be reassigned to other duties. Notifies the nurse of abnormalities and changes in the resident's condition that require further assessment.
14. Document the procedure and your observations.	Ongoing progress and care given are documented. Provides a legal record. Informs other members of the interdisciplinary team of the care given.

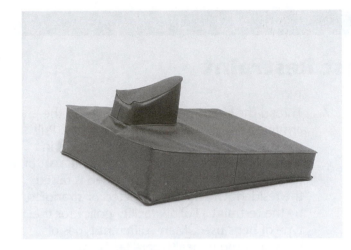

Figure 7-14 The pommel cushion keeps the resident's hips back and prevents sliding forward. (Courtesy of Skil-Care Corporation, Yonkers, NY; (800) 431-2972)

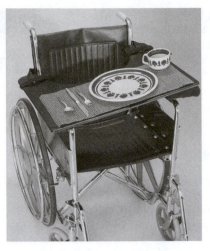

Figure 7-16 Nonslip matting is cut from a roll and has many useful purposes. The matting can be rinsed and reused, but should not be used when wet. (Courtesy of Skil-Care Corporation, Yonkers, NY; (800) 431-2972)

to the back of the seat (Figure 7-14). The pommel in the center prevents the resident from sliding forward. It is used for residents who slide forward on the seat of the chair.

- A vinyl wedge cushion can be used for residents who slide forward (Figure 7-15). It is also useful to prevent residents from rising in the chair. The cushion makes standing difficult because the hips are lower than the knees when the wedge is in place.

- Nonslip matting is sometimes called *gripper* or *dycem* (Figure 7-16). It has many purposes. It can be used as a placemat for residents whose dishes slide away from them when they eat. It can be used alone on the seat of a wheelchair to prevent a resident from sliding. It can also be placed

under a wedge cushion for extra security for residents who slide. This product comes on a roll, and a section of the correct size is cut off. The matting may be rinsed with water if it becomes soiled. Hang the matting to dry. The surface of the matting becomes slippery when wet, so do not use it until it is completely dry.

- Support the resident's feet when he is seated in the chair. Dangling freely is painful for the legs, and complications may develop. Sometimes the resident's legs are too short to touch the floor or the footrests of the wheelchair. In this case, a footrest extender pad may be used (Figure 7-17). The footrest also provides a firm base of support and makes it more difficult for the resident to tip the chair.

- Side rails can be considered a restraint. If a resident tries to get out of bed by climbing over the rail, he is at high risk of injury. Bed control bolsters may be

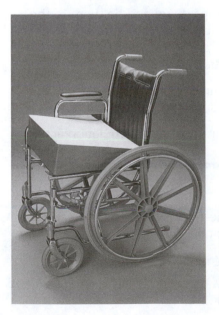

Figure 7-15 The vinyl wedge keeps the hips lower than the knees, making it difficult to stand. The cushion also prevents sliding forward in the chair. When using a wedge cushion, make sure the resident's feet are supported on footrests or the floor. (Courtesy of Skil-Care Corporation, Yonkers, NY; (800) 431-2972)

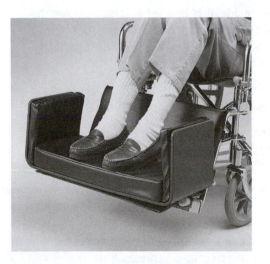

Figure 7-17 The feet must be supported at all times when the resident is up in a chair. If the resident's legs are too short to reach the footrests, an elevator pad may be added to prevent pain and deformity. (Courtesy of Skil-Care Corporation, Yonkers, NY; (800) 431-2972)

5 Applying a Vest Restraint

1 Obtain a restraint of the proper type and size.

2 Get help if necessary.

3 Perform your beginning procedure actions.

4 Slip the resident's arms through the arm-holes of the vest.

5 Make sure that the clothing under the restraint is not wrinkled and that the vest fits smoothly.

6 Cross the vest in the front and thread the straps through the slots on the sides of the vest. If a vest is used on a female resident, be sure that the breasts are not under the straps.

7 Thread the straps *between* the seat and the armrest if the resident is in a wheelchair. Pull the straps back securely. If the resident is in bed, attach the straps to the moveable part of the bed frame. (This way, if the bed is raised, the resident will not be restricted or strangled by the restraint.) Follow facility policy for the type of beds used. Many different types of beds are used in health care facilities.

8 Finish tying the restraint in a slipknot under the chair or to the bed frame. Refer to the specific manufacturer's directions for the restraint you are using.

9 Insert three fingers under the restraint and check to be sure that it is not too tight.

10 Perform your procedure completion actions.

6 Applying a Belt Restraint

1 Perform your beginning procedure actions.

2 Get help from another nursing assistant, if necessary.

3 If the resident is in a wheelchair, move the hips as far back as possible, position the footrests to support the feet, and lock the brakes.

4 Place the belt around the waist. Cross the straps through the loops behind the resident.

5 After the straps are threaded through the loops, tighten the belt securely around the waist.

6 Insert the straps between the seat and arm-rest, or between the seat and backrest, according to the manufacturer's recommendations for the type of restraint you are using.

7 Bring the straps down and tie them to the kickspurs of the wheelchair, using a quick-release knot, according to the manufacturer's directions.

8 Insert three fingers under the restraint and check to be sure that it is not too tight.

9 Perform your procedure completion actions.

used alone or in pairs. They keep the resident from rolling off the bed and serve as a reminder not to get up. The bolsters are half the length of the bed. They can also be used as a prop to keep the resident in good body alignment. Residents who are restless benefit from the use of bolsters because they protect the resident from injury caused by striking the side rails.

Other restraint alternatives include:

• Sensor bracelets that set off alarms if the resident tries to leave the facility

- Self-releasing seat belts similar to the lap belts used in a car
- "Lap buddies" or foam cushions placed on the resident's lap when he is in the chair
- Special chairs designed to make it more difficult for the resident to get up; other types of chairs are used for residents with special positioning needs
- Participation in activity programs that keep residents busy
- Increased personal attention that the staff gives to the resident

As a nursing assistant, you spend more time with the residents than the other members of the interdisciplinary team. If you have an idea that could be used to eliminate or reduce restraints, share this information with the interdisciplinary team. If you observe a problem, such as too much noise in the environment that causes a behavior problem in a resident, sharing this information is important. If all team members work together, keeping most residents safe and secure without using restraints is possible.

Many excellent alternatives to restraints are available. However, you must remember that any device is a restraint if the resident does not have the physical or mental ability to remove it.

FIRE SAFETY

Your facility will have special fire safety procedures. All staff must watch for fire hazards and report them immediately to the proper authority. Because fire safety is extremely important, most states have laws requiring long-term care facilities to have frequent fire drills. Know where the alarms and fire extinguishers are in your facility and how to use them. Know your facility evacuation plan in case of fire (Figure 7-18).

Major Causes of Fire in Long-Term Care Facilities

Fires often are caused by:

- improper or unsupervised use of smoking materials
- defects in the heating system
- improper trash disposal
- misuse of electrical equipment
- spontaneous combustion
- lint buildup in dryers

In order for a fire to occur, three things must be present (Figure 7-19):

- material that burns
- flame or spark
- **oxygen** in the air

Fire safety is very important when oxygen is being used. A tiny spark from turning on a hair dryer or a cigarette ash can cause a fire when oxygen is present in larger amounts than is normally present in the air. Special procedures must be followed when oxygen is used. Follow your facility policy for use of oxygen, oxygen signs, and modifications in procedures you must take when a resident is using oxygen.

Actions to Take When You Discover a Fire

If you discover a fire, take these actions:

- Follow the facility's procedures.
- Alert and assist residents who have vision and hearing impairments.
- Follow facility policy for getting **immobile** residents out of dangerous areas. This may include placing the resident on a blanket on the floor and

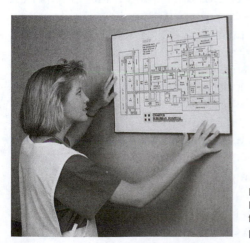

Figure 7-18
Know your facility evacuation plan.

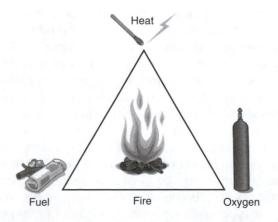

Heat

Fuel   Fire   Oxygen

Figure 7-19 The fire triangle, representing the three elements needed to start a fire

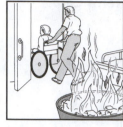
Remove

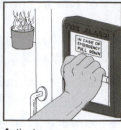
Activate

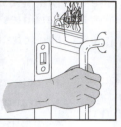
Contain or

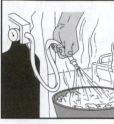
Extinguish or

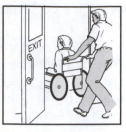
Evacuate

Figure 7-20 The RACE system

pulling the resident, or moving the entire bed with the resident in it. Nursing facility doors are required to have fire ratings. Close the doors to place a barrier between the resident and the fire.

The RACE System

Many facilities use the R A C E system (Figure 7-20) as a general guideline in fire safety.

- **R**emove residents who are in immediate danger.
- **A**ctivate the alarm to alert others.
- **C**ontain the fire by closing doors.
- **E**xtinguish the fire, if possible or **E**vacuate, if so instructed.

EMERGENCY MEASURES

There may be times when **emergency** measures must be performed. Your facility will have a specific policy for emergency procedures. Your responsibility is to tell the nurse immediately and follow the nurse's instructions. Knowing some emergency procedures is important. You might want to take a CPR and first aid course offered by a community organization.

CHOKING

An **obstructed airway** occurs when food or an object becomes lodged in the throat, cutting off the airway. Some residents have difficulty swallowing. The best measure is to prevent choking, but even with the best care, some residents may choke on food or other objects. Facility policies vary, but there may be times when you have to help a resident who is choking.

Choking often occurs when residents are eating, drinking, laughing, or talking at the same time. The food or foreign object goes into the throat. It is usually too far down for the fingers to reach. The foreign body obstructs the airway so that the resident is not able to speak or breathe. The resident may put one or both hands on the neck. This is the universal sign for choking.

If you suspect that the resident is choking, ask the resident, "Are you choking?" If the resident signals yes, you must do something right away. The **Heimlich maneuver** is the common name for the procedure done to remove a foreign object from an obstructed airway.

CARDIOPULMONARY RESUSCITATION

Cardiopulmonary resuscitation (CPR) is a basic, lifesaving procedure given to a person whose heart has stopped beating. This is called cardiac arrest. The techniques of CPR must be taught by a certified instructor. The following outline provides an overview of the CPR procedure. It does not replace a CPR course.

1. Gently shake the resident's shoulder and shout, "Are you O.K.?" Call for help.
2. Position the resident on his back.
3. Open the airway by tilting the resident's head backward and lifting the chin. Look, listen, and feel for breath.
4. Pinch the nose, cover the resident's mouth with a barrier device, and give two full breaths into the mouth.
5. Feel the neck for the carotid pulse. Begin chest compression if there is no pulse.
6. Place the heel of one hand on the breastbone in the center of the chest. Place the other hand on top. Use an imaginary line between the nipples as your landmark. Keep your elbows straight. Interlace your fingers.
7. Compress the breastbone downward 1½ to 2 inches at a rate of 100 a minute. Use the heels of your hands. Keep the fingers off the chest.
8. Do 30 compressions, then 2 breaths. Repeat.
9. Continue the procedure until the resident recovers, help arrives, or you are exhausted and unable to continue.

PERFORMANCE PROCEDURE

7   Clearing an Obstructed Airway (Heimlich Maneuver)

Clearing an Obstructed Airway in a Conscious Resident

1 Ask the resident, "Are you choking?" or "Can you speak?" (If so, encourage the resident to try to cough the object out. Stay with the resident and assist if the cough is weak or the resident is in distress.) Call for the nurse immediately.

2 Tell the resident that you will help. If the resident is sitting or standing, stand behind him.

3 Wrap your arms around the resident's waist, above the hips.

4 Make a fist with one hand.

5 Place the thumb side of your fist against the resident's abdomen, just above the navel and below the tip of the breastbone (Figure 7-21A).

6 Grasp the fist with the other hand.

7 Pull inward and upward on the abdomen with a quick thrust (Figure 7-21B).

8 Repeat the thrusts until the foreign body comes out or the resident loses consciousness. If the resident begins to cough, wait and see if he can expel the object.

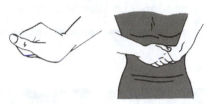

Figure 7-21A Position your hands slightly above the navel. Turn your thumb inward.

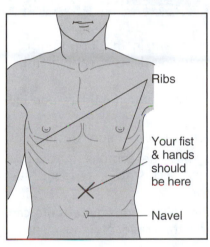

Ribs

Your fist & hands should be here

Navel

Figure 7-21B Grasp your bottom hand with the top hand and deliver inward, upward thrusts. Avoid resting your forearms on the ribs.

Clearing an Obstructed Airway in an Unconscious Resident

It is important that you know your facility's policy regarding this procedure. This procedure may be the responsibility of the nurse. The procedure is listed here for your general understanding only.

1 Call for help, but do not leave the resident alone.

2 Wear gloves during this procedure and apply standard precautions.

3 Lower the resident to the floor and position him on his back.

4 Open the airway by doing a head tilt chin lift maneuver.

5 Look in the mouth. If you see a foreign body, try to remove it. Take care to avoid pushing the object farther down the throat.

6 Open the airway again by using the head tilt chin lift maneuver. Attempt to ventilate. If the breath does not go in, reposition the head and attempt to ventilate again. Use a pocket mask or other barrier, according to facility policy.

Note: Follow your facility policy for mouth-to-mouth ventilation. To prevent the transmission of disease, standard precautions should be used. This means that gloves are worn for the finger sweep. A ventilation barrier mask with a valve that prevents the backflow of secretions, or a resuscitation face shield, should be placed between your mouth and the resident's mouth for ventilations. Familiarize yourself with the devices in your facility. CPR classes are offered to teach you how to use ventilation devices correctly. Attending a CPR class will benefit you personally and professionally.

(continued)

7 *continued*

7 Check for a pulse and begin CPR.

8 Assist the nurse, code team, or emergency medical services (EMS), as appropriate.

9 Discard gloves and face shield, or disinfect reusable ventilation device according to facility policy.

10 Perform your procedure completion actions.

11 Observe and report to the nurse:
   • exact time the choking and unconsciousness started and stopped
   • the procedures done and the time that you started and stopped
   • the resident's response
   • factors related to the cause of choking, if known

KEY POINTS IN THIS CHAPTER

▲ Safety is very important in the long-term care facility because many residents are at high risk of accidents or injuries.

▲ Accident and injury prevention is the responsibility of the entire staff.

▲ Falls are a frequent cause of injury to residents.

▲ Incident reports must be completed when an accident or injury occurs to a resident, staff member, or visitor.

▲ Residents who are restrained require more care and take more time than residents who are not in restraints.

▲ Residents should be free from restraints whenever possible.

▲ Restraints may be used only when other means of protecting residents have not been successful.

▲ Restraints require a doctor's order and must be released at least every 2 hours for 10 minutes for exercise and care.

▲ Fire safety is so important that most states require frequent fire drills for long-term care facilities.

▲ In an emergency, you must follow facility policies.

REVIEW QUIZ

1. Which of the following residents has the highest risk of falls?
   a. A resident with Alzheimer's who wanders about using a walker with a slow, steady gait.
   b. An alert resident who uses a wheelchair and transfers herself onto and off the toilet.
   c. A resident who wears glasses and is ambulatory, but is very impatient.
   d. A newly admitted resident with a history of two recent falls at home.

2. Which is the safest way to prevent residents from having contact with hazardous substances, such as cleaning supplies and medications?
   a. Label containers with the poison sign.
   b. Tell residents to stay away from hazardous materials.

   c. Lock cabinets where hazardous materials are stored.
   d. Tell alert residents to watch confused residents.

3. Which of the following floor conditions poses a threat to resident safety?
   a. a shiny surface
   b. spilled liquids
   c. beige-colored tile
   d. a carpeted surface

4. If the resident begins to fall while you are walking with him, you should:
   a. gently ease the resident to the floor.
   b. ask another resident to help you.
   c. quickly go and get the nurse.
   d. get a pillow for the resident immediately.

5. What must be done when an event that is not part of the normal routine happens?
   a. An incident report must be completed.
   b. The nursing assistant should call the administrator of the facility.
   c. The resident must be restrained.
   d. All staff must report to the scene of the incident.

6. Which is true regarding the use of restraints?
   a. Restraints may be applied when the nursing staff is busy.
   b. Restraints are applied to all confused residents to keep them safe.
   c. Restraints may be applied to any resident who will not stay in bed.
   d. Restraints may be applied only if necessary to protect the resident from harm.

7. Restraints should be released at least:
   a. once every shift.
   b. every two hours.
   c. every three hours.
   d. every four hours.

8. Which of the following rules should you follow when using restraints?
   a. Restraints should be the proper size to fit the resident.
   b. Restraints must always be tied in a square knot.
   c. Visually check the restrained resident every 60 minutes.
   d. Avoid waking sleeping residents to release restraints.

9. For a fire to occur, what must be present?
   a. oxygen and material
   b. flame, oxygen, and smoke
   c. oxygen, material, and spark
   d. flame and oxygen

10. In case of fire, what should be done first?
    a. Call the fire department.
    b. Remove residents in danger.
    c. Alert other staff.
    d. Announce the location of the fire over the intercom.

11. When an emergency occurs in the long-term care facility, your responsibility as a nursing assistant is to:
    a. follow the directions of your supervisor.
    b. notify the family immediately.
    c. contact the physician for instructions.
    d. stay out of the way.

12. The universal sign for choking is:
    a. coughing.
    b. clutching the throat.
    c. shouting.
    d. waving arms about.

13. If a resident is coughing and able to breathe, you should:
    a. perform the Heimlich maneuver.
    b. use finger sweeps to remove the object.
    c. stay with the resident and let him continue coughing.
    d. give the resident oxygen.

14. The correct procedure for clearing an obstructed airway in an unconscious adult is to place the heel of your hand:
    a. on the chest.
    b. below the navel.
    c. above the navel.
    d. on the back.

15. One of the most frequent causes of accidents to residents in long-term care facilities is:
    a. falls.
    b. smoking.
    c. choking.
    d. poisoning.

16. Accident prevention is the responsibility of the:
    a. safety committee.
    b. maintenance department.
    c. nursing department.
    d. entire staff.

17. You are assigned to care for Jeffrey Greene, a 54-year-old resident with Alzheimer's disease. Mr. Greene is very confused and restless. The care plan states that he is to use a vest restraint when he is in the wheelchair. You get Mr. Greene up and apply the vest restraint. Before leaving the room you should:
    a. tie the restraint securely in a knot so that the resident cannot untie it.
    b. ask Mr. Greene to behave himself until you come back in two hours.
    c. move Mr. Greene's wheelchair away from the other furniture so that he does not get hurt.
    d. place the signal cord so that Mr. Greene can reach it.

18. You are assigned to work in the dining room during the evening meal. You are passing food trays when you notice that Mrs. Hernandez is sitting at the table with her hands on her throat. You should:
    a. continue passing trays, as you are not assigned to care for Mrs. Hernandez.
    b. go immediately to Mrs. Hernandez and ask her if she is choking (can speak).
    c. leave the dining room immediately and get the nurse.
    d. help Mrs. Hernandez to the floor and perform abdominal thrusts.

19. You are working the 10:00 p.m. to 6:00 a.m. shift on C wing. As you walk down the hallway,

you look into Mr. Griffin's room and notice that he is on the floor next to the bed. You should:

a. call for the nursing assistant who is assigned to care for Mr. Griffin.

b. go and get the nurse.

c. continue walking and pretend that you did not see the resident.

d. go into the room and check the resident.

20. You are assigned to straighten the drawers in Mr. Atkins's room. Mr. Atkins is a confused resident with Alzheimer's disease. When you open the drawer to the nightstand you find a comb, a wrapped candy bar, a roll-on deodorant, an electric razor, a toothbrush, a package of denture cleaning tablets, and an emesis basin. Which of these items is most likely to cause harm to Mr. Atkins?

a. the razor

b. the denture tablets

c. the roll-on deodorant

d. the comb

CHAPTER 7
CROSSWORD PUZZLE

Directions: Complete the puzzle using these words found in Chapter 7.

airway	immobile	oxygen
CPR	impairment	restraint
emergency	incident	spark
gait	material	transfer
geriatric	protective	
hazard	obstructed	

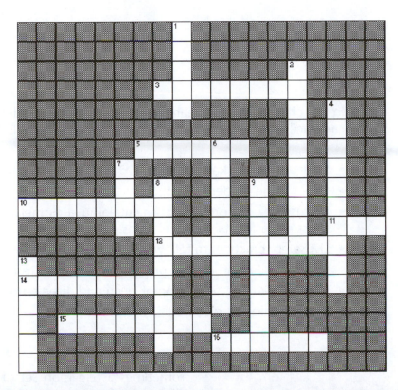

CHAPTER 7
PUZZLE CLUES

ACROSS

3. A device that the nursing assistant uses to assist a resident when moving from the bed to a chair is a _____ belt.
5. A source of potential danger
10. Unable to move
11. Cardiopulmonary resuscitation
12. Something that hinders proper function
14. An unusual occurrence or event
15. In order for a fire to start, you need oxygen, a spark, and _____ that will burn.
16. A colorless, odorless, tasteless gas in the air

DOWN

1. A sudden quick light
2. A type of restraint that is used to keep a resident from harm is called a _____ device.
4. The Heimlich maneuver is done if a resident has an _____ airway.
6. A device that is applied to the resident to restrict freedom of movement
7. A _____ belt is used to assist residents in walking.
8. A _____ chair is a chair with wheels and a tray that is a type of restraint.
9. An event that calls for immediate action
13. The breathing passage in the throat

The Resident's Unit

OBJECTIVES

In this chapter, you will learn how to care for the resident's unit in a long-term care facility. After reading this chapter, you will be able to:

- Spell and define key terms.
- Care for the resident's unit.
- Discuss the importance of maintaining a homelike environment and respecting residents' personal items.
- List safety practices to follow in residents' units.
- Describe infection control practices to follow in residents' units.
- Demonstrate the separation of clean and dirty items in residents' units.
- Make the unoccupied bed.

KEY TERMS

bedside stand: a nightstand or table for personal possessions and equipment used for personal care of the resident

gatch handles: the handles at the end of some beds used to raise the head, foot, or height of the bed

low bed: a bed on which the frame extends only 6 to 8 inches from the floor.

overbed table: a narrow table on wheels; the height of the table is adjustable

resident's unit: the space for one resident in a long-term care facility

THE RESIDENT'S UNIT

When we speak of the **resident's unit,** we are referring to the area that is for a resident's personal use. The items in the unit are a bed, chair, overbed table, bedside stand, dresser, wastebasket, closet, and sometimes a television set or radio. Many facilities allow some furniture items from the resident's former home. The nursing assistant must realize that the long-term care facility is now the resident's home. Caring for the resident includes some care of the unit.

The OBRA legislation emphasizes the importance of maintaining a homelike environment. The unit should be comfortable and attractive in appearance. The resident's personal items should be used to decorate the room whenever possible (Figure 8-1). These items are important because they bring back memories of the past. The items brought to the nursing facility are often the most important to the resident and may be the only possessions that she has left in the world. Handling these items with respect and care shows the resident that you care. Showing respect for personal belongings is one way you can help the resident with grief and loss issues.

The resident has a right to expect her unit to be treated with respect and dignity. This includes knocking on closed doors and giving the resident

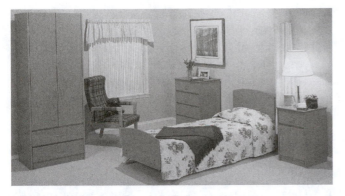

Figure 8-1 Make the room as homelike and comfortable as possible by displaying the resident's belongings. (Courtesy of Medline Industries, Inc. Mundelein, IL. 1-800-MEDLINE).

and visitors the right to privacy when requested. When giving the resident personal care, you must close the door, pull the privacy curtain, and close the drapes on the window, even if you are alone in the room with the resident.

Unit Safety and Infection Control

Think safety each time you enter and leave the resident's room. Check the resident's unit each day for safety.

The Bedside Stand

The **bedside stand** is an important piece of equipment for resident care. The bedside stand is used to store personal items and articles used by the nursing assistant to deliver care to the resident. Bedside stands vary in design. Most have at least one drawer at the top. The lower portion of the stand may have a cupboard-type door or several drawers. Follow your facility policy for storage of items in the bedside stand. Clean and dirty items must be kept separate. For example, the drawer in the top of the bedside stand is often used to store the resident's toothbrush, hairbrush, and comb. It is important that these items do not come into contact with each other for the following reasons:

- Hair is a magnet for germs, which is why nurses formerly wore caps.
- Hair gets in the toothbrush.
- Germs from brush and comb get in toothbrush.

The lower part of the bedside stand often contains the washbasin and bedpan or urinal. The washbasin is considered a clean item. It should not come into contact with the bedpan and urinal, which are considered dirty. In the cupboard-type

✓ Guidelines for Caring for the Resident's Unit

- ☐ Check side rails to be sure they are secure. These are used by the resident to prevent falling and assist with turning in bed.
- ☐ Check the call signal. Make sure the signal is working and within the resident's reach at all times, even if the resident is confused.
- ☐ If the resident is confined to bed or chair in the room, make sure that water, tissues, and other needed personal items are within reach.
- ☐ Keep the unit tidy. Major cleaning is the job of other departments. However, the nursing assistant may be responsible for caring for the resident's personal items.
- ☐ Keep the top of the **overbed table** clean at all times. The overbed table is used when giving personal care, such as a bed bath. The height of the table can be adjusted to a high or low position. The resident uses the overbed table for drinking water and meal trays. You may need to wipe this table frequently throughout the shift so that it is kept clean at all times.
- ☐ You may be responsible for changing the resident's drinking water one or more times during your shift. Most facilities collect the water pitchers and drinking glasses and wash them in the dishwasher at least once a day.
- ☐ Always respect the resident's choices. Ask her how and where she wants items, if possible.
- ☐ Respect the resident's right to privacy when you straighten closets and drawers.
- ☐ Check for items on the floor that the resident and staff could trip or slip on.
- ☐ If you notice personal items in the room that you feel may be unsafe for the resident, check with the nurse regarding what to do with them.
- ☐ If an electrical or mechanical safety hazard exists, follow your facility policy for having the equipment removed or repaired.
- ☐ Check the unit for sharp items, chemicals, improperly stored food items, medications, and other items, such as aerosol cans, that may not be kept in the room according to your facility policy or state law.

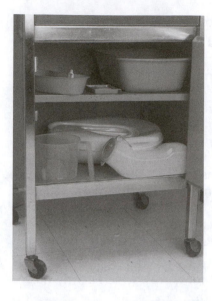

Figure 8-2 Separate clean and soiled items on shelves in the bedside stand.

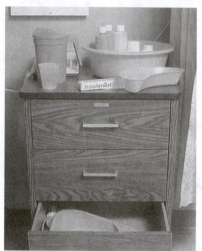

Figure 8-3 Store clean and soiled items in separate drawers of the bedside stand.

bedside stand, the inside is typically divided by two shelves. Many facilities keep the washbasin on the top shelf and the bedpan on the bottom shelf so that they are separated (Figure 8-2). In bedside stands with drawers, these items may be stored in separate drawers (Figure 8-3). Follow your facility's infection control policies for separation of clean and dirty personal care articles in the bedside stand.

THE HOSPITAL BED

The hospital bed is the most important piece of furniture in the resident's unit. As a nursing assistant, you must learn to meet all basic personal care needs for bedfast residents. This may mean adapting some normal procedures, such as bathing. For the bedfast resident, the hospital bed becomes the focal point for care. There will be some type of privacy barrier around the bed, such as a curtain or screen. This barrier must be closed when personal care is being provided, even if you are alone in the room with the resident.

The hospital bed may be electric or manual. Specialty (therapeutic) beds may be used for medical treatments, such as pressure ulcer management. You must learn the purpose of the specialty beds used in your facility and how to operate them.

The head and knee area can be raised or lowered in all regular hospital beds. Changing the angle of the head or knee of the bed is done for resident comfort, and to meet medical needs. Most beds also have a high-low function that raises and lowers the height of the bed. This feature has no therapeutic benefit for residents. Always keep the height of the bed in the lowest horizontal position for resident use. Using the high-low feature makes your job easier and reduces the risk of injury to your back when you are working at the bedside. Raise the height of the bed when you are providing care, or performing a procedure such as making the bed. Lower it immediately when you are finished. You must learn to operate the hospital beds used in your facility. General considerations for all hospital beds are:

- The **gatch handles** are used to change the height of manually operated beds. The gatch handles are at the foot of the bed (Figure 8-4A). They are turned clockwise to raise the bed and counterclockwise to lower the bed. The handle on the left raises and lowers the head of the bed. The handle on the right raises and lowers the foot of the bed. The center handle is used to control the horizontal height of the bed. Use this handle to adjust bed height so it is in a comfortable working position for you. To prevent injuries to residents and staff, always fold the gatch handles under the bed when not in use (Figure 8-4B).

- Wheels on the hospital bed enable you to move the bed, if necessary. Make sure that all four wheels are locked in place, except when the bed is actually being moved.

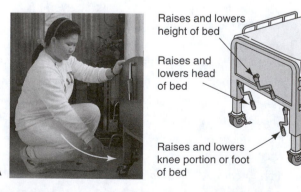

Raises and lowers height of bed

Raises and lowers head of bed

Raises and lowers knee portion or foot of bed

Figure 8-4 (A) The handle on the left raises and lowers the head of the bed. The handle on the right raises and lowers the foot of the bed. (B) For safety, tuck the gatch handles under the foot of the bed when not in use, to prevent injury to residents and staff.

- Hospital beds are designed to be used with side rails. Some beds have a full-length rail on either side of the bed. Others have two small half-rails on each side, one at the head and one at the foot. You must elevate the rails when you are caring for the resident with the bed in the highest horizontal position. Lower the rail only when you are at the bedside providing care. Raise it if you must step away, even for a moment. Keep the rail up on the opposite side of the bed. Some residents pull on the bed rails when positioning and turning in bed. Aside from these two situations, side rails may not be used for some residents. Check the care plan for instructions for each of your assigned residents. Safe use of side rails is also discussed in Chapter 7.

- Many facilities use electric beds. Switches are used to change the position of the head, knee, and horizontal bed height. In some beds, these controls are permanently mounted on the bed rail.

- Always check the bed carefully for lost items before removing the linen. Items such as dentures, glasses, and hearing aids are commonly left on the bed. These items are very expensive and will not survive a trip through the washer and dryer.

Low Beds

Low beds (Figure 8-5) are commonly used in health care facilities for residents who are at risk of falls and for whom use of side rails is not desirable. The bed frame is 4 to 6 inches from the floor to the top of the frame deck. These beds reduce the risk of injury if the resident falls from the bed. Some facilities place pads on the floor next to the bed to further reduce the risk of injury.

Low beds are wonderful tools for reducing resident injuries, but the nursing assistant must use good body mechanics and common sense to prevent back injuries when lifting, moving, and caring for residents, and when making these beds. Some low beds have high-low features, but many are stationary, which increases the risk of back injury. If the bed you are using has a high-low feature, use it whenever caring for the bedfast resident, transferring the resident, or making the bed. A mat on the floor reduces the risk of injury when a resident falls, but it can also be a trip hazard. Move slowly and carefully when working near a floor mat. Avoid entering the room in the dark. Leave a nightlight on, or turn the light on when entering. Squat or kneel on the floor mat when caring for the resident, to reduce back strain caused by bending at the waist. Use good body mechanics, a transfer belt, or a mechanical lift when assisting residents into and out of low beds, to prevent back injuries. The care plan will provide resident-specific instructions. Avoid bending at the waist when moving the resident.

Making the Resident's Bed

The nursing assistant is responsible for making the resident's bed each day. When the resident is out of bed, you will use the unoccupied bedmaking procedure. Facilities use many different types of linen for bedmaking. Some use flat sheets. Many use a fitted sheet on the bottom. Some facilities use draw sheets. Some use plastic or rubber draw sheets on the bed if the resident is incontinent or uses the bedpan or urinal when in bed. Other facilities use large disposable or reusable underpads in place of rubber sheets. Many types of bedspreads can be used to make the resident's room appear homelike and attractive.

When making the bed, raise it to a comfortable working height for you. Avoid walking around the bed many times. Make one side of the bed first, then go to the other side and complete the bedmaking procedure. By raising the height of the bed

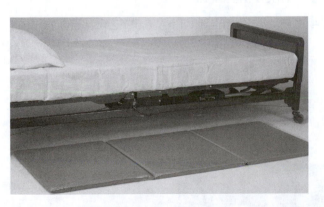

Figure 8-5 Low beds may be used for residents who are at risk of falls. Plan resident care and organize the bedmaking procedure carefully to avoid injury to your back. Remove the mat when the resident is out of bed, to prevent falls.

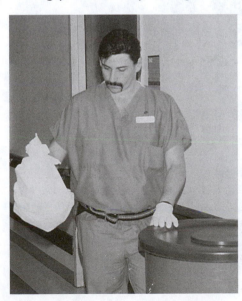

Figure 8-6 Always keep the lid to the soiled linen hamper tightly closed.

and making one side of the bed at a time, you will reduce fatigue and prevent injury to your back.

Knowing your facility policy for placement of clean and dirty linen when making the bed is important. Always wash your hands before handling clean linen. Wash your hands again after discarding soiled linen, even if you were wearing gloves. Carry clean and dirty linen away from your uniform. Most facilities have specific locations where clean linen should be placed. Soiled linen should never be placed on the floor. Know and follow your facility policy for placing soiled linen until it can be placed in the linen hamper (Figure 8-6). When placing soiled linen in the hamper, secure the lid tightly. Linen should not overflow the top of the hamper. Never allow clean and dirty linen to touch each other.

PERFORMANCE PROCEDURE

8 Making the Unoccupied Bed

1 Wash your hands. Gather supplies needed: two large sheets (or one flat and one fitted sheet), a linen draw sheet (if used), plastic or rubber draw sheet (if used), pillowcase, laundry bag or hamper, and clean bedspread, if needed. Stack the linen in the order in which it will be used. Obtain disposable gloves if the old linen is soiled with blood or any moist body fluid.

2 Perform your beginning procedure actions.

3 Carry the clean linen away from your uniform (Figure 8-7).

4 Place the linens on a clean area near the bed in the order of use, from bottom to top.

5 Elevate the bed to a good working height for you.

6 Position the bed so that it is flat.

7 Remove and fold the bedspread if you are reusing it.

8 Apply gloves if linen to be removed is soiled.

9 Remove the linen from the bed by rolling it in a ball. Do not let it touch your uniform.

10 Place soiled linen in a laundry bag, or dispose of it according to facility policy. If gloves were used, remove them and dispose of them according to facility policy. Check the mattress to be sure it is in good repair. Wash your hands before handling clean linen, even if gloves were worn.

11 Follow your facility policy for wiping the mattress. Some facilities require that the mattress be wiped with disinfectant if the linen was soiled with excretions or secretions. (Wear gloves for this task.)

12 Place the bottom sheet on the bed, centering the lengthwise middle fold of the sheet in the middle of the bed.

13 Open the sheet.

14 Place the sheet with small hem even with the foot edge of the mattress (Figure 8-8).

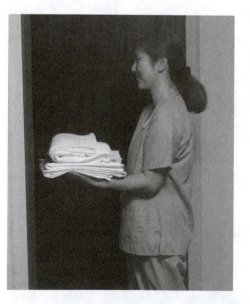

Figure 8-7 Carry clean linen away from your uniform.

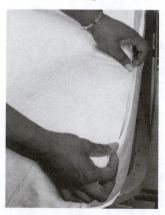

Figure 8-8 Align the hem of the bottom sheet even with the end of the mattress.

8   *continued*

15 Tuck the top of the sheet under the top of the mattress.

16 Miter the corner of the sheet at the head of the bed on the side where you are working (Figure 8-9).

OR

Secure upper and lower corners of fitted sheet.

17 Tuck in the bottom sheet on the side of the bed, working from head to foot.

18 Place the plastic draw sheet, if used, over the middle one-third of the bed.

19 Place the linen draw sheet over the plastic sheet, covering the entire plastic sheet.

20 Tuck the edge of the plastic sheet and draw sheet under the mattress (Figure 8-10).

21 Place the top sheet on the bed, centering the lengthwise middle fold in the center of the bed.

22 Position the sheet with the top edge even with the top of the mattress (Figure 8-11).

23 Tuck the bottom of the sheet under the mattress at the foot of the bed.

24 Place the bedspread on the bed.

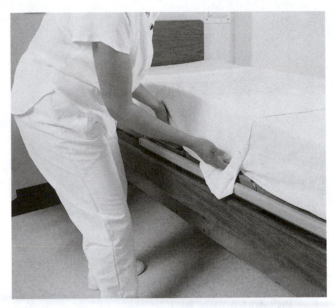

Figure 8-10 If a draw sheet is used, position it so it will be under the resident's shoulders to below the hips.

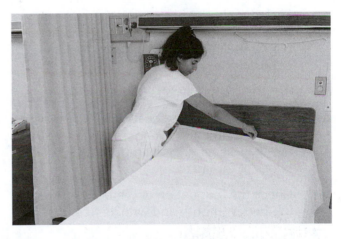

Figure 8-11 Position the hem of the top sheet even with the top of the mattress, then fold it down.

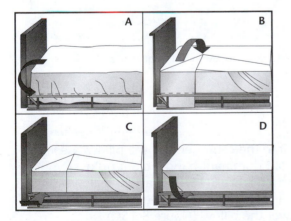

Figure 8-9 Making a mitered corner. (A) The sheet is hanging loose at the side of the bed. (B) Pick up the sheet about 12 inches from the head of the bed to form a triangle. (C) Tuck in the sheet at the head of the bed. Pick up the triangle and place your other hand at the edge of the bed, near the head of the bed, to hold the edge of the sheet in place. Bring the triangle over the edge of the mattress and tuck it smoothly under the mattress. (D) Tuck in the rest of the sheet along the side of the mattress. Tighten the sheet to make sure it is wrinkle-free.

25 Position the bedspread about 4 inches above the top edge of the mattress.

26 Miter linens at the foot of the bed.

27 Move to the other side of the bed.

28 Pull and smooth out the bottom sheet.

29 Tuck the bottom sheet under the mattress at the head of the bed, pulling tight.

30 Miter the corner of the sheet at the head of the bed.

8   *continued*

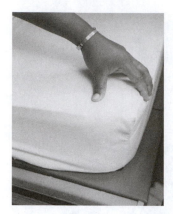

Figure 8-12 Tuck the fitted sheet securely under the mattress.

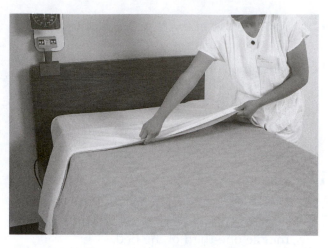

Figure 8-13 Fold the top sheet and spread down, forming a cuff.

OR

Secure upper and lower corners of the fitted sheet (Figure 8-12).

31   Pull and tightly tuck the side of the bottom sheet under the mattress.

32   Pull the plastic sheet tight.

33   Tuck the plastic sheet under the mattress, pulling and tucking from the middle of the plastic sheet first. Then pull and tuck the edges of the sheet.

34   Pull the linen draw sheet tight.

35   Tuck the linen draw sheet under the mattress, pulling and tucking from the middle of the draw sheet first. Then pull and tuck the edges of the sheet.

36   Check the foundation of the bed. Make sure the bed is smooth and wrinkle-free.

37   Pull and smooth the top sheet.

38   Pull and smooth the spread.

39   Tuck the sheet and spread under the foot of the mattress.

40   Miter the top linens at the foot of the bed.

41   Fold the spread back about 30 inches.

42   Make a cuff on the top sheet by folding it back about 4 inches at the top edge of the sheet (Figure 8-13).

43   Place the pillow on the bed.

44   Fold the pillow in half lengthwise and insert the zippered end of the pillow in the pillowcase toward the closed end (Figure 8-14).

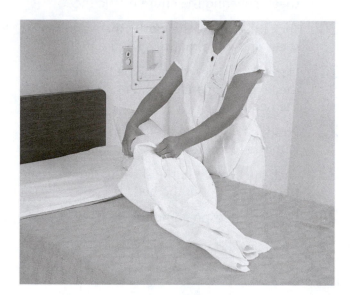

Figure 8-14 Fold the pillow in half lengthwise and slip it into the pillowcase.

OR

Grab the center end of the pillowcase with your dominant hand. Fold it up over your arm (Figure 8-15A). Grab the pillow with this hand (Figure 8-15B). Unfold the pillowcase over the pillow (Figure 8-15C).

45   Straighten the pillowcase on the pillow.

46   Place the pillow at the head of the bed with the open end facing away from the door.

47   Cover the pillow with the bedspread.

48   Perform your procedure completion actions.

8   *continued*

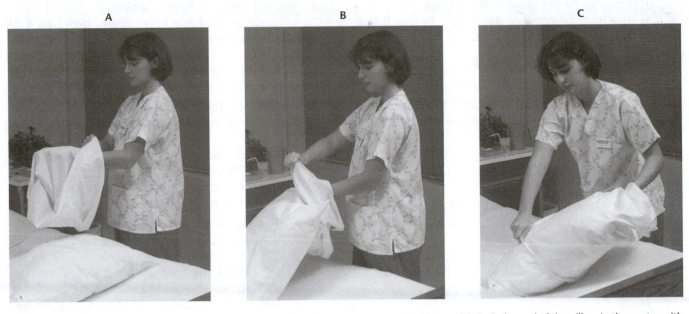

Figure 8-15 (A) Grasp the pillowcase at the seam and fold it back and over your wrist, inside out. (B) Grab the end of the pillow in the center with your pillowcase-covered hand. If the pillow has a tag, grasp the end with the tag on it. (C) Unfold and smooth the pillowcase over the pillow.

Making the low bed.   The bedmaking procedure for low beds is the same as for hospital beds. However, you must protect your back and reduce your risk of injury. To make this task easier:

- Mentally plan and prepare yourself for the procedure.
- Organize your work well to reduce the total number of motions required to complete the task.
- Make sure you have everything you need before entering the room.
- Place linen and needed items on the resident's chair or within close reach.
- Elevate the height of the bed, if possible. Avoid twisting. If you are unable to raise the bed to a comfortable working height, you may consider kneeling or squatting on a plastic mat on the floor during the bedmaking procedure. Maintain a neutral posture and bend from the legs and hips, not the waist.

- Slowly remove the bed linen several pieces at a time. Avoid trying to remove all the linen in one bundle. The weight of the linen and your posture increase the risk of back injury.
- Make one side of the bed at a time. This is faster and more efficient, and conserves energy.
- Use a fitted bottom sheet to reduce the number of movements necessary for making the bed, thereby reducing the risk of back strain.
- If a plastic mat is used on the floor when the resident is in bed, fold it and move it out of the way so that no one trips on it.

KEY POINTS IN THIS CHAPTER

▲ The resident's unit is an area for personal use.

▲ The OBRA legislation promotes a homelike environment.

▲ Respect residents' rights when performing care and handling their possessions.

▲ You show respect for residents by treating their possessions with care.

▲ *Think safety* each time you enter and leave a resident's room.

▲ Follow your facility infection control policies for linen handling and separation of clean and dirty items in the resident's room.

REVIEW QUIZ

1. The resident's personal unit includes:
   a. the floor or wing of the facility in which the resident's room is located.
   b. the nurse's station.
   c. the resident's room and furnishings.
   d. the dining area closest to the room.

2. The nursing assistant's responsibility for daily care of the resident's unit includes:
   a. washing the bed.
   b. mopping the floor.
   c. cleaning the bathroom.
   d. checking for safety.

3. The resident's room should appear:
   a. homelike.
   b. institutional.
   c. like a hospital.
   d. neat and impersonal.

4. When entering and leaving the resident's room, you should *always*:
   a. pull the privacy curtain.
   b. think safety.
   c. leave the door open so others know where you are.
   d. be as quiet as possible.

5. When cleaning the resident's bedside stand, you should:
   a. remove all food items and throw them away.
   b. keep clean and dirty items separated.
   c. remove the bedpan and washbasin, as they do not belong there.
   d. place the toothbrush and hairbrush together in the emesis basin.

6. If the resident is in a bed that is elevated, you should:
   a. always leave the side rails up.
   b. always leave the side rails down.
   c. leave the gatch handle out at the foot of the bed so that you can adjust the bed quickly.
   d. always elevate the knee rest to make the resident more comfortable.

7. When making the unoccupied bed, you should always:
   a. put the soiled linen on the floor.
   b. wear gloves when handling clean linen.
   c. wear gloves if you anticipate contact with blood or moist body fluid.
   d. keep the bed at the lowest possible height.

8. You will prevent fatigue if you:
   a. walk around the bed several times to tuck the sheets in.
   b. make the bed before the resident gets up.
   c. change the resident's linen once a month.
   d. make one side of the bed at a time.

9. You show respect for the resident when you:
   a. call the resident "sweetie," "honey," or "dear."
   b. keep the door to the resident's room closed at all times.
   c. handle the resident's belongings with care.
   d. make the resident's bed each day.

10. The gatch handles of the bed should be:
    a. tucked under the foot of the bed when not in use.
    b. left out at the foot end of the bed so they can be quickly located.
    c. left out if the resident is in bed all the time.
    d. tucked under the bed only if the resident is ambulatory.

11. You are assigned to straighten Mrs. Hillyer's room. When you enter the room, you introduce yourself and tell Mrs. Hillyer what you are going to do. The resident instructs you to "Leave my things alone." You should:
    a. continue straightening the room as you were instructed to do.
    b. tell the resident that her room is messy and that you were told to clean it.
    c. do as the resident requests and report what she said to the nurse.
    d. tell the resident that you will have to report her to the administrator.

12. Mrs. Jaffe is a 93-year-old bedfast resident. She is alert and uses the bedpan independently. You enter her room and find a full bedpan on the overbed table touching the water glass. You should:
    a. move the bedpan away from the glass and pour fresh water.
    b. scold the resident for not calling for help with the bedpan.
    c. remove the bedpan and tell the resident not to do that again.
    d. remove the bedpan, wipe the table, and get a clean glass.

CHAPTER 8
CROSSWORD PUZZLE

Directions: Complete the puzzle using these words found in Chapter 8.

bed	home	signal
chair	overbed	stand
clean	respect	unit
dirty	safety	unoccupied
gatch	side	

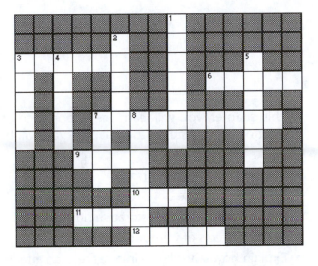

CHAPTER 8
PUZZLE CLUES

ACROSS

3. Check the call _____ every day to be sure it works properly.
6. The piece of equipment the resident sits on
7. The type of bedmaking procedure used when the resident is not in the bed
9. Check the _____ rails every day to be sure that they work properly.
10. The piece of equipment that the resident sleeps on
11. The resident's room should appear _____ like.
12. Separate clean and _____ items.

DOWN

1. Handling the resident's belongings with care shows _____.
2. Articles used for resident care that are not dirty
3. The table next to the bed that contains personal items and articles used for personal hygiene is the bedside _____.
4. The handles at the foot of the bed are _____ handles.
5. Think _____ when you enter and leave the room.
7. The resident's room is also called the resident's _____.
8. The adjustable table that is used for resident care and for serving food trays is the _____ table.

Body Alignment and Activity Needs

OBJECTIVES

In this chapter, you will learn the importance of proper positioning, moving, and lifting. After reading this chapter, you will be able to:

- Spell and define key terms.
- State the purpose of restorative nursing.
- List the principles of restorative nursing.
- List the effects of immobility.
- Explain how a weakness in one area can affect the resident's functioning and well-being.
- Demonstrate the principles of body mechanics.
- Demonstrate good body alignment.
- Move and position the resident.
- Ambulate the resident using a gait belt, cane, or walker.
- Transfer the resident.
- Help the resident do range-of-motion exercises.

KEY TERMS

abduction: moving an extremity *away from* the body

adduction: moving an extremity *toward* the body

ADLs: activities of daily living that include bathing, dressing, grooming, eating, and moving about

alignment: proper position, as in good posture

ambulate: to walk

atrophy: wasting away of muscle

body mechanics: proper use of the body to attain the most strength and reduce injury and fatigue

contracture: abnormal tightening or shortening of muscles from lack of sufficient exercise

contraindicated: not indicated, improper or undesirable

edema: swelling in the tissues often seen in legs, ankles, feet, and hands

extension: straightening out of a joint

flaccid paralysis: loss of muscle tone and absence of tendon reflexes

flexion: bending of a joint

Fowler's position: sitting with the head of the bed elevated 45 to 60 degrees with the knees bent

friction: rubbing and chafing against the resident's skin so that the skin becomes irritated

hemiplegia: condition in which one half (right or left side) of the body is paralyzed

high Fowler's position: same as the Fowler's position, but with the head of the bed elevated 90 degrees

immobility: inability to move

lateral position: lying on one side

paraplegia: paralysis of the lower half of the body, including both legs; bowel and bladder control are also lost

paralysis: loss of ability to move a part or all of the body

pressure ulcers: red or open areas on the skin caused by prolonged pressure

prone position: lying on the abdomen (stomach)

prosthesis: artificial body part

range-of-motion (ROM) exercises: exercises that move each muscle and joint

rehabilitation: a process designed to restore and maintain a resident's highest level of ability

restorative nursing care: nursing care designed to promote health and restore as much independence as possible

semi-Fowler's position: similar to Fowler's position, but with the head elevated 30 to 45 degrees and the knees lower

semiprone position: a modified prone position in which the body is supported on pillows to relieve pressure from most of the bony prominences

semisupine position: a modified side-lying position in which the body is supported on pillows to relieve pressure from most of the bony prominences

shearing: stretching the skin between the bone inside and the bed or another surface outside the body

Sims' position: lying on the left side with the top knee flexed and supported on a pillow. This position is used for enemas and examinations

spastic paralysis: a paralytic condition in which the extremities move in an involuntary pattern, similar to muscle spasms. The resident is aware of the movements, but cannot stop them

supine position: lying on one's back

tetraplegia: paralysis affecting the arms and legs. *Quadriplegia* is an older term for this condition. Residents with tetraplegia are more likely to exhibit spastic paralysis

transfer: moving from one surface to another, as in moving a resident from bed to wheelchair

REHABILITATION AND RESTORATION

Rehabilitation is the process designed to help a resident restore and maintain the highest possible level of physical and mental ability. As a nursing assistant, you will have a major role in the resident's rehabilitation program. The care plan will describe your responsibilities. Other members of the rehabilitation team include the nurse, physical therapist, occupational therapist, speech therapist, and the activities department (Figure 9-1). Rehabilitation programs are based on the resident's physical condition and ability and desire to cooperate.

Restorative nursing care is given by the nursing team to help the resident restore health and maintain and improve his level of function and independence. Some people use the terms *rehabilitation* and *restoration* interchangeably. However, they are not the same. Rehabilitation involves skilled care given by therapists and other licensed health care professionals. Restoration, or restorative nursing, involves nursing procedures that are designed to maintain or improve the resident's condition. If a resident does not use his abilities, he may eventually lose them. For example, a resident who sits in a wheelchair all the time may lose the ability to walk. A resident who is spoon-fed by staff may lose the ability to feed himself. Rehabilitation and restorative nursing programs are designed to prevent declines such as these.

The OBRA legislation requires us to assist all residents to achieve and maintain their highest level of function. Rehabilitation and restorative care should be part of the care of each resident. We recognize that residents' independence affects their self-esteem. Residents who are totally dependent on others may feel as if they are not worthwhile. Sometimes we perform care that residents can do themselves because it is faster. Realizing that this goes against the intent of OBRA and is not good for

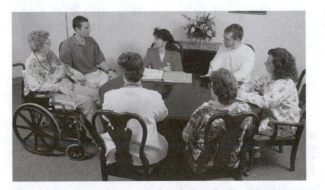

Figure 9-1 Members of the interdisciplinary team meet to plan rehabilitation and restorative nursing care.

residents is important. Learn to organize your work so that you can enable residents to do as much for themselves as possible. Perform other duties while the resident is performing self-care. When the resident is unable to complete a procedure, the nursing assistant should step in and assist as appropriate. Before physically assisting the resident, use verbal cues. This means that you tell the resident how to do the task in simple terms. If the resident does not respond to your cues, using hand-over-hand technique may be necessary. This is done by placing your hand on top of the resident's hand and doing the skill. If this is ineffective, you must complete the task for the resident. Sincerely compliment the resident for the part of the task that he was able to complete.

Principles of Rehabilitation and Restorative Nursing

The principles of rehabilitation and restorative nursing care are the same:

- Emphasize the resident's ability, not his disability. For example, stress what the resident can do, not what he cannot.

- Use the resident's strengths to help him overcome weaknesses.

- Prevent further disability.

- Begin treatment as early in the illness or injury as possible.

- Treat the whole person. Look at the resident as a whole, not just the condition causing the disability. Look at the resident as a complete individual with many complex needs. A weakness in one area can affect all areas of the resident's life. For example, if the resident becomes depressed, he may refuse therapy. This refusal can affect many other areas of the resident's physical and mental condition.

- Praise the resident's accomplishments.

Considerations for care.   Some points to remember in any rehabilitation or restorative program include:

- Encourage self-care with **ADLs** by using adaptive equipment such as a shoe horn or gripper. By using adaptive equipment, the resident may be able to perform a procedure independently. Enabling the resident to be independent promotes good self-esteem.

- Emphasize the resident's abilities.

- Encourage the resident in active **range-of-motion (ROM) exercises.** During this exercise, the resident moves all limbs freely. If the

resident is not able to move all extremities, the nursing assistant should do passive range-of-motion exercises (PROM) on the limbs that the resident is unable to move.

- Encourage the resident to be as independent as possible.

- Follow the care plan for a resident using a **prosthesis** such as an artificial leg or arm.

IMMOBILITY EFFECTS

Immobility affects residents' physical and psychosocial needs. Try to understand how frustrated residents must feel when they always need help to move. Some residents will not be able to move at all without your help. Besides the mental frustrations, there are medical effects of inactivity on the body.

Physical Effects of Immobility

Some physical problems seen in all body systems because of inactivity:

- Circulatory system
  - Blood in vessels may pool, causing blood clots.
  - Poor blood flow may cause **edema** (swelling) in the tissues.
  - The heart has to work harder.

- Respiratory system
  - The resident has more difficulty expanding the lungs.
  - Fluid accumulates in the lungs and respiratory tract.
  - The risk of lung infection increases.

- Urinary system
  - Without gravity, urine may be retained in the bladder, causing urinary tract infection.
  - Kidney stones may develop.

- Digestive system
  - The resident loses his appetite.
  - Constipation may occur.

- Musculoskeletal system
  - Calcium loss increases when stress is not placed on bones.
  - **Contractures** are deformities. They result from shortening and tightening of muscles and occur in muscles that are not used.

— **Atrophy,** or wasting of muscle tissue, results in weakness of muscle.

- Integumentary System
  — **Pressure ulcers** develop easily and quickly reach deeper tissues, including muscle, tendon, and bone.

Mental and Social Effects of Immobility

Inactivity leads to loss of self-esteem, poor body image, sensory deprivation, and increased dependence on others. Inactivity is often a factor leading to depression. Most residents feel better if they have some interaction with others. The resident who cannot move should be helped to get out of the room and spend time near activity. Inactivity and immobility can lead to withdrawal, isolation, and loneliness. Instructions to help the immobile resident are found on the care plan.

BODY MECHANICS

Body mechanics refers to the correct use of the muscles, to help use your strength properly and to avoid fatigue and injury to yourself or others (Figure 9-2). Using proper body mechanics is one of the safest things you can to do prevent injury to residents and to yourself. Nursing assistants move, lift, and turn residents often. Using proper body mechanics can prevent injuries and lessen strain and fatigue. Proper body mechanics involves:

- Using good posture and balance. Use the strongest muscles of the body to do the work.

- Using a back support belt, if this is your preference or the policy of your facility. The back support belt does not make you stronger, and you should not lift more weight than you would if you were not wearing it. Back injuries are very common in health care workers. Many nursing assistants feel better if they are wearing a belt for support. Several studies have shown that workers who use a back support have fewer back injuries. Other studies have shown that there is no difference in the rate of injuries. The belt reminds you to keep your back straight and to use good body mechanics. Using improper body mechanics when wearing the belt is difficult. For this reason alone, the belt may prove beneficial. You are less likely to become injured if you use good body mechanics. Tighten the belt immediately before a lifting or moving procedure. Release the belt when you are not lifting and moving.

- Correctly using your own body and that of the resident.

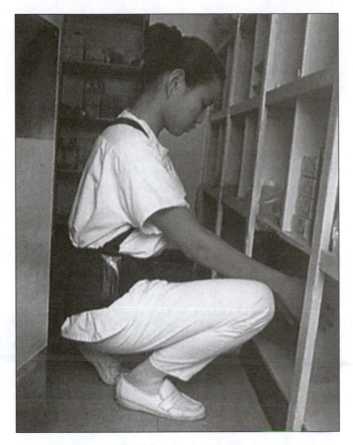

Figure 9-2 Make good body mechanics a habit.

- Enhancing the safety, comfort, and confidence of residents.

- Using pillows, props, and other supports to maintain the resident's body in good alignment.

BODY ALIGNMENT

The correct positioning of the resident's body is called body **alignment.** The resident should be positioned in good posture when sitting or lying. Always follow instructions from the supervising nurse or the resident's care plan. The following points refer to proper body alignment and positioning techniques.

Fowler's Position

The **Fowler's position** (Figure 9-3) is used when the resident is sitting in bed. The headrest of the bed is elevated 45 to 60 degrees, and the knee area of the bed is raised slightly. The **high Fowler's position** is similar, but the head of the bed is elevated 90 degrees. In the **semi-Fowler's position,** the head of the bed is elevated 30 to 45 degrees. Follow these guidelines:

- Have the resident lie on his back with the head of the bed and knees elevated.

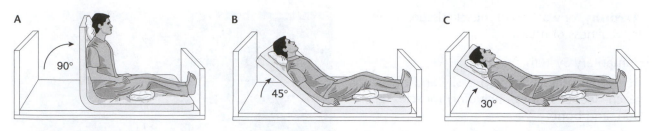

Figure 9-3 (A) High Fowler's position is used for meals and for residents who have difficulty breathing. (B) Fowler's position (C) Semi-Fowler's position

- Make sure the resident's hips are at the bend of the bed.
- If necessary, move the resident up in bed at intervals.
- Support the resident's arms with pillows, if necessary.

- Remember that this position increases pressure on the buttocks, increasing the risk of pressure ulcer development. The resident should not be left in this position for prolonged periods. Follow your facility policy or the resident's care plan for the time frame.

✔ GUIDELINES for Using Proper Body Mechanics

☐ Check the care plan before moving residents. The care plan will list special instructions for moving, positioning, and transferring each resident.

☐ Plan what you are going to do.

☐ Know what the resident can do to assist.

☐ Explain the procedure to the resident.

☐ Ask for the resident's help.

☐ Ask for help from others if you are not sure whether you can move a resident or lift an object.

☐ Face your work.

☐ Keep your back straight.

☐ Have a wide base of support. Place your feet 12 to 14 inches apart.

☐ Move close to the resident. Do not reach from a distance.

☐ Use both hands when lifting and moving heavy objects.

☐ Keep heavy objects as close to your body as possible when lifting, moving, and carrying.

☐ Avoid lifting heavy objects that are above your shoulder height.

☐ Use your "internal girdle." Tighten your abdominal muscles upward and your buttock muscles downward before lifting.

☐ Squat to move or lift an object. Bend at the knees and hips. Keep your back straight.

☐ Lift by using your thigh muscles.

☐ Use smooth, even movements instead of quick, jerking motions.

☐ Match your movements when working with a partner.

☐ Avoid twisting at the waist. If you must turn, pivot instead. If you must change direction, take a few short steps. Turn your entire body instead of twisting your back or neck.

☐ Do not lift when you can push or pull.

☐ When giving bedside care, raise the height of the bed to a comfortable height for your body so you will not have to bend at the waist. When finished, remember to lower the bed to the lowest horizontal position.

☐ Use lifting aids when appropriate, such as mechanical lifts and lift sheets.

☐ Always use a transfer belt for moving residents from one place to another, unless **contraindicated.** The care plan will state when a belt should not be used for moving a resident because of a specific medical condition. A *transfer belt* is a heavy canvas belt used for lifting and moving residents. The same belt is also called a *gait belt* when it is used for helping residents to ambulate.

Sitting in a Chair

Proper positioning in the chair is important so that the resident can breathe correctly. Good positioning promotes resident comfort and a sense of well-being. Follow these guidelines:

- Place the resident's feet flat on the footrests of the wheelchair, the floor, or a stool. The feet should not dangle.
- Position the hips and knees at right angles.
- Rest the buttocks firmly against the back of the chair. You may wish to pad the seat of the chair for the resident's comfort and to prevent skin breakdown.
- Position the spine straight against the back of the chair.
- Position the resident's head directly over the shoulders.
- Support the forearms and elbows on the armrests of the chair.
- If necessary, prop the resident with pillows or pads to maintain good alignment.

Proper position at mealtime is important to prevent choking. Position the resident upright, using pillows or props for support, if necessary. The elbows should be below wrist level when the resident is eating. Pay attention to table height. If the table is too high for the resident, he will have more difficulty eating. Seating the resident on a cushion may help. Likewise, make sure that the resident is close to the table. Residents who are seated in wheelchairs may be too far away. After meals, residents should remain upright for at least 30 to 60 minutes, if possible.

Supine Position

The **supine position** (Figure 9-4) is used when the resident is lying on the back.

- Place a small pillow under the resident's head. This allows better alignment than a large pillow. If a large pillow is used, extend it down past the

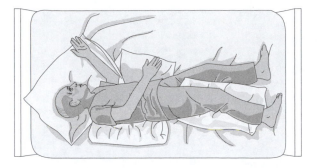

Figure 9-5 The semisupine position is a very comfortable position that relieves pressure from all major bony prominences.

neck so that it supports both the shoulder area and the head.

- Keep the feet in proper alignment and prevent foot drop with a footboard or other device specified on the care plan.
- Use positioning devices, such as handrolls, splints, foam, or firm wedges, as indicated on the care plan to maintain position.

The **semisupine position** (Figure 9-5) is also called the *tilt position*. Do not confuse it with the lateral position. The resident in the lateral position is lying on his side. This increases pressure on the bony prominences of the ear, shoulder, elbow, hip, and ankle. The resident in the semisupine position is on his side, but is tilted at an angle. When used correctly, this position relieves pressure from all bony prominences and keeps the spine straight. The resident is positioned so that he is leaning against a pillow for support. The legs are straight, with the top leg slightly behind the bottom leg. A pillow is placed under the top leg to keep it even with the hip joint. The lower shoulder is pulled forward. This causes pressure to be distributed across the back, not the shoulder joint. The arms can be at the sides or folded across the abdomen.

Lateral Position

The **lateral position** (Figure 9-6) is used when the resident is to lie on the side.

- Support the upper arm and leg with pillows.
- Position the upper leg so that its weight does not rest on the lower leg.
- Place a pillow lengthwise to support the resident's back and maintain the position.

Sims' Position

The **Sims' position** is commonly used when an enema is given or when the physician is doing an examination.

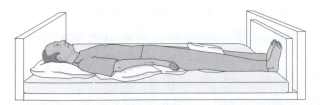

Figure 9-4 When the resident is in the supine position, pillows may be placed behind the knees and under the arms for comfort.

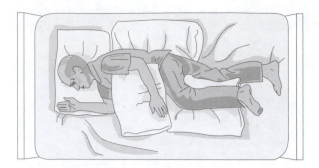

Figure 9-6 Use pillows to support the resident in the lateral position. Make sure the bottom shoulder is pulled forward slightly to prevent pain and pressure on the joint.

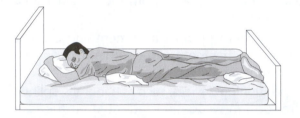

Figure 9-7 Check the resident frequently when using the prone position. Use this position only if permitted by your facility. Hang the feet over the end of the mattress or elevate the shins with pillows to prevent pressure on the toes.

- The resident is positioned on the left side.
- The left arm is positioned behind the back and extended.
- The right arm is flexed and brought forward, supported on a pillow.
- The right knee is flexed and supported on a pillow.
- A small pillow is placed under the resident's head.

Prone Position

The **prone position** (Figure 9-7) is used when the resident is lying on the abdomen. Use this position

Sheepskin

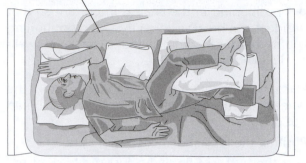

Figure 9-8 The semiprone position is very comfortable for the resident. Use this position only if permitted by your facility.

for residents only if directed to do so by the care plan. Check the resident every 15 to 30 minutes, or according to facility policy, when in the prone position.

- Turn the resident's head to one side when he is lying prone.
- Place a small pillow under the resident's abdomen near the waist.
- Flex (bend) the resident's arms and position them near the head.
- Place the resident's feet in the space between the mattress and the foot of the bed.

The **semiprone position** (Figure 9-8) is the opposite of the semisupine position. It is a very comfortable position for the resident. Like the semisupine position, it eliminates pressure on the bony prominences, reducing the risk of pressure ulcers. To place the resident in this position, begin by turning the resident prone. Lift the shoulder and chest on the side closest to you. Support them with a pillow. Position the opposite arm behind the resident. The legs and spine are straight. Fold a second pillow in half and

---

PERFORMANCE PROCEDURE

9 Positioning the Resident in the Supine Position

1 Perform your beginning procedure actions.

2 Position the resident so that he is lying on his back.

3 Place the resident's arms at his sides in a comfortable, functional position, supporting them with pillows if necessary.

4 Check for good body alignment.

5 Pad bony prominences of elbows and heels if indicated.

6 Elevate the knees slightly for comfort, if desired.

7 Perform your procedure completion actions.

10 Moving the Resident to the Side of the Bed

1 Perform your beginning procedure actions.

2 Stand on the side of the bed opposite from the one on which the resident will lie.

3 Use proper body mechanics to move the resident.

4 Place the resident's arms across his chest. Cross the resident's legs at the ankles.

5 Remove the pillow.

6 Place one of your arms under the resident's shoulder. Place the other arm under the back.

7 Move the upper part of the resident's body toward you.

8 Place one of your arms under the resident's waist and the other arm under the resident's thighs.

9 Move the resident's midsection toward you.

10 Move the resident's legs toward you. Uncross the ankles. Straighten the resident's arms.

11 Replace the pillow.

12 Begin positioning or transferring the resident, or go to the next step of this procedure.

13 If the resident is to be left in this position, straighten the linen and raise the side rails if ordered.

14 Perform your procedure completion actions.

11 Moving the Resident to the Side of the Bed Using a Draw Sheet

1 Perform your beginning procedure actions.

2 Use proper body mechanics to move the resident.

3 Place the resident's arms across his chest. Cross the resident's legs at the ankles.

4 Remove the pillow.

5 Roll the sides of the draw sheet toward the resident until they touch the body.

6 Using an overhand grip, place one hand at the upper end of the draw sheet, by the resident's shoulders. Place the lower hand on the draw sheet in the hip area.

7 The nursing assistant on the side of the bed to which the resident will be moved does most of the work and calls the signals.

8 Move one foot about 12 inches forward to give you a broad base of support. Place your weight on this foot.

9 Flex your knees and keep your back straight.

10 On the count of three, both nursing assistants lift and pull the sheet toward the side of the bed.

11 Uncross the resident's ankles and straighten his arms.

12 Replace the pillow and unroll the draw sheet.

13 Begin positioning or transferring the resident, or go to the next step of this procedure.

14 If the resident is to be left in this position, straighten the linen and raise the side rails, if ordered.

15 Perform your procedure completion actions.

12   Assisting the Resident to Move Up in Bed

1   Perform your beginning procedure actions.

2   Lower the head of the bed.

3   Remove the pillow and lean it against the headboard.

4   Stand next to the bed.

5   Ask the resident to bend his knees and put his feet flat on the mattress.

6   If the resident is able, ask him to bend his arms at his sides and place his hands on the bed. Ask him to push when told to do so.

7   Slide one hand and arm under the resident's upper back and shoulders.

8   Slide the other arm under the resident's hips and buttocks.

9   Instruct the resident to push with his hands and feet on the count of three.

10   On the count of three, move the resident to the head of the bed. Repeat as necessary until the resident is correctly positioned.

11   Replace the pillow.

12   Check to see if the resident is in good alignment.

13   Perform your procedure completion actions.

place it under the top leg. Turn the resident's head to either side. Use a small pillow for comfort.

Moving a Resident with a Draw Sheet

Some residents are too weak, ill, or large for you to move by yourself. Sometimes moving the resident with your arms causes pain for the resident. Using a draw sheet to move and turn the resident prevents **friction** and **shearing** between the resident's skin and the sheets. Another advantage of moving the resident with a draw sheet is that it reduces the risk of a back injury in the nursing assistant. The following

13   Moving the Resident to the Head of the Bed Using a Draw Sheet

1   Perform your beginning procedure actions.

2   Place the resident's arms across his chest.

3   Remove the pillow.

4   Roll the sides of the draw sheet toward the resident until they touch his body.

5   Using an overhand grip, place one hand at the upper end of the draw sheet, by the resident's shoulders. Place the lower hand on the draw sheet in the hip area.

6   Both nursing assistants stand with feet apart, one foot ahead of the other.

7   Bend your knees and keep your back straight.

8   On the count of three, both nursing assistants shift their weight from one foot to the other while lifting the draw sheet and moving it toward the head of the bed.

9   Straighten the resident's arms.

10   Replace the pillow and unroll the draw sheet.

11   Straighten the linen and leave the resident comfortable.

12   Perform your procedure completion actions.

✔ **GUIDELINES for Lifting and Moving Residents**

The nursing assistant does a great deal of lifting and moving. Wear uniforms that fit loosely enough to allow you to move comfortably without tearing. Wear nonskid shoes so you do not slip. Use a back support if this is your preference or facility policy. Plan your moves to include the following:

☐ Refer to the care plan for specific instructions.
☐ Explain the procedure to the resident, making certain that he understands what is to be done and how he should help.
☐ Use a transfer belt to prevent injury to yourself and the resident.
☐ Use lifting devices, if indicated.
☐ Position the bed in the lowest possible position.
☐ Get assistance if you are not sure whether the resident can safely move, position, or transfer.

Be alert to safety:

☐ If you will be transferring the resident into a wheelchair, position the small front wheels so the large part is facing forward before beginning the transfer.
☐ Lock the brakes on beds, wheelchairs, and lifts.
☐ Make sure that lifting and moving devices are in good working condition.
☐ When transferring a resident, move the resident toward his stronger side.
☐ Support the resident's weaker side during transfers.
☐ Be alert to catheters and other tubing so that tubes are not accidentally pulled or dislodged.
☐ Have the resident wear nonskid shoes or footwear.
☐ Apply artificial limbs and braces properly.
☐ Avoid lifting the resident under the arms. This can cause pain and dislocate the resident's shoulders.
☐ The resident should not use your neck for support.
☐ Support body parts when turning the resident.
☐ When ambulating residents, approach corners slowly and watch for approaching traffic.
☐ Check the rubber tips of canes and walkers before using them, to be sure they are not too worn.

Observe and report changes:

☐ change in color, paleness, sweating
☐ dizziness, unsteadiness
☐ shortness of breath or difficulty breathing
☐ changes in vital signs
☐ signs of skin irritation
☐ resident's comments and concerns

Also be aware of these psychosocial concerns:

☐ Let the resident help as much as possible if consistent with the care plan.
☐ Encourage the resident to be in charge of moving.
☐ Ask the resident to count to three.
☐ Offer the resident choices, such as where and when to be moved.
☐ Realize that the inability to move is a great loss of the resident's independence.
☐ Know the resident's fears, such as falling or being left alone.

procedure assumes that a draw sheet is left on the bed at all times for lifting and moving the resident. In this procedure, you will need a coworker to help you.

Moving the Resident to the Head of the Bed Using a Draw Sheet

Using a draw sheet to move the dependent resident prevents friction and shearing between the resident's skin and the sheets. This procedure assumes that a draw sheet is left on the bed at all times for lifting and moving the resident. In this procedure, you will need a coworker to help you.

TRANSFERRING AND AMBULATING THE RESIDENT

You will be transferring, or moving, residents out of beds and wheelchairs several times a day. It is important that you do this correctly to avoid injury to the resident and to yourself. It is always good to practice these skills with another nursing assistant. Practice will reinforce and help you learn the rules of safety. Another task you will be expected to perform is to **ambulate,** or walk with, residents. Using a transfer belt or gait belt helps assure safety for both the resident and you.

Using the Transfer (Gait) Belt

A gait belt and a transfer belt are the same piece of equipment. The belt is called a *transfer belt* when it is used to **transfer** the resident. It is called a *gait belt* when it is used to ambulate the resident. It should be worn around the nursing assistant's waist when it is not being used on a resident. In some facilities, a belt is left with each resident and the nursing assistant uses only this belt for transferring the resident. Know and follow your facility policy.

A transfer belt is a heavy canvas belt placed closely around the resident's waist (Figure 9-9). You can hold onto it while moving the resident instead of pulling the resident under the arms. When using the transfer belt, always grasp it with an underhand grasp for good control. While ambulating the resident, a firm underhand grasp on the transfer belt helps you ease the resident to the floor in case of a fall. Never use the resident's own belt or the waistband of clothing in place of the transfer belt.

Contraindications for use of the transfer belt.
Before using the transfer belt on any resident, check with the nurse or care plan. The transfer or gait belt

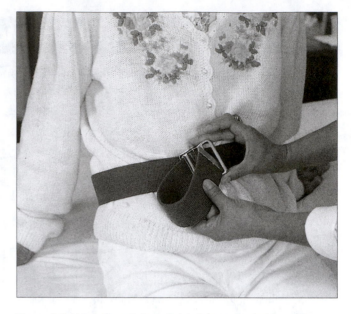

Figure 9-9 Using the gait (transfer) belt keeps both the resident and the nursing assistant safe.

is contraindicated in residents with these medical conditions:

- colostomy
- a gastrostomy tube
- recent abdominal surgery or a fresh incision
- severe cardiac or respiratory disease
- fractured ribs
- pregnancy
- an abdominal pacemaker. This is a surgically implanted device that regulates the rate of the heartbeat. Most commonly, it is placed in the chest, but occasionally the abdomen is used. The device is visible beneath the skin surface.
- implanted medication pump. Some residents have implanted medication pumps under the skin of the abdomen. These are not always visible, although an incision will be present over the implant. The care plan, nurse, or resident will inform you if such a device is present. If the surgical site is well healed, it is probably safe to use the gait belt. However, you should always follow the care plan or check with the nurse before using a gait belt to move a resident who has any type of implanted device.
- abdominal aneurysm. An *aneurysm* is a ballooning of the wall of an artery due to a structural weakness. If the aneurysm ruptures, the resident will die.

PERFORMANCE PROCEDURE

14   Using a Transfer (Gait) Belt

1 Perform your beginning procedure actions.

2 Assist the resident to sit on the side of the bed.

3 Assist the resident to put on clothing and shoes or other footwear with nonslip soles.

4 Explain to the resident that the transfer belt is a safety device that will prevent pulling and tugging on the resident. Explain that it will be removed when the resident has been transferred.

5 Always apply the belt over the resident's clothing.

6 Place the belt around the resident's waist and buckle it in the front. Take care with female residents to ensure that the breasts are not under the belt.

7 Thread the belt through the teeth side first. Place the end of the belt through both openings so that it is double-locked.

8 The belt should fit snugly, but you should check it by slipping your fingers comfortably underneath to be sure it is not too tight. Monitor female residents to be sure that the breasts are not under the belt.

9 Using an underhand grasp, insert your hands under the belt on each side and assist the resident to stand.

10 Complete the transfer or ambulation procedure.

11 Perform your procedure completion actions.

Transferring the Resident into a Wheelchair

If you will be transferring the resident into a wheelchair, you must position the chair and lock the brakes before beginning the transfer. Remove the footrests or push them up and out of the way during the transfer. (If you remove the legrests, make sure to replace them.) Before beginning the transfer, position the wheelchair at a 45° to 60° angle to the surface from which you are transferring. If the resident has a strong side, position the chair so the strongest leg moves toward the chair. Pay very close attention to the small, front caster wheels of the wheelchair. These wheels allow the chair to move in all directions. The large part of the wheel faces back when the chair is moving. During transfers, position the large part of the small front wheels facing forward (Figure 9-10). This changes the center of gravity of the chair and reduces the risk of tipping. To reposition the wheels, back the chair up, then move it forward until the wheels are in good alignment, then lock the brakes.

The resident must be able to move to the side of the bed or front edge of the chair before standing, and for most transfers. Sitting in this position moves the center of gravity over the base of support in the feet, making standing easier and safer. Several methods can be used for moving the resident forward. If

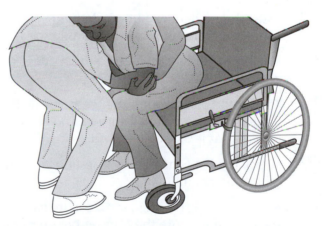

Figure 9-10 Position the small, front caster wheels so that the large part of the wheel faces forward. Lock the brakes. This changes the center of gravity of the chair and reduces the risk of tipping the chair.

he cannot scoot forward independently, the care plan will list the method to use.

Paralysis and Spinal Cord Injuries

Some residents are admitted to the facility because of conditions resulting in **paralysis.** This is loss of movement and impairment of various parts of the body. In spinal cord injury, paralysis develops immediately below the level of injury. Strokes, brain tumors, and other medical problems may also cause paralysis.

15   Transferring the Resident from Bed to Wheelchair—One Person

1   Perform your beginning procedure actions.

2   Position the wheelchair so the resident's stronger side will be closest to the wheelchair when the resident is sitting on the edge of the bed. Place the wheelchair within one foot of the bed at a slight angle. Position the large part of the front wheels facing forward.

3   Raise or remove the wheelchair footrests.

4   Lock the wheelchair brakes.

5   Raise the head of the bed.

6   Lock the wheels of the bed.

7   Lower the bed to the lowest position. Lower the side rail.

8   Assist the resident to sit on the side of the bed.

9   Assist the resident to put on clothing and shoes or other footwear with nonslip soles.

10   Place the transfer belt around the resident's waist and buckle it in the front.

11   Thread the belt through the teeth side first. Place the end of the belt through both openings so that it is double-locked.

12   Check the fit of the belt by inserting your fingers underneath it.

13   Make sure that the resident's feet are flat on the floor. If not, use the transfer belt to move the resident to the side of the bed until his feet touch the floor (Figure 9-11).

14   Instruct the resident to push off the bed with his hands on the count of three.

15   Using an underhand grasp, insert your hands under the belt on each side, count to three, and assist the resident to stand.

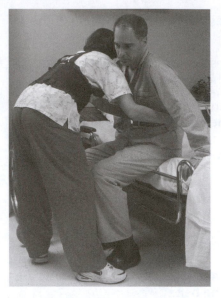

Figure 9-11 Maintain a wide base of support and use good body mechanics when transferring residents.

16   Support the resident's weaker side.

17   Pivot and turn the resident with his back to the wheelchair.

18   Continue to hold the transfer belt, and guide the resident backward until he can feel the edge of the wheelchair seat with the back of his legs.

19   Tell the resident to place his hands on the wheelchair arms. Seat the resident in the chair.

20   Remove the transfer belt.

21   Adjust the wheelchair footrests.

22   Cover the resident's lap with a lap blanket or other covering, if needed. Be sure that the blanket does not become caught in the wheels.

23   Perform your procedure completion actions.

16   Transferring the Resident from Bed to Wheelchair—Two Persons

1   Perform your beginning procedure actions.

2   Position the wheelchair so the resident's stronger side will be closest to the wheelchair when the resident is sitting on the edge of the bed. Place the wheelchair within one foot of the bed at a slight angle. Position the large part of the front wheels facing forward.

3   Raise or remove the wheelchair footrests.

4   Lock the wheelchair brakes.

5   Raise the head of the bed.

6   Lock the wheels of the bed.

7   Lower the bed to the lowest position. Lower the side rail.

8   Assist the resident to sit on the side of the bed.

9   Assist the resident to put on clothing and shoes or other footwear with nonslip soles.

10   Place the transfer belt around the resident's waist and buckle it in the front.

11   Thread the belt through the teeth side first. Place the end of the belt through both openings so that it is double-locked.

12   Check the fit of the belt by inserting your fingers underneath it.

13   Use the transfer belt to move the resident to the edge of the bed until his feet are flat on the floor. Each nursing assistant places the hand closest to the resident at the back of the belt and the other hand at the front of the belt and slides the resident forward.

14   On the count of three, both nursing assistants move the resident at the same time. Coordination of movement is very important.

15   Each nursing assistant places the hand closest to the resident through the belt with an underhand grasp behind the resident.

16   The nursing assistant closest to the chair, on the resident's stronger side, stands in a position so that he can pivot and move away, allowing the resident access to the chair. This nursing assistant should stand with the left leg further back than the right leg.

17   The other nursing assistant should use her left knee to support the resident's weaker leg. This nursing assistant's right leg is positioned further back than the left one.

18   Instruct the resident to lean forward and push off the bed, using the palms of his hands, on the count of three.

19   The resident's knees should be spread apart. Tell the resident to put both feet back, with the stronger foot behind the weaker foot.

20   Both nursing assistants should bend their knees, squat slightly, and spread their feet to provide a broad base of support.

21   On the count of three, the resident stands. The nursing assistants pivot the resident slowly and smoothly by pivoting their feet, legs, and hips toward the chair until the resident can feel the wheelchair with the back of his legs (Figure 9-12).

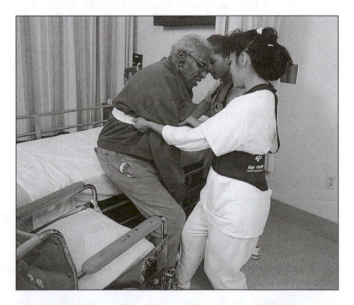

Figure 9-12 On the count of three, both nursing assistants lift and pivot the resident.

(continues)

16 *continued*

22 Tell the resident to place both hands on the armrests of the chair and lean forward slightly.

23 Both nursing assistants bend their knees and lower the resident into the chair (Figure 9-13).

24 Remove the transfer belt.

25 Adjust the wheelchair footrests.

26 Cover the resident's lap with a lap blanket or other covering, if needed. Be sure that the blanket does not become caught in the wheels.

27 Perform your procedure completion actions.

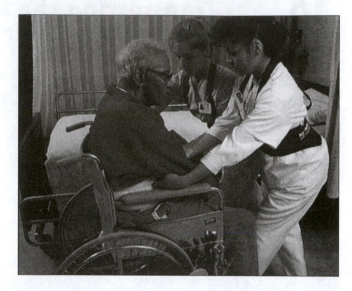

Figure 9-13 Keep your back straight and gently lower the resident into the chair.

PERFORMANCE PROCEDURE

17 Ambulating the Resident with a Gait Belt

1 Perform your beginning procedure actions.

2 Assist the resident to sit on the side of the bed.

3 Assist the resident to put on shoes or other footwear with nonslip soles.

4 Explain to the resident that the gait belt is a safety device that will prevent pulling and tugging on the resident. It allows you to guide and support the resident during the ambulation procedure.

5 Always apply the belt over the resident's clothing.

6 Place the belt around the resident's waist and buckle it in the front.

7 Thread the belt through the teeth side first. Place the end of the belt through both openings so that it is double-locked.

8 The belt should fit snugly, but you should check it by slipping your fingers comfortably underneath to be sure it is not too tight. Monitor female residents to be sure that the breasts are not under the belt.

9 Using an underhand grasp, insert your hands under the belt on each side and assist the resident to stand.

10 Walk behind and slightly to one side of the resident during ambulation. Maintain a firm, underhand grasp at the center back of the gait belt.

11 Encourage the resident to use handrails in the hallway.

12 Walk the distance recommended by the care plan or the nurse's instructions.

13 Monitor the resident for signs of fatigue. If this occurs, assist the resident to sit in a chair.

14 After ambulating the resident, return to the resident's room.

15 Assist the resident to sit in the chair or return to bed.

16 Remove the gait belt.

17 Perform your procedure completion actions.

18 Ambulating the Resident with a Cane or Walker

1 Perform your beginning procedure actions.

2 Assist the resident to sit on the side of the bed.

3 Assist the resident to put on shoes or other footwear with nonslip soles.

4 Check the tips of the cane or walker for safety.

5 Place the gait belt around the resident's waist and check the fit.

6 Place the cane in the resident's hand or the walker in front of the resident.

7 Help the resident stand. Grasp the gait belt underhand at the resident's sides.

8 When the resident is standing and is balanced, ask if he feels dizzy or weak.

9 Walk behind and slightly to one side of the resident during ambulation. Maintain a firm, underhand grasp at the center back of the gait belt.

10 Walk the distance recommended by the care plan or the nurse's instructions.

11 Monitor the resident for signs of fatigue. If this occurs, assist the resident to sit in a chair.

12 After ambulating the resident, return to the resident's room.

13 Assist the resident to sit in the chair or return to bed.

14 Remove the gait belt.

15 Perform your procedure completion actions.

19 Transferring the Resident from Wheelchair to Toilet

1 Perform your beginning procedure actions.

2 Make sure the bathroom is empty.

3 Bring the resident in a wheelchair to the bathroom.

4 Close the bathroom door.

5 Position the wheelchair at right angles to the toilet.

6 Place the transfer belt around the resident's waist.

7 Lock the wheelchair brakes.

8 Tell the resident to push up from the wheelchair while you lift her with the transfer belt. Count to three to match movements.

9 Ask the resident to hold the bathroom grab bar.

10 Help the resident stand, giving her time to get balanced.

11 Pivot the resident so that she is standing in front of the toilet, facing you.

12 Lower the resident's pants and underwear.

13 Help the resident sit on the toilet.

14 Be sure the call signal is close to the resident. Instruct the resident to call when she is finished.

15 Wash your hands and leave the bathroom if doing so is safe for the resident. Close the door behind you.

(continues)

19   *continued*

16 Return when the resident calls.

17 Put on gloves if helping the resident wipe excess urine or bowel movement is necessary.

18 Remove the gloves and discard according to facility policy.

19 Wash your hands.

20 Assist the resident to stand by using the gait belt. Tell the resident to hold onto the bathroom grab bar and pull herself up. Match movements on the count of three.

21 Pull the resident's pants and underwear up.

22 Smooth the resident's clothing.

23 Pivot and seat the resident in the locked wheelchair. Flush the toilet. If abnormalities are noted in the urine or stool, do not flush. Save the specimen for the nurse to see.

24 Help the resident wash her hands.

25 Remove the resident from the bathroom.

26 Remove the transfer belt.

27 Perform your procedure completion actions.

Paralysis affects sensation and voluntary movement below the level of injury. Residents with this condition are at great risk for developing pressure ulcers and other skin injuries. Because sensation is impaired, they will not feel the pain that serves as a warning sign when the skin begins to break down. If not promptly identified and treated, pressure ulcers worsen rapidly and may cause other serious complications. Pressure ulcers are always easier to prevent than to treat. Take preventive skin care very seriously in residents with paralysis.

Paraplegia is paralysis of the lower half of the body, including both legs. Bowel and bladder control are also lost. **Tetraplegia** is paralysis affecting the arms and the legs. *Quadriplegia* is an older term for this condition. **Hemiplegia** is paralysis on one side of the body, such as the right arm and leg. **Flaccid paralysis** involves loss of muscle tone and absence of tendon reflexes. Some residents have **spastic paralysis.** These residents have no voluntary movement. The extremities move in an involuntary pattern, similar to muscle spasms. The resident is aware of the movements, but cannot stop them. The type of paralysis is determined by the level of injury and cause of the problem. Residents with tetraplegia are more likely to exhibit spastic paralysis.

Independence.   Most dictionaries define the term *independent* as self-reliant or self-supporting. In reality, it includes much more than this. People who are independent move about and complete ADLs at will,

without assistance. In some ways, independence is a state of mind. It is freedom to do what we want, when we want, within the constraints of personal ethics and the law. Independence is a tangible thing that most people take for granted. We do not realize how greatly we value it until we lose it. Loss of independence is an enormous loss. People who were suddenly paralyzed lost their independence in seconds. Imagine the shock of living normally one minute, then developing an injury or medical condition that renders you completely unable to care for yourself. Imagine the loss of your income. Imagine the inability to earn a living, then having to wait for months for government assistance to be approved. Imagine the shame of having to ask for it in the first place! People with paralysis have experienced devastating losses. Because of this, some seem to have an attitude or behavior problems. Be honest and sincere with the resident. Allow him to direct the care that you give. This gives the resident a measure of control, and improves self-esteem.

Positioning and spasticity.   When positioning residents with paralysis, move the extremities slowly and gently. Rapid, rough movements will cause spasticity. If a resident's extremities move into a position of **flexion,** gently move them into extension. If the extremities move into a position of **extension,** position them in flexion. Spasticity can be very strong. Avoid forcing the extremity into position, as this may break a bone or cause other injuries. Positioning devices may be necessary to maintain position. However, attention to proper positioning is important. This is a major key to preventing contractures and deformities in these high-risk residents.

Moving and positioning the resident.   Residents with spinal cord injury can provide limited to no assistance with positioning, moving, and transfers. Allow the resident to verbally direct you. Elevate the bed to the high position when giving care (make sure the rail is up on the opposite side of the bed). To prevent injury to your back, never move a resident who has a spinal cord injury by yourself. Make sure that another assistant is available to help you. Using lift sheets, mechanical lifts, and other adjunctive devices makes moving the resident easier for both the resident and the nursing assistant.

The Mechanical Lift

A mechanical lift is used when a resident is heavy, helpless, unbalanced, or has a condition, such as amputated legs or paralysis, that makes transfer with a belt difficult or impossible. Many facilities use beds with frames that are 4 to 6 inches above the floor. If the resident falls from bed, the chance of injury is lower than with a fall from a regular hospital bed. Unfortunately, transferring residents into and out of such low beds increases the risk of back injuries for nursing assistants. Using a mechanical lift for this type of transfer reduces the risk of injury. Know and follow your facility policy for use of the mechanical lift. Most facilities require two or more nursing assistants to operate the lift safely.

The mechanical lift is a hydraulic unit. Always check the floor near the lift before using it. If an oily substance is on the floor, do not use the lift until it is checked and repaired. Always check the sling, release mechanisms, straps, and chains for safety problems before using the lift. If anything is in need of repair, do not use it. Follow your facility policy for removing the lift from service. Obtain safe equipment before taking the lift to the resident's room.

PERFORMANCE PROCEDURE

20   Transferring the Resident Using a Mechanical Lift

Supplies needed:

- mechanical lift
- straps or chains for mechanical lift
- seat for mechanical lift
- disposable underpad for lift seat, if needed
- disposable exam gloves if contact with body fluids, secretions, or excretions is likely

1   Perform your beginning procedure actions.

2   Place the wheelchair at right angles to the foot of the bed, facing the head. Lock the wheelchair and elevate or remove the footrests.

3   Elevate the bed to a good working height for you. Lock the wheels of the bed.

4   Lower the side rail on the side nearest you.

5   Roll the resident on his side (Figure 9-14A).

6   Position the lift seat under the resident's body so that it supports the resident's shoulders, buttocks, and thighs. Smooth out the sling.

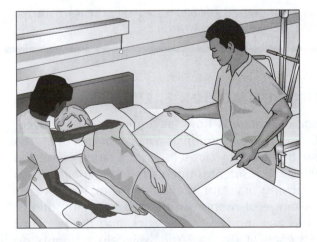

Figure 9-14A Position the sling between the shoulder blades and thighs.

(continues)

20   *continued*

7   Roll the resident back onto the sling and properly position it on the other side.

8   Position the frame of the lift over the bed. Spread the legs of the lift to the widest open position to maintain a broad base of support.

9   Attach the suspension straps or chains to the sling. The "S" hooks should face *away* from the resident's body, to prevent injury (Figure 9-14B).

10   Position the resident's arms comfortably inside the sling.

11   Attach the straps or chains to the lift frame.

12   While talking to and reassuring the resident, slowly raise the boom of the lift until the resident is above the bed.

13   Slowly guide the lift away from the bed.

14   Position the lift over the chair.

15   The second nursing assistant holds the sling and helps lower the resident slowly into the chair, keeping the hips back, while the first nursing assistant slowly lowers the lift (Figure 9-14C).

16   Monitor the location of the resident's feet and arms to prevent injury.

17   Unhook the straps or chains and remove the lift.

18   Support the resident's feet with footrests.

19   Perform your procedure completion actions.

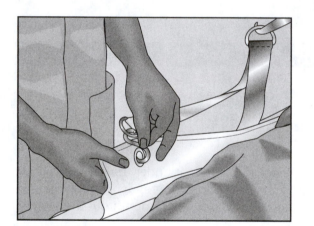

Figure 9-14B Center the lift over the resident and fasten the straps with the "S" hooks facing outward.

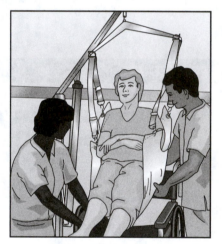

Figure 9-14C Slowly lower the lift while monitoring the resident's legs and arms and guiding the hips back into the chair.

RANGE-OF-MOTION EXERCISES

Range of motion is how far a joint can be moved. Active range of motion is when the resident can move the joints by himself. Passive range of motion is when the resident is unable to move the joints, so the nursing assistant moves them for him. A person's range of motion is affected by many things, such as age, body size, genetics, and the presence or absence of disease. You will help residents do range-of-motion exercises each day. Follow the directions on the care plan. Ask for help if you are not certain how to perform this procedure.

You must become familiar with several terms regarding range-of-motion exercises. **Abduction** is moving the resident's extremity away from the body. **Adduction** is moving an extremity toward the body. Flexion is bending a joint. Extension is straightening a joint.

Purpose of Range-of-Motion Exercises

Range-of-motion exercises are done for residents who are unable to move their own joints. There are several reasons for these exercises. Muscles that are not used atrophy, become weak, and develop contractures. Contractures are deformities that cannot always be reversed.

Reasons for passive range-of-motion exercises include:

- preventing deformities
- preventing pain
- maintaining normal joint function
- increasing joint motion
- improving circulation
- promoting a sense of well-being

✔ GUIDELINES for Doing Range-of-Motion Exercises

- ☐ Follow the care plan instructions.
- ☐ Explain the procedure to the resident.
- ☐ Use good body mechanics.
- ☐ Expose only the part of the body being exercised.
- ☐ Know your facility policy for exercising the head and neck. This is not done without a doctor's order in some facilities.
- ☐ Support the limbs above and below the joint being exercised.
- ☐ Do not push the joint past the point of pain or resistance.
- ☐ Watch the resident's face for an indication of pain or discomfort.
- ☐ Stop at the end of each motion before repeating it again.
- ☐ Do each exercise three to five times, or as indicated in the care plan.
- ☐ Encourage the resident to help with the exercises as indicated on the care plan.
- ☐ Report and record how the resident tolerated the procedure, the degree of joint movement, which extremity was exercised, and type of exercise.

PERFORMANCE PROCEDURE

21 Giving Passive Range-of-Motion Exercises

1 Perform your beginning procedure actions.

2 Position the resident in the supine position.

3 Exercise the extremities as indicated on the care plan, supporting the extremity at the closest joints.

Head and Neck

Perform range of motion in this area only if it is your facility policy or if you have a physician's order.

1 Lean the head forward, bringing the chin to the chest.

2 Lean the head backward, with the chin up.

3 Turn the head from side to side.

4 Turn the head back and forth in a circular motion.

Shoulders, Arms, and Elbows

1 Move the arm over the head, with arm touching the top of the head.

2 Return the arm to the side.

3 Move the arm across the chest.

4 Return the arm to the side.

5 Move the arm straight up.

6 Return the arm to the side.

7 Bring the arm away from the body at the side to the shoulder level.

8 Return the arm to the side.

9 With the arm straight out at the side, bend at the elbow and rotate the shoulder.

10 Return the arm to the side.

(continues)

21 *continued*

11 Bend at the elbow and bring hand to chin (Figure 9-15A).

12 Return the arm to the side.

Wrists, Fingers, and Forearms

1 Bend the hand backward at the wrist (Figure 9-15B).

2 Bend the hand forward at the wrist.

3 Clench the fingers and thumb slightly, as if making a fist.

4 Extend the fingers and thumb.

5 Move fingers and thumb together and then apart.

6 Flex and extend joints in the thumb and fingers.

7 Move each finger in a circular motion.

8 Extend the arm along the side of the body with the palm facing upward.

9 Rotate the forearm with the palm facing upward, then downward.

Legs, Hips, and Knees

1 Stretch the leg out from the body. Return the leg to the other leg, crossing over the other leg only at the ankle.

2 Bend and straighten the knee (Figure 9-15C).

3 Roll the knees inward and outward.

Ankles, Feet, and Toes

1 With the leg straight on the bed, push foot and toes toward the front of the leg (Figure 9-15D).

2 Push the foot and toes out straight. Point toward the foot of the bed.

3 With the leg straight, turn the foot and ankle from side to side.

4 Curl toes downward and upward.

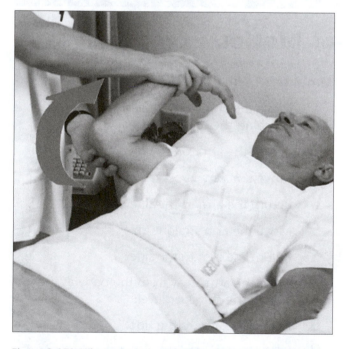

Figure 9-15A When exercising the elbow, support the arm above and below the joint.

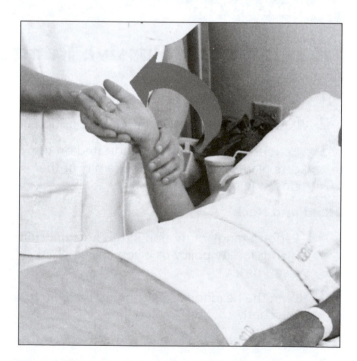

Figure 9-15B Range-of-motion exercises for the wrist

(continues)

21 *continued*

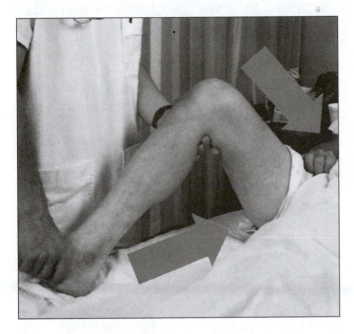

Figure 9-15C Range-of-motion exercises for the hip and knee. Support the knee joint during this activity.

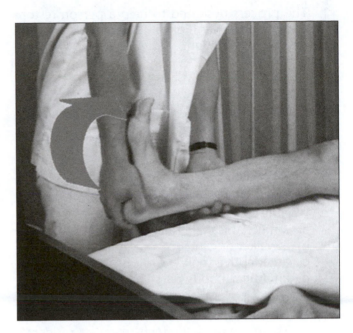

Figure 9-15D Range-of-motion exercises for the foot and toes

5 Spread the toes and move each toe away from the second toe, then toward the second toe.

6 Repeat each exercise as indicated on the care plan.

7 Note the resident's response to exercise.

8 Perform your procedure completion actions.

KEY POINTS IN THIS CHAPTER

▲ Rehabilitation and restorative nursing are designed to restore and maintain the resident's highest possible level of function.

▲ Immobility leads to complications in all body systems.

▲ Proper body alignment is necessary for the resident while sitting or lying down.

▲ Using a transfer belt helps prevent injury to the nursing assistant and the resident.

▲ Always follow the care plan when moving and lifting residents.

▲ Range-of-motion exercises are done to prevent deformities and increase circulation and joint motion.

▲ Safety is important when moving or lifting residents.

REVIEW QUIZ

1. The process designed to help a person restore and maintain her highest level of ability is:
   a. range of motion.
   b. rehabilitation.
   c. activities of daily living.
   d. assistance.

2. Maintenance, prevention, and restoration of abilities are the principles of:
   a. adaptive devices.
   b. nursing care.
   c. rehabilitation.
   d. activity therapy.

3. What is a prosthesis?
   a. a mechanical lift
   b. a walker or cane
   c. an adaptive tool
   d. an artificial body part

4. All of the following are true statements *except*:
   a. Immobility affects the resident physically.
   b. There are mental effects from the resident's inability to move about.
   c. Only the circulatory system is affected by immobility.
   d. Residents may feel frustrated when they must rely on others to move about.

5. An effect of immobility on the circulatory system may be:
   a. swelling of the tissues due to poor blood flow.
   b. constipation and loss of appetite.
   c. development of a bladder infection.
   d. loss of calcium in the bones.

6. Proper body mechanics includes:
   a. having a wide base of support.
   b. using the strong back muscles to lift.
   c. keeping the feet close together when lifting.
   d. keeping the object to be lifted at arm's length from the body.

7. Using good body mechanics does all of the following *except*:
   a. prevent fatigue in the nursing assistant.
   b. reduce injury to the nursing assistant.
   c. reduce the risk of injury to the resident.
   d. increase the resident's strength.

8. Body alignment is:
   a. lifting and moving residents.
   b. positioning the body correctly.
   c. comfortable positioning for the nursing assistant.
   d. using the muscles the best way.

9. What is the correct positioning for the resident when sitting in a chair?
   a. The feet should be dangling.
   b. The hips should be at right angles in the chair.
   c. The knees should be extended.
   d. The spine should be slanted as much as possible.

10. A resident in the supine position is lying on the:
    a. side.
    b. abdomen.
    c. back.
    d. side with pillows supporting the spine.

11. When a resident is in the prone position, he is lying on the:
    a. abdomen.
    b. side.
    c. back.
    d. back and side.

12. When moving a resident up in bed, ask the resident to help by:
    a. pulling on the side rails.
    b. pushing the pillow up.
    c. straightening the legs and pushing with the feet.
    d. bending the knees, placing feet flat on the bed, and pushing.

13. Using a draw sheet when moving residents helps prevent:
    a. infections.
    b. friction and shearing.
    c. contractures.
    d. atrophy.

14. When moving a resident up in bed, the pillow should be:
    a. placed against the headboard.
    b. placed on the chair.
    c. kept at the foot of the bed.
    d. left under the resident's head.

15. A belt that is placed around the resident's waist to assist with moving is called a:
    a. lifting belt.
    b. transfer or gait belt.
    c. mechanical lifter.
    d. lifting and moving belt.

16. Which of the following is *not* true regarding lifting and moving residents?
    a. There is no need to explain procedures to confused residents.
    b. Refer to the care plan for special instructions.

c. Make sure the equipment used for lifting and moving is working properly.
d. Get help, if necessary.

17. When the resident has a weak side, it is best to move him:
a. weak side first.
b. with either side moving first.
c. toward the weaker side.
d. toward the stronger side.

18. Before assisting a resident to ambulate with a cane or walker, you should:
a. do range-of-motion exercises.
b. place a gait belt loosely around the resident's waist.
c. make sure that the resident has on shoes with nonslip soles.
d. have the resident rest in bed.

19. Passive range-of-motion exercises are done for the resident:
a. who is up and about.
b. who can move well without help.
c. who cannot exercise himself.
d. by licensed professionals only.

20. What are your major concerns when lifting or moving a resident?
a. how good the resident looks when you are finished
b. safety of the resident and nursing assistant
c. how quickly you can do the task
d. wearing gloves and using standard precautions

21. Mr. Macmillan is a 66-year-old resident who is 6 feet tall and weighs 210 pounds. He has had a stroke and requires total care. You have never transferred this resident before. The nurse assigns you to get this resident up in the chair for 2 hours after his bath. You should:
a. do as you are told without asking questions.
b. check the care plan for instructions on how to transfer the resident.
c. tell the nurse that the resident is too big for you to move.
d. report the nurse to the director of nursing for giving you such a difficult assignment.

22. You are assigned to care for Dr. Stuart, a 77-year-old retired professor. Dr. Stuart has had a respiratory infection and fever. She is taking antibiotics and has been in bed for three days. The nurse tells you in report that the resident's fever is normal and that it is time to get Dr. Stuart up in the chair for an hour. When it is time to get

Dr. Stuart up, she tells you, "Sick people must stay in bed." Your best response is to:
a. inform Dr. Stuart that the nurse insists that she get up.
b. leave Dr. Stuart in bed.
c. advise Dr. Stuart that getting out of bed may help her to get well faster.
d. call the resident's daughter and inform her that her mother will not cooperate.

23. You are assigned to bathe Michael Cleary, a 72-year-old resident with diabetes. Mr. Cleary walks about the facility at will. When you hand him the washcloth and ask him to wash his face, he says, "I am paying you to wash my face." Your best response is to:
a. wash the resident's face.
b. ignore what Mr. Cleary said and leave the room.
c. tell him that you are not paid to wash his face.
d. consult the care plan or ask the nurse for advice.

24. You are caring for Mrs. Kaiser, an 88-year-old resident who is confined to bed. The nurse instructed you in report to make sure that the resident is turned every 2 hours. Mrs. Kaiser has a large pressure ulcer on her buttocks. You do not know whether you should position her on her back or not. You should:
a. turn her on her back anyway because the nurse did not give you special instructions.
b. ask another nursing assistant what to do.
c. consult the care plan or ask the nurse for advice.
d. leave Mrs. Kaiser on her side for 4 hours because you cannot turn her on her back.

25. Mrs. Ashe is a newly admitted resident whose daughter has been caring for her in the home. You are assigned to transfer Mrs. Ashe from the bed to the chair by using the transfer belt. When you explain the procedure to Mrs. Ashe, she says that her daughter always put her hands under her arms and lifted her. She says she does not think the belt is necessary. You should:
a. place your hands under Mrs. Ashe's arms and lift her into the chair.
b. continue to explain to Mrs. Ashe why the transfer belt is the safest method to use.
c. tell Mrs. Ashe that her daughter transferred her improperly.
d. leave Mrs. Ashe and care for the other residents you are assigned to.

CHAPTER 9
CROSSWORD PUZZLE

Directions: Complete the puzzle using these words found in Chapter 9.

ADL	flex	pressure
alignment	Fowler's	prone
ambulate	friction	prosthesis
atrophy	hemiplegia	range
contracture	immobility	rehabilitation
contraindicated	lateral	restorative
edema	mechanics	shearing
extend	paralysis	supine

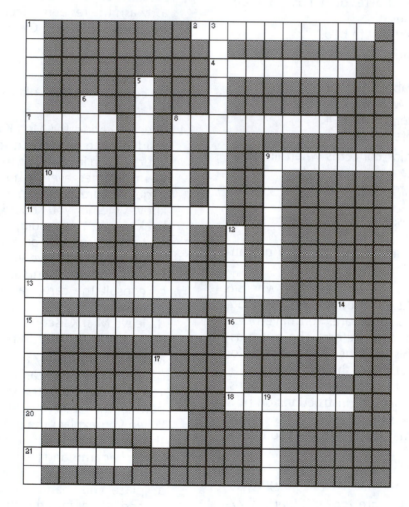

CHAPTER 9
PUZZLE CLUES

ACROSS

2. An artificial body part
4. Stretching the skin between the bone inside and the bed on the outside of the body is _____.
7. Swelling
8. Loss of ability to move
9. Sitting in bed with the head elevated and knees bent is the _____ position.
10. Activities of daily living
11. Abnormal tightening or shortening of a muscle
13. Designed to restore and maintain the resident's highest level of ability
15. Inability to move
16. Side lying
18. Muscle wasting
20. Proper position in good posture
21. To straighten

DOWN

1. Lying on the back
3. Nursing care designed to assist the resident by restoring health and promoting independence is _____ nursing.
5. Proper use of the body is good body _____ .
6. To walk
8. Areas of skin redness or breakdown are _____ ulcers.
9. Rubbing on the resident's skin in a manner that irritates it
11. Improper or undesirable
12. Paralysis on one side of the body
14. To bend
17. Lying on the abdomen
19. Exercises that move muscles and joints are _____ of motion.

Personal Care Needs

OBJECTIVES

In this chapter, you will learn the importance of giving personal care to residents. After reading this chapter, you will be able to:

- Spell and define key terms.
- Describe the goals of skin care.
- Identify pressure ulcers and describe how they are caused and prevented.
- List guidelines for personal care of the resident.
- Perform oral hygiene for the resident.
- Bathe the resident.
- Perform perineal care.
- Help groom the resident.
- Describe care of a resident with a prosthesis.
- Demonstrate care of the hair and nails.
- Apply support hosiery.
- Make an occupied bed.

KEY TERMS

abrasion: a rubbing away or scraping of the skin

anti-embolism stockings: elastic stockings that improve circulation by compressing the veins in the legs

anus: the outlet for the rectum

axilla: the armpit

decubitus ulcer (plural: decubiti): a pressure sore, pressure ulcer, or bedsore

dentures: artificial teeth; may be partial or complete, upper or lower dentures

genital area: the area that includes the external sex organs and anus

incontinent: unable to control the discharge of urine or stool

perineal (peri) care: cleansing the genital area

waterless bathing: a method of washing that uses prepacked, premoistened cloths instead of soap and water

SKIN CARE

The skin is the largest organ of the body, and it performs several necessary functions. The skin is an outer covering that protects a person from infection

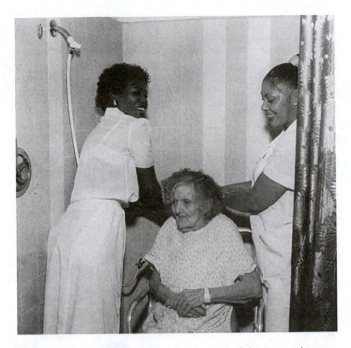

Figure 10-1 Nursing assistants provide most of the personal care to residents.

and injury. The skin also removes water, salt, and waste through sweat. At certain places the skin joins with mucous membranes to line body openings. The hair and nails are considered part of the skin system.

As a nursing assistant you will give skin care to residents (Figure 10-1). Knowing the changes caused by aging is important for you.

Age-Related Changes in the Skin

As in every body system, aging brings some changes in the skin, hair, and nails. The changes vary due to heredity and individual lifestyle, but generally the age-related changes in the skin are as follows:

- Skin becomes drier, scaly, thin, and wrinkled.
- Skin loses elasticity.
- The fatty tissue under the layer of skin decreases.
- Less oil and sweat are produced.
- Skin tags and moles are more common.
- The skin becomes less sensitive to heat, cold, and pain.
- The skin becomes fragile; it is easily damaged, bruised, and torn.
- Fingernails and toenails become thicker and brittle, cracking more easily.
- Skin injuries heal slowly.

Goals of Skin Care

The resident's care plan will state specific skin care goals, but some general goals are important to observe when giving skin care.

An elderly person's skin produces less oil, so the skin is often dry and flaky. Therefore, having a full bath every day is not necessary for most elderly persons. In fact, bathing every day often makes the skin drier. Most residents will have a partial bath at least once a day, but a full bath or shower is usually given only two or three times a week. The resident's care plan states the bathing schedule. In residents with dry skin, the care plan may direct you to apply a moisturizing lotion.

When a person perspires, or sweats, the drops on the surface of the skin can pick up dirt and dust that mix with tiny flakes of skin. Some diseases also cause flaking and cracking of the skin. Some residents are incontinent of bowel and bladder. These excretions are very irritating to the skin. The warm, dark, damp skin area gives bacteria the chance to grow and spread. Therefore, cleaning the resident's skin is one of your major responsibilities. Know the major goals of bathing or cleaning the resident.

- Cleanliness
  - removes bacteria on the skin
  - removes sweat and other body secretions
  - removes body odors
  - promotes a sense of well-being

- Stimulation of circulation
  - Warm water on the surface of the skin increases blood flow.
  - Light skin stroking during washing helps blood flow.
  - Massage soothes and stimulates the skin.

- Mild exercise for the resident
  - Moving the body, trunk, arms, and legs is mild exercise.
  - Mild exercise gives the resident the opportunity to do range-of-motion exercises.

- Observation. Bath time is an opportunity to inspect the resident's skin. Report:
  - irritation
  - texture change
  - color change
  - lumps under the skin or areas of new growth
  - injury
  - pressure ulcers
  - drainage
  - rashes
  - any resident complaint

- Other benefits of bathing
  - Bath time provides the nursing assistant an opportunity to have personal, therapeutic communication with the resident.
  - The feeling of being clean and attractive is refreshing and adds to the dignity, self-worth, and sense of well-being of the resident.

PRESSURE ULCERS

Bedsores are called pressure sores, pressure ulcers, **decubitus ulcers,** or decubiti. The most accurate name for this problem is *pressure ulcer*. Pressure ulcers develop quickly in the immobile, elderly resident because of prolonged pressure and lack of blood flow to an area. The name "bedsore" is deceiving. Pressure ulcers can develop anytime the resident has pressure on the skin. Pressure ulcers may develop even when the resident is sitting up in a chair. Your observation and reporting skills must be very sharp in this area. A reddened area can progress to a deep ulcer very quickly (Figure 10-2). Deep ulcers are painful and difficult to heal. Infections and other complications may develop. Prevention is the best treatment for pressure ulcers. Pressure ulcers frequently develop over areas of bony prominences (Figure 10-3):

- back of head
- side of head
- ears
- shoulder blades
- elbows
- breasts in women
- spine

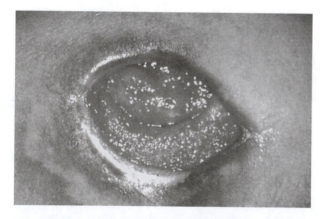

Figure 10-2 A pressure ulcer can progress from a reddened area to a deep, serious ulcer very quickly. (Permission to reproduce this copyrighted material has been granted by the owner, Hollister, Incorporated.)

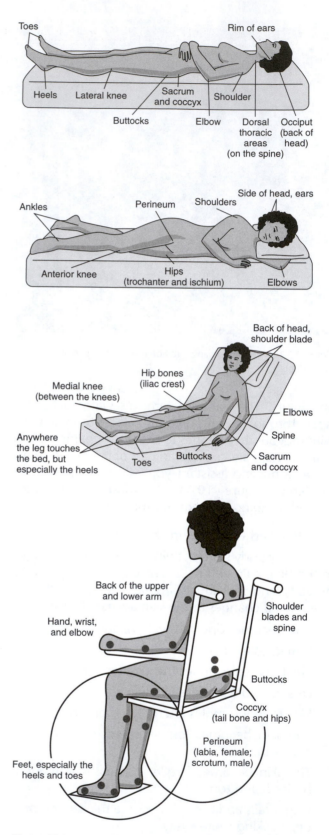

Figure 10-3 Common areas of pressure ulcer development in bed and chair

✔ GUIDELINES for Preventing Pressure Ulcers

Use the following approaches to prevent pressure ulcers from beginning:

☐ Keep the resident up and walking as tolerated.

☐ Change all residents' positions every 2 hours, more often if the care plan indicates, or if the resident is uncomfortable. Remember that this applies to residents sitting in chairs and those in bed.

☐ Keep residents' skin clean and dry. Prolonged moisture causes the skin to break down. Wash the resident immediately after each episode of incontinence. Use a cleansing agent that reduces skin irritation. Be sure to rinse and dry well.

☐ Use facility-approved moisture lotions if the resident's skin is dry.

☐ Help residents drink enough liquids and eat correctly.

☐ Keep linens free of wrinkles and crumbs.

☐ Avoid friction and shearing when moving residents.

☐ Use lifting devices to move residents whenever possible.

☐ If residents are sitting in chairs, teach them to shift their weight every 15 minutes.

☐ Use pressure-relieving pads in beds and wheelchairs.

☐ Position and pad the resident so that the skin at bony areas, such as the knees and ankles, does not rub together.

☐ If the resident is in bed with the head elevated, do not allow the resident to sit in this position for more than 2 hours.

☐ Follow the nurse's or care plan instructions for special treatment of pressure ulcers.

☐ Apply the principles of standard precautions when providing care.

- hips and buttocks
- sacrum and coccyx
- genitalia in men
- thighs in contact with catheter tubing
- knees
- ankles
- heels
- toes

Stages of Pressure Ulcers

Pressure ulcers progress in four stages:

- *Stage I.* Redness that does not go away within 30 minutes of the time that pressure is relieved. In a dark-skinned person, this may appear as a blue or black discoloration.
- *Stage II.* Partial skin loss, a blister, or a shallow crater.
- *Stage III.* A full layer of skin is lost, extending down into the subcutaneous fat layer.
- *Stage IV.* A full layer of skin is lost, and the damage extends down to muscle, tendon, and bone.

Observation and Reporting

Report immediately:

- redness of the skin that does not go away within 30 minutes after the pressure is relieved

- blisters
- skin tears or **abrasions**
- pain or tenderness
- bruises
- rashes
- any skin color changes

Use devices that reduce friction and shearing, such as:

- sheepskin pads
- heel and elbow protectors

Use devices that reduce pressure, such as:

- pillows
- foam wedges (Figure 10-4)
- alternating-pressure mattresses
- special gel-, water-, and foam-filled mattresses, cushions, and overlays
- low-air-loss and other therapeutic beds (Figure 10-5)
- other devices used by your facility

Follow the care plan when using these devices. Although the resident may be using a pressure-reducing device, changing position is still necessary.

Nursing Measures

Certain nursing measures are used to prevent pressure ulcers from developing. These include changing

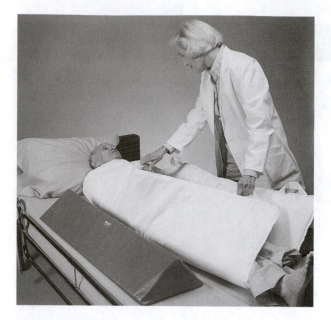

Figure 10-4 The bed positioning system is used for moving the resident. The positioning pad is inserted to maintain position, then Velcro fasteners are used to attach the pad to the bolster cushion. (Courtesy of Skil-Care Corp., Yonkers, NY; (800) 431-2472)

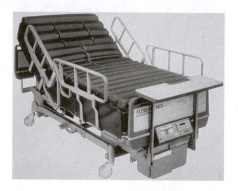

Figure 10-5 Low-air-loss therapy beds are beneficial for residents who have severe skin breakdown. Residents using these beds must be turned regularly because breakdown can occur. (Courtesy of Hill-Rom)

the resident's position every 2 hours, or more often if necessary, and assisting the resident to maintain good nutrition and hydration.

PERSONAL CARE

Personal care of the resident includes care of the mouth, teeth, hair, nails, and feet. It also involves bathing, dressing, and grooming the resident. You will be responsible for helping the resident with these activities of daily living. A well-groomed appearance affects the resident's self-esteem.

The resident has done her own care all her life. It may take longer to let the resident wash her own face and brush her own teeth, but you will add to the resident's self-worth by helping the resident, rather than doing it for her. Helping the resident be as independent as possible is one goal of restorative nursing care. Refer to the guidelines for personal care.

ORAL HYGIENE

Oral hygiene is the cleaning of the mouth, teeth, gums, and tongue. The purpose of oral hygiene is to remove food particles and reduce the amount of bacteria in the mouth. One of your responsibilities is to provide good mouth care and cleanliness for the resident. A clean mouth helps prevent mouth odor and tooth decay. A feeling of well-being is created when a person has good oral hygiene.

Another purpose of providing oral hygiene is observation. While brushing the resident's teeth, you have an opportunity to observe the mouth. Remember when giving oral hygiene:

- Encourage self-care if consistent with the care plan.
- Let the resident brush her own teeth. Get supplies ready, and take the resident into the bathroom in a wheelchair.
- Wear gloves when doing oral hygiene.
- Observe and report to the nurse any signs of irritation, sores, loose teeth, and pain.

Special Situations

Some residents need frequent mouth care because of special medical problems. These include residents who are receiving tube feedings and those who are in a coma. Many of these residents breathe through the mouth. The mucous membranes of the mouth and nose dry out quickly. The mouth should be cleaned frequently to keep it moist, prevent caking of secretions, and make breath feel and smell fresh. Follow your facility policy and the care plan for cleaning and moisturizing the resident's mouth. Some comatose residents require mouth care as often as every one or two hours. These points are important to remember when giving special mouth care:

- Always explain the procedure to the resident even if the resident appears unresponsive.
- Turn the resident's head to the side when cleaning the mouth of an unconscious resident, to avoid getting liquids into the lungs.
- Moisten the resident's lips with lip balm or other lubricant according to facility policy.

DENTURE CARE

Many residents in a long-term care facility have **dentures** (false teeth). Dentures may be the entire set of teeth or only a few teeth. Dentures are necessary for eating, retaining the shape of the face and jaw, and for giving the resident a sense of well-being.

✔ GUIDELINES for Providing Personal Care

☐ Bathing should be a good cleaning of the body in a pleasant, relaxed area. Refer to the care plan for special bathing instructions.

— If you will be using liquid soap from a wall dispenser, avoid putting the soap directly into the bath water. Dispense some soap into a small cup and carry it to the bedside. Pour the liquid soap onto the washcloth as needed.

— In some facilities, bar soap is not permitted. If refillable liquid soap bottles are used, each resident should have a bottle labeled with his name. The soap from that bottle is used for that resident only.

— If you wash the resident's hair in the shower, placing cotton in the ears will prevent problems if the spray is misdirected. Bring an extra towel and wrap the resident's head after rinsing the shampoo.

☐ Assist the resident with toileting before beginning a procedure.

☐ Give the resident choices. Schedule time for personal care according to the resident's needs and desires.

☐ Independence promotes positive self-esteem. Allow the resident to do as much self-care as possible. Follow the care plan.

☐ Use adaptive devices that promote independence, such as:

— long-handled shoehorn

— long-handled grippers

— adaptive brushes and combs

— other devices used by your facility to promote independence

☐ Protect the resident's privacy.

— Close the door, window curtain, and privacy curtain.

— Expose only the part of the body on which you are working.

☐ Dress the resident in appropriate clothing. Clothing should be appropriate for the season and the resident's age, and be color-coordinated. Clothing should be of the proper size and fit and in good repair.

☐ Avoid cold or exposure.

— Make sure the room is warm enough.

— Use a bath blanket to keep the resident covered if the body will be exposed. This is a modesty and dignity issue, in addition to providing warmth.

— A shower bath is commonly given in the long-term care facility. Keep the spray of warm water on the resident's body during the entire procedure to prevent chilling.

☐ Avoid the overuse of powders or talc. Too much powder is not good for the skin. Know and follow your facility policy. Some facilities do not allow the use of body powder unless the resident requests it.

☐ Dry the resident well.

— Pay special attention to skin folds, creases, and the skin between the toes.

— Drying the resident helps prevent infection and skin breakdown. Do not rub the resident vigorously. Pat and gently rub the skin dry.

☐ Be alert to safety concerns.

— Use a transfer belt to move the resident.

— Test the temperature of the bath water.

— Use safety belts on tub lifts and shower chairs.

— Make certain that bath mats are secure.

— Help residents in and out of the tub and shower.

— Stay with the resident in the tub and shower.

— Observe the resident for shortness of breath or complaints of feeling dizzy.

— Report anything unusual to the nurse.

— Record the procedure according to facility policy.

(continues)

✓ GUIDELINES for Providing Personal Care (continued)

☐ Be alert to infection control issues.

— Apply the principles of standard precautions when providing personal care.

— Always wash from the cleanest area to the dirtiest.

— Change water, washcloth, and gloves after washing a contaminated or dirty area.

— After using a washcloth or towel below the waist, avoid using it above the waist.

— The handheld shower spray should be placed on the hook when not in use. Do not let it hang down or touch the floor, which is always considered dirty.

— Disinfect the tub, shower chair, or whirlpool after each use.

— Handle soiled towels and linen properly.

PERFORMANCE PROCEDURE

22   Brushing the Resident's Teeth

Supplies needed:
- toothbrush
- toothpaste
- water
- mouthwash
- straw
- emesis basin
- towel
- disposable exam gloves

1   Perform your beginning procedure actions.

2   Place a towel across the resident's chest.

3   Help the resident in self-care, if possible.

4   Moisten the toothbrush. Apply toothpaste.

5   Brush the resident's teeth using a circular motion on all surfaces. Brush gums, tongue, sides, and roof of the mouth (Figure 10-6).

6   Let the resident rinse the mouth with water or mouthwash.

7   Hold the emesis basin while the resident spits.

8   Wipe the mouth with a towel.

9   Check the mouth for sores, redness, or irritation.

10   Perform your procedure completion actions.

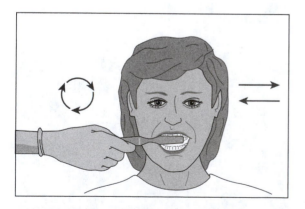
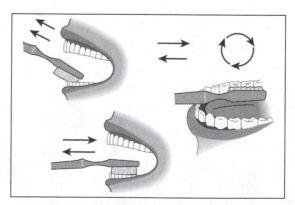

Figure 10-6 Gently brush all surfaces of the teeth and gums.

PERFORMANCE PROCEDURE

23   Special Oral Hygiene

Supplies needed:
- special mouth applicators or swabs used by your facility
- water
- plastic bag
- lubricant for lips
- emesis basin
- two towels
- disposable exam gloves

1   Perform your beginning procedure actions.

2   Cover the pillow with a towel and turn the resident's head to the side. Position the head forward so that any fluid and secretions will not run down the resident's throat.

3   Place the emesis basin against the resident's chin.

4   Gently open the resident's mouth.

5   Dip the premoistened applicators into water, mouthwash, or solution used by the facility. Press the applicator against the inside of a glass to remove excess liquid.

6   Wipe the gums, teeth, and inside of the mouth with applicators.

7   Discard the used applicators in the plastic bag.

8   Apply lubricant to the resident's lips.

9   Perform your procedure completion actions.

PERFORMANCE PROCEDURE

24   Denture Care

Supplies needed:
- disposable gloves
- emesis basin
- denture cup
- denture brush or toothbrush
- denture paste or powder
- towel
- tissues
- disposable cup
- straw
- paper towels
- mouthwash
- gauze sponges, if you will be removing the dentures
- small plastic bag for trash

1   Perform your beginning procedure actions.

2   Drape the towel across the resident's chest.

3   Line the emesis basin with paper towels.

4   Ask the resident to remove the dentures, if able, and place them in the emesis basin.

5   Offer the resident a tissue to wipe her mouth after removing the dentures.

6   If the resident is unable to remove the dentures, cover your gloved fingers with a gauze sponge. Grasp the center of the upper denture with your thumb and index finger. Gently move the denture up and down to break the seal. Pull the denture out of the mouth and place it in the emesis basin. Discard the gauze sponge in the plastic bag.

7   To remove the lower denture, cover your gloved fingers with a gauze sponge. Gently grasp it with your thumb and index finger. Turn it to the side slightly and lift it from the mouth. Place it in the emesis basin. Discard the gauze sponge in the plastic bag.

8   Line the bottom of the sink with paper towels and fill the sink half full of cool water so the dentures will not break if they drop.

9   Rinse the dentures well under cool running water to remove food particles and other debris.

10 Wet the toothbrush and apply the denture paste or powder.

(continues)

24   *continued*

11   Hold the dentures securely and brush all surfaces.

12   Rinse the dentures well under cool running water. Place them in the denture cup.

13   Return to the bedside.

14   Let the resident brush her gums and tongue, then clean and rinse her mouth with a solution of equal parts water and mouthwash before replacing dentures.

15   Hold the emesis basin under the chin and allow the resident to spit out the solution.

16   Hand the resident the denture cup and ask her to insert the dentures, if able. Some residents may ask for denture paste or powder to hold the dentures in place. Apply it according to the directions on the package.

17   If the resident is unable to insert the dentures, grasp the middle front of the upper denture firmly with your thumb and index finger. Raise the upper lip with your other hand and slide the denture into the mouth. Place both index fingers in the mouth on each side of the upper denture and press firmly to ensure that the denture is in place.

18   Grasp the middle front of the lower denture securely with your thumb and index finger. With your other hand, pull the lower lip down and slide the denture into the mouth. Place both index fingers in the mouth on each side of the denture and press firmly to ensure that it is in place.

19   Remove the towel and discard according to facility policy.

20   Rinse and dry the denture cup and return it, with your other supplies, to the top drawer of the bedside stand. If the resident does not want the dentures in the mouth, they are stored in the cup in the bedside stand. Some dentures are stored dry, but most should be kept moist. Ask the resident how the dentures should be stored. If in doubt, fill the cup with clean, cool water and place the dentures in it. Cover the cup and place it in the bedside stand.

21   Perform your procedure completion actions.

Losing teeth is depressing to some people. Many residents will try to keep others from seeing them without their dentures in place. Always respect the resident's privacy when giving denture care. Be very careful when handling dentures. Dentures are very expensive and can break easily if dropped. Follow these important considerations in caring for dentures:

- Wear gloves and apply the principles of standard precautions.

- Remove dentures carefully. Let the resident remove them, if possible. Place the dentures in an emesis basin lined with a paper towel.

- Fill the sink with water and line the bottom of the sink with a paper towel or washcloth so that the dentures do not break if they slip.

- Rinse the dentures well under cool running water to remove food particles and other debris.

- Brush dentures very well with a denture brush and the cleaning agent used by your facility. Hold them securely.

- Rinse the dentures under cool, running water.

- Check the dentures for cracks, chips, or loose teeth.

- Let the resident clean and rinse the mouth before replacing dentures.

- Store dentures in a marked denture cup according to facility policy. Some facilities store dentures dry. Others put water or denture cleaning tablets in the cup.

- Always respect the resident's privacy during this procedure.

BATHING RESIDENTS

The residents in a long-term care facility usually need help bathing. Most residents receive a full bath or shower two or three times a week. A partial bath is given at least once a day. The care plan and assignment sheet will tell you what type of bath to give the resident and when to give the bath. Bathing assignments may be flexible depending on resident requests and needs.

Types of Baths

Residents who are able will get a tub, shower, or whirlpool bath. Many long-term care facilities have a bathroom that has a whirlpool tub, which cleans as well as tub or shower bathing and is very relaxing for the resident. A special shower chair is used for residents who are getting showers. A shampoo is often given as part of the bathing procedure. Refer to the care plan if the resident is to have the hair washed while having a bath.

Follow your facility policy for transporting residents to the tub or shower room. Make sure that they are not exposed while being transported in the hallway.

Residents who are either too weak or ill to receive a tub bath or shower are given a bed bath. A nursing assistant cleans the resident's entire body, one part at a time while the resident remains in bed.

A partial bath is usually given to residents at least once a day. A partial bath includes washing the face, hands, underarms, back, and genital area. The procedures for giving a bed bath and partial bath follow later in this chapter. Most facilities also assist residents to wash their face and hands before and after meals.

Waterless Bathing

When residents are bathed in bed, a basin of water and soap were traditionally used. Over the past few years, a newer system of bathing, developed by a nurse, has become popular. This system is called **waterless bathing.** It may also be called basinless bathing or "bag bath." The waterless bathing system is prepackaged. A package of moistened washcloths is used in place of the water basin and soap. The package may be used at room temperature, or heated in the microwave or commercial warmer, according to facility policy and resident preference. Advantages of the waterless bathing system include:

- Faster and more economical for the facility; each bath takes approximately 8 to 10 minutes

- Less fatiguing for the resident
- Conserves moisture, reduces drying, and is gentler to skin than soaps
- Less friction, because the cloths are softer than regular washcloths and towels, and the need for drying is eliminated

The procedure is similar to a bed bath, with cleansing done in the same order:

- face and neck
- far arm and hand
- near arm and hand
- chest and abdomen
- far leg and foot
- near leg and foot
- back and buttocks
- perineum

Discard used cloths properly, according to facility policy. *Avoid flushing them down the toilet.* A plastic bag at the bedside works well for cloth disposal.

Perineal Care

Perineal care is also called **peri care** and refers to the thorough washing of the **genital area.** In the female, the genital area includes the urinary opening, the vaginal area, and the rectum. In the male, the penis, scrotum, and rectum are included. For the resident who is **incontinent,** peri care must be given frequently. Urine or stool on the skin causes the already frail skin of the elderly person to break down more quickly. Practice peri care keeping these considerations in mind:

- Apply the principles of standard precautions during this procedure.

✔ GUIDELINES for Bathing Residents with the Waterless Bathing System

☐ The cloths in the package are for single use only.

☐ The waterless bathing products are designed to be used for one bath. A full-size kit contains eight cloths. Smaller kits containing four cloths are also available for partial baths and perineal care. The package may be resealed if some cloths are not used. If you seal a package, date it and discard after 72 hours, immediately if the cloths are dry, or according to facility policy.

☐ The washcloths may be used at room temperature, but many facilities warm them for resident comfort. Monitor the temperature carefully to prevent overheating and hot spots that could injure the resident.

☐ Peel the label back or open the package before heating it to keep it from bursting in the microwave.

☐ Follow the manufacturer's directions for heating the package. Thirty seconds to one minute is usually sufficient to warm the contents.

- Realize that many older people are modest and may be embarrassed by having others clean the genital area.

- Protect the resident's modesty by giving privacy and exposing only the body part you are cleaning. Cover the resident with a bath blanket and be sure that the privacy curtain, window curtain, and door are closed during this procedure.

- With the female resident, keep the labia separated as much as possible during the procedure. Avoid placing your fingers on an area after washing it. You may need several washcloths to perform the procedure without contamination. (Some states and facilities require a second, clean washcloth for rinsing; the used cloth is not put back into the water basin).

- If using a mitt is difficult for you, an alternate method is to fold the washcloth in fourths. One edge will have corners that can be folded down separately. Wet the washcloth and squeeze out excess water. Place a drop of liquid soap on each corner of the edge. Fold these corners back, one at a time, to expose a clean area of the cloth with each stroke. Turn the cloth around and use the other area of the washcloth to cleanse the perineum.

- If you are applying barrier cream after perineal care, remove your gloves, wash your hands, and apply new gloves. Your gloves become contaminated during the peri care procedure, and you must use new (clean) gloves to apply barrier cream.

- Wash properly, using warm soapy water or the perineal cleansing product used by your facility. Always wash the cleanest area first. This means that you always wash from the front to the back of a female. In the male resident, begin at the end of the penis and move down toward the body, under the scrotum, then back to the rectum. Do not rub back and forth. Rinse and dry thoroughly. Some nursing facilities may use special products for peri care. Follow your facility policy.

- For the catheterized resident, wash the catheter gently to remove urine, stool, or mucus.

- Wash away from the resident's body. Begin at the urinary meatus and wash downward on the catheter for at least three inches. Do not rub back and forth.

- You will be expected to give perineal care to both male and female residents in most cases.

PERFORMANCE PROCEDURE

25   Giving a Bed Bath

Supplies needed:
- washbasin
- soap
- washcloth
- bath blanket
- two or more towels
- clean gown or clothing
- lotion
- comb or brush
- deodorant
- disposable exam gloves

1 Perform your beginning procedure actions.

2 Remove the bedspread and blanket. Fold them and place on the chair.

3 Place the bath blanket over the top sheet. Remove the sheet without exposing the resident. Place the soiled sheet in the hamper or dispose of it according to facility policy.

4 Remove the resident's gown.

5 Raise the side rail.

6 Fill the basin with warm water. Check the temperature with a thermometer. It should be 105°F. Changing the water during the procedure may be necessary. Add more hot water if it becomes too cool.

7 Return to the bedside and lower the side rail.

8 Place a towel under the resident's chin.

9 Offer the resident the washcloth to wash her own face, if possible.

10 Make a mitten by folding the washcloth around your hand.

11 Wash the resident's eyelids from the inner side of the eye to the outer side of the eye,

(continues)

25 *continued*

using plain water without soap. The eyes have a mucous membrane, so you should wear gloves during this part of the procedure.

12   Rinse the washcloth.

13   Dry the washed area.

14   Wash the remainder of the resident's face, neck, and ears. Ask the resident if she prefers to use soap. Some elderly residents do not use soap on the face.

15   Place a towel under the resident's arm farthest from you.

16   Hold the resident's arm up. Wash the whole arm from the shoulder to the wrist and fingertips.

17   Rinse and dry the arm.

18   Wash, rinse, and dry the **axilla** or armpit.

19   Repeat for the other arm.

20   If possible, place the resident's hands in water. Wash, rinse, and dry hands, fingers, and nails.

21   Place the towel across the chest. Pull the bath blanket down to the abdomen.

22   Move the towel to expose half of the chest.

23   Wash, rinse, and dry the chest. In the female resident, dry the area under the breasts well. Repeat for the other side of the chest.

24   Cover the chest with the towel.

25   Pull the bath blanket down to expose the abdomen.

26   Wash, rinse, and dry the abdomen.

27   Return the bath blanket to the resident's shoulders.

28   Remove the towel from under the blanket.

29   Uncover the leg farthest from you. Place the towel under the leg.

30   Wash, rinse, and dry the leg from the groin area to the toes.

31   Repeat for the other leg.

32   If possible, place feet in a basin one at a time.

33   Wash, rinse, and dry the feet. Make sure that you dry well between the toes.

34   Cover the legs with the bath blanket.

35   Raise the side rail.

36   Empty the basin and refill with clean water.

37   Lower the side rail.

38   Ask the resident to turn with her back toward you. Assist if necessary.

39   Wash, rinse, and dry the back.

40   Put lotion on back, massaging the entire back.

41   Use gloves to wash the genital area. Wash from the front of the genital area to the rectal area.

42   Dispose of soiled linen according to facility policy.

43   Remove gloves and dispose of them according to facility policy.

44   Put the side rail up.

45   Wash your hands.

46   Return to the bedside and put the side rail down.

47   Help the resident into a clean gown or other clothing of choice.

48   Comb the resident's hair. Help with other grooming requests.

49   Replace bed linens, if indicated, or straighten the bed.

50   Perform your procedure completion actions.

PERFORMANCE PROCEDURE

26   Giving a Partial Bath

Supplies needed:
- washbasin
- soap
- washcloth
- two towels
- clean gown or clothing
- bath blanket
- lotion
- comb or brush
- deodorant
- disposable exam gloves

1   Perform your beginning procedure actions.

2   Place a towel under the resident's chin.

3   Offer the resident the washcloth to wash her own face, if possible.

4   Make a mitten by folding the washcloth around your hand.

5   Wash the resident's eyelids from the inner side of the eye to the outer side of the eye, using plain water without soap. Wash the eye on the opposite side first, then the eye closest to you. The eyes have mucous membranes, so you should wear gloves for this part of the procedure.

6   Rinse the washcloth.

7   Dry the washed area.

8   Wash the remainder of the resident's face, neck, and ears. Ask the resident if she prefers to use soap. Some elderly residents do not use soap on the face.

9   Dry the washed area.

10   Place the towel under the hand farthest from you.

11   If possible, place the resident's hand in the basin. Wash, rinse, and dry hand.

12   Repeat for the other hand.

13   Wash, rinse, and dry axilla (armpit).

14   Repeat for the other axilla.

15   Ask the resident to turn with her back toward you. Assist if necessary.

16   Wash, rinse, and dry the back.

17   Put lotion on back, massaging the entire back lightly.

18   Use gloves when washing the genital area. Wash from the front of the genital area to the rectal area.

19   Put side rail up.

20   Remove gloves and dispose of them according to facility policy.

21   Wash your hands.

22   Return to the bedside and put side rail down.

23   Help the resident into a clean gown or other clothing of choice.

24   Comb the resident's hair. Help with other grooming requests.

25   Replace bed linens, if indicated, or straighten the bed.

26   Perform your procedure completion actions.

Perineal care is a skills testing procedure in most states. Great emphasis is placed on using proper technique, and certain errors result in automatic failure of the skills test. This is understandable, as urinary tract infection is the most common infection seen in long-term care facility residents. Infection may be difficult to treat and often leads to more serious complications. *Each state has its own sequence* *for this skill that may vary from the procedure listed here.* In some states, you will begin at the center of the labia, then move to the far side, then the near side. In many states, you must use a new section of the washcloth for each downward stroke. Your instructor will guide you in the procedure steps and sequence that is used in your state.

PERFORMANCE PROCEDURE

27   Female Perineal Care

Note: The guidelines and sequence for this procedure vary slightly from state to state. Your instructor will inform you if the sequence in your state differs from the procedure listed here. Know and follow the required sequence for your state.

Supplies needed:
- washbasin
- washcloth(s)
- clean gown or clothing
- disposable exam gloves
- soap
- two towels
- bath blanket
- bed protector

1   Perform your beginning procedure actions.

2   Remove the bedspread and blanket. Fold them and place on the chair.

3   Place the bath blanket over the top sheet. Fanfold the sheet to the foot of the bed without exposing the resident. If the sheet is soiled, dispose of it according to facility policy.

4   Ask the resident to raise her hips while you place a bed protector under her buttocks. Remove the soiled bed protector, if present. (Apply the principles of standard precautions during this activity.)

5   Raise the side rail.

6   Fill the basin with warm water.

7   Return to the bedside and lower the side rail.

8   Position the bath blanket so that only the area between the legs is exposed.

9   Ask the resident to separate and bend her knees.

10   Put on disposable gloves.

11   Wet the washcloth and make a mitten out of it.

12   Apply soap to the washcloth. Use caution. Too much soap can be irritating.

13   With one hand, separate the labia.

14   With the other hand:
  a   Wash the far side of the labia from top to bottom, using a single downward stroke (Figure 10-7).
  b   Rinse and turn the washcloth.
  c   Wash the near side of the labia from top to bottom, using a single downward stroke.
  d   Rinse and turn the washcloth.
  e   Wash the center of the labia from top to bottom, using a single downward stroke.
  f   Turn the washcloth. Rinse the area well with the washcloth.
  g   Gently pat the area dry with a towel.

15   Turn the resident away from you. Flex the upper leg slightly, if possible.

16   Wet the washcloth and make a mitt. Apply soap.

17   Expose the **anus.**

18   Wash the area, stroking from the perineum to the coccyx.

19   Rinse the area well with the washcloth.

20   Gently dry the area with a towel.

21   Return the resident to her back.

22   Remove and dispose of the bed protector according to facility policy.

23   Raise the side rail.

24   Dispose of soiled linen according to facility policy.

25   Remove gloves and dispose of them according to facility policy.

26   Wash your hands.

27   Lower the side rail. Replace the top covers and remove the bath blanket.

28   Help the resident into a clean gown or other clothing of choice.

29   Perform your procedure completion actions.

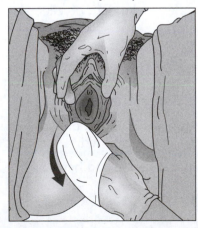

Figure 10-7 Wash the labia from top to bottom using downward strokes. Avoid rubbing back and forth.

Perineal care is a skills testing procedure in most states. Great emphasis is placed on using proper technique, and certain errors result in automatic failure of the skills test. This is understandable, as urinary tract infection is the most common infection seen in long-term care facility residents. Infection may be difficult to treat and often leads to more serious complications. *Each state has its own sequence for this skill that may vary from the procedure listed here.* In many states, you must use a new section of the washcloth for each cleansing stroke. Your instructor will guide you in the procedure steps and sequence that is used in your state.

PERFORMANCE PROCEDURE

28   Male Perineal Care

Note: The guidelines and sequence for this procedure vary slightly from state to state. Your instructor will inform you if the sequence in your state differs from the procedure listed here. Know and follow the required sequence for your state.

Supplies needed:
- washbasin
- soap
- washcloth(s)
- two towels
- clean gown or clothing
- bath blanket
- bed protector
- disposable exam gloves

1   Perform your beginning procedure actions.

2   Remove the bedspread and blanket. Fold them and place on the chair.

3   Place the bath blanket over the top sheet. Fanfold the sheet to the foot of the bed without exposing the resident. If the sheet is soiled, dispose of it according to facility policy.

4   Ask the resident to raise his hips while you place a bed protector under his buttocks. Remove the soiled bed protector, if present. Apply the principles of standard precautions during this activity.

5   Raise the side rail.

6   Fill the basin with warm water.

7   Return to the bedside and lower the side rail.

8   Position the bath blanket so that only the area between the legs is exposed.

9   Ask the resident to separate and bend his knees.

10   Put on disposable gloves.

11   Wet the washcloth and make a mitten out of it.

12   Apply soap to the washcloth. Use caution. Too much soap can be irritating.

13   With one hand, grasp the penis gently and wash. Begin washing at the urinary meatus and wash the penis in a circular motion toward the base of the penis (Figure 10-8).

14   If the resident is not circumcised, pull the foreskin back to wash it. Rinse the penis, dry, and replace the retracted foreskin.

15   Wash the scrotum, then gently lift it and wash the perineum.

16   Rinse the washcloth, make a mitten, and rinse the entire area, beginning with the penis.

17   Gently dry the area with a towel.

18   Ask the resident to turn so his back is facing you. Assist if necessary.

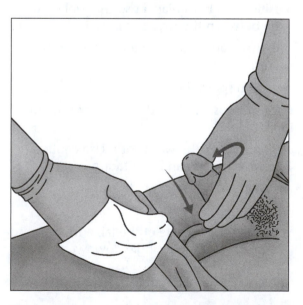

Figure 10-8 Wash from the tip of the penis down to the scrotum, then underneath the scrotum.

(continues)

28   *continued*

19 Expose the anus.

20 Wash the area, stroking from the perineum to the coccyx.

21 Rinse the area well with the washcloth.

22 Gently dry the area with a towel.

23 Return the resident to his back.

24 Remove and dispose of the bed protector according to facility policy.

25 Raise the side rail.

26 Dispose of soiled linen according to facility policy.

27 Remove gloves and dispose of them according to facility policy.

28 Wash your hands.

29 Return to the bedside and lower the side rail.

30 Replace the top covers and remove the bath blanket.

31 Help the resident into a clean gown or other clothing of choice.

32 Perform your procedure completion actions.

APPLYING LOTION TO THE RESIDENT

Another part of good skin care is massaging the skin with lotion. Always refer to the care plan. If indicated, massage the resident's skin with light, smooth strokes. Massage can stimulate circulation and is often recommended. It is soothing and refreshing to the resident. If the resident uses lotion on the legs, pat it in gently. Do not massage the legs. Massaging the legs may cause complications due to blood clots. Avoid applying lotion between the toes.

29   Giving a Backrub

Supplies needed:
- basin of water (105°F)
- soap
- washcloth
- towel
- disposable exam gloves
- lotion of resident's choice

1 Perform your beginning procedure actions.

2 Place the bottle of lotion in the basin of water to warm it.

3 Expose the resident's back and upper buttocks.

4 Wash, rinse, and dry.

5 Pour a small amount of lotion into one hand.

6 Warm the lotion by rubbing it between your hands, if necessary.

7 Apply lotion to the resident's back.

8 Rub the back with gentle but firm strokes with both hands in a circular motion from buttocks to shoulders:

  a Begin at the base of the spine and rub up the center of the back with long, soothing strokes (Figure 10-9).

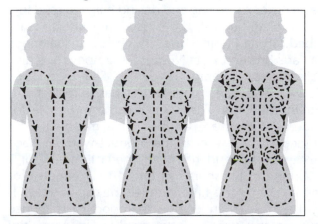

Figure 10-9 Rub the resident's back using gentle, circular motions.

(continues)

29 *continued*

b Use a circular motion with your hands as you bring them down from the shoulders back to the buttocks.

c Repeat this procedure for three to five minutes.

9 Remove excess lotion from the back.

10 Straighten and tighten the bottom sheet and draw sheet.

11 Change the resident's gown, if necessary.

12 Perform your procedure completion actions.

GROOMING THE RESIDENT

Grooming the resident includes combing hair, shaving, caring for nails, and putting glasses or hearing aids in place. Self-esteem is increased when one is well groomed. Follow these rules for grooming residents:

- Give the resident choices, if possible.
- Encourage self-care, if possible.
- Provide privacy.
- Dress and groom residents appropriately.
- Do not share grooming items with other residents.
- Clean all grooming items after using them: razor, comb, brush.
- Help the resident clean eyeglasses. Handle the glasses with care.
- Care for the resident's hearing aid, if necessary.

Shampooing the Resident's Hair

Follow your facility policy for washing the resident's hair. Some facilities require a doctor's order for this procedure. If permitted, the hair can be washed in the tub or shower. Some ladies have their hair done in the beauty shop (weekly is common). If this is the case, check with the nurse before washing the hair. Offer the resident a washcloth or towel to hold over the face when washing and rinsing hair. For residents on complete bedrest, this procedure must be done in bed. Some facilities use dry chemical shampoos that are brushed out. No-rinse shampoos are also available for bedfast residents. Shampoo caps (Figure 10-10) are a popular alternative for bathing bedfast residents. These are most comfortable for residents if they are warmed in a microwave for 30 seconds or less, or in the product warmer. Place the cap on the resident's head, then rub gently for 1 to 2 minutes for short hair and 4 to 5 minutes for long hair. After this time, remove the cap and towel-dry the hair, then comb. Shampoo caps reduce tangling and do not leave residue like some dry chemical products.

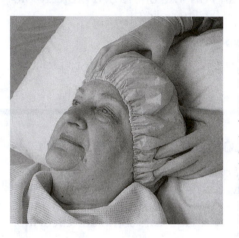

Figure 10-10 Shampoo caps simplify the hairwashing procedure for bedfast residents. The products leave the hair feeling clean and reduce tangles. (Courtesy of Medline Industries, Inc.; (800) MEDLINE)

Care of African American residents' hair. African American residents have special hair care needs. With these residents, hair texture can vary from soft and silky to coarse and thick. Residents with coarse hair need special care to prevent damage, tangling, and breaking. Asking the resident or family how to care for the hair is not offensive. In fact, it shows that you care about meeting the resident's needs. They have been caring for the hair for years, and are experts at it. They also know what products work and which do not.

In general, avoid using hair products designed for Caucasian persons. Most of these are designed to eliminate oil. Eliminating the oil from the hair is one of the worst things to do when caring for a person of color. Use a shampoo marketed specifically for African American hair. In most cases, the resident or family will provide or specify a desired product. Wash the hair once every week or two, as specified on the care plan. Washing more often than this dries the hair and causes breakage. If a special shampoo is not available, baby shampoo works best. Use a detangling conditioner according to product directions. After washing the hair, gently towel it dry. Cover the resident's shoulders with a dry towel. Use a wide-toothed comb or pick to comb through the damp hair. Be gentle and patient. It may take time to work through the tangles.

30 Combing the Resident's Hair

Supplies needed:
- towel
- comb
- hair brush

1 Perform your beginning procedure actions.

2 Cover the pillow with a towel. If the resident is sitting in a chair, place the towel over the shoulders.

3 Section the resident's hair with one hand between the scalp and the ends of the hair.

4 Brush the hair thoroughly.

5 Have the resident turn so that you can comb and brush the back of the hair.

6 If the hair is tangled, use the comb to separate it. Take a small section of hair. Beginning at the end, comb downward. Support the hair above where you are combing with the fingers of your other hand so that you do not pull on the resident's scalp. Continue working upward until you reach the scalp.

7 Ask the resident how she wants the hair styled, or arrange the hair attractively and in a style appropriate for the resident's age. If the resident has long hair, consider braiding it or putting it up. Coarse, tightly curled hair may require special treatment.

8 Perform your procedure completion actions.

Persons of color need additional oil on the hair at all times. Some residents use products they refer to as hair "grease." If the resident does not have a product preference, apply baby oil *to the scalp, not the hair*. Then, using a soft brush, brush from the scalp to the ends of the hair until all the hairs are covered with oil. You may need to apply this heavily. If it is too oily, wipe the excess with a towel. If you use enough, the hair will appear shiny.

The resident's hair can be braided while damp. Run the wide-toothed comb through the hair to remove tangles, following the guidelines in Procedure 30. Gently twist the hair and apply a hair tie. Avoid using rubber bands, if possible. These cause breakage and damage hair. If a rubber band must be used, apply hair grease or baby oil liberally to your fingers. Roll the rubber band around in the hair grease until it is well coated, then apply it to the hair. Style the hair in a pony tail, then section and braid it. When you get to the end, apply more grease. Wrap the ends around a barrette and snap it shut, or use a hair tie or grease-coated rubber band.

Shaving the Male Resident

Men should be shaved every day as part of the morning care procedure. Honor the resident's preference to grow a mustache or beard. Because the probability of contacting blood during this procedure is fairly high, you should wear gloves.

31 Shaving the Resident

Supplies needed:
- washcloth
- towel
- electric or safety razor
- shaving cream or preshave lotion
- basin of water (105°F)
- mirror
- aftershave lotion
- disposable exam gloves

1 Perform your beginning procedure actions.

2 Cover the resident's chest with the towel.

3 Soften the resident's beard by placing a warm washcloth over it for 2 to 3 minutes. Moisten the face with water and apply shaving cream.

4 Put on disposable gloves.

(continues)

31 *continued*

5 Beginning in front of the ear, hold the skin taut.

6 Bring the razor down from the cheek to the chin in one-half- to one-inch increments. Continue until the entire cheek has been shaved. Rinse the razor between strokes.

7 Repeat with the other cheek.

8 Ask the resident to tighten his upper lip. Shave from the nose to the upper lip in short, downward strokes.

9 Ask the resident to tighten his chin. Shave the chin in downward strokes in one-half- to one-inch increments.

10 Ask the resident to tip his head back.

11 Apply shaving cream to the neck area.

12 Hold the skin taut. Shave the neck area in smooth, upward strokes in one-half- to one-inch increments.

13 Wash the resident's face and neck. Dry the area well.

14 Apply aftershave lotion if resident prefers.

15 Perform your procedure completion actions.

✓ GUIDELINES for Applying Support Hosiery

☐ Follow the care plan regarding when the stockings are to be put on and for how long the resident is to wear the hosiery.

☐ Put stockings on the resident before she gets out of bed in the morning. Elevate the legs before applying the hosiery.

☐ Anti-embolism stockings come in several sizes. The resident is measured with a tape measure to find the correct size. The hose must fit well to be effective.

☐ The stockings must be applied smoothly, with no wrinkles.

☐ Follow your facility policy for washing anti-embolism stockings. These must be hand-washed and drip-dried. The hose are damaged by the commercial washers and dryers used in the health care facility.

☐ To preserve the life of the stockings, avoid contact with lotions, ointments, or oils containing lanolin or petroleum products. These products deteriorate the elastic.

☐ Do not apply the hosiery over open areas, fractures, or deformities. If the resident has an open or abnormal skin area, fracture, or deformity on the legs or feet, inform the nurse.

☐ Check the stockings periodically to be sure the tops have not rolled or turned down. Keep the fabric straight.

☐ Most elastic stockings have a hole in the toe end to allow access for circulation checks. In some stockings, the hole is on the top of the foot, and on others it is on the bottom. As long as the heel is centered, the hole will be in the correct place.

☐ Monitor circulation in the resident's toes every 4 hours, or as specified on the care plan. Note color, sensation, swelling, temperature, and ability to move. Report abnormalities to the nurse.

☐ The care plan will specify the wearing schedule for the stockings, according to physician orders and facility policies. For most residents, the hosiery is applied during the day and removed at bedtime.

PROSTHESIS CARE

A *prosthesis* is an artificial body part. Prosthetic devices, such as artificial legs, arms, or breasts, can make life much more enjoyable for the person who uses the device. You will find some residents in the long-term care facility who wear a prosthesis.

Understand these considerations when caring for a resident who uses a prosthesis:

• Refer to the care plan for special instructions.

• Remember that this is part of the resident's body and should be respected and cared for as such.

Be aware of confidentiality issues. The resident may not want others to know of the prosthesis.

- Keep the prosthesis clean.
- Be alert to pressure areas under the prosthesis. Check for redness, irritation, and blisters. Listen carefully to resident complaints of discomfort.
- Keep the skin under the prosthesis clean and dry.
- Dress the resident wearing the prosthesis properly. A stockinette may be worn under artificial limbs.
- Report to the nurse if you feel that the prosthesis needs repair.
- An artificial eye is usually cared for by the nurse. If you are instructed to care for a resident with an artificial eye, handle the eye carefully. The eye socket and the artificial eye must be cleaned as indicated on the care plan. Apply the principles of standard precautions during this procedure.
- Maintain a professional attitude when caring for a resident who uses a prosthesis.

FOOT CARE

Special care is sometimes part of caring for the resident's feet. Because poor blood circulation to the feet is common, the skin on the resident's feet heals slowly if injured. Injury prevention is often the best treatment in caring for the feet. Know and follow your facility policy for foot and toenail care. Many facilities do not allow the nursing assistant to trim toenails. In these facilities, the nursing assistant is responsible for keeping the feet clean and dry. Report to your supervisor if the nails need to be cut or if other abnormalities are noted. Note these considerations in giving foot care:

- Follow the care plan.
- Soak the feet often.
- Dry the feet well, especially between the toes.
- Apply lotion to clean feet, but do not put lotion between the toes.
- Follow your facility policy for clipping toenails.

PERFORMANCE PROCEDURE

32   Hand and Fingernail Care

Supplies needed:
- soap
- towel
- bed protector
- basin of water (105°F)
- lotion
- nail clippers
- orange stick
- nail file or emery board
- disposable exam gloves if contact with non-intact skin is likely

1 Perform your beginning procedure actions.

2 Adjust the height of the overbed table and place it in front of the resident. Cover the overbed table with the bed protector.

3 Place the basin of water on the table.

4 Instruct the resident to place hands in the water (Figure 10-11A).

5 Soak the hands for approximately 10 minutes. Cover the resident's hands and the basin with a towel to keep the water warm. Add more warm water if necessary.

6 Wash the resident's hands. Push the cuticles back gently with the washcloth or an orange stick.

7 Lift the resident's hands out of the water and dry them with the towel.

8 Clip the nails if permitted by facility policy (Figure 10-11B):
- Cut the nails straight across.
- Do not trim the nails below the fingertips.

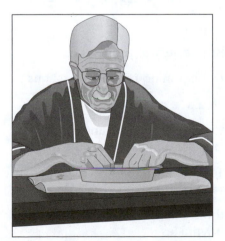

Figure 10-11A Soak the resident's hands in warm water.

(continues)

32   *continued*

- Keep the nail clippings on the bed protector to be discarded later.

9 Shape the nails with the nail file or emery board (Figure 10-11C). Apply fingernail polish if requested by a female resident.

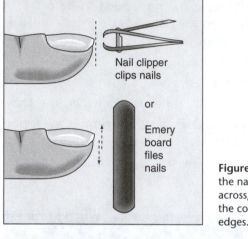

Figure 10-11B Clip the nails straight across, then smooth the corners and edges.

10 Pour a small amount of lotion into your hands and rub it into the resident's hands.

11 Perform your procedure completion actions.

12 Disinfect the clippers according to facility policy after each use.

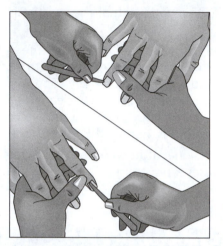

Figure 10-11C Gently clean under the nails.

APPLYING SUPPORT HOSIERY

Support hosiery are for the resident who has circulation problems. The hose provide some pressure on the legs, which helps increase the blood flow. These stockings are made of stretchable elastic and fit very closely. Support stockings may be knee length or cover the entire leg. These types of hosiery are called **anti-embolism stockings,** and are often referred to by the brand name, such as TED® Hose.

PERFORMANCE PROCEDURE

33   Applying Support Hosiery

Supplies needed:
- anti-embolism hosiery of proper size

1 Perform your beginning procedure actions.

2 Expose one leg at a time.

3 Grasp the stocking with both hands at the top opening and roll or gather toward the toe end.

4 Apply the stocking to the leg by rolling or pulling upward over the leg.

5 Make sure the stocking is on evenly. Be sure there are no wrinkles.

6 Expose the other leg.

7 Grasp the stocking with both hands at the top opening and roll or gather toward the toe end.

8 Apply the stocking to the leg by rolling or pulling upward over the leg.

9 Make sure the stocking is on evenly. Be sure there are no wrinkles.

10 Perform your procedure completion actions.

MAKING THE OCCUPIED BED

There may be times when you must change the sheets or make the entire bed while the resident is in it. This is done for residents restricted to bedrest; that is, those who are too weak or ill to get out of bed. Other times you will change only some linens while the resident remains in bed. Follow your facility infection control policies and procedures for placement of clean and dirty linen. Apply the principles of standard precautions during this procedure.

PERFORMANCE PROCEDURE

34　　Making the Occupied Bed

Note: The guidelines for this procedure vary slightly from state to state. Your instructor will inform you if the procedure in your state differs from the one listed here. Know and follow the required procedure for your state.

Supplies needed:
* two large sheets
* linen draw sheet, if used
* plastic or rubber draw sheet, if used
* bed protector, if used
* pillowcase
* bath blanket
* laundry bag or hamper
* clean bedspread and blanket, if needed
* disposable exam gloves

1 Perform your beginning procedure actions.

2 Remove the bedspread and blanket. Fold them and place on the chair.

3 Place the bath blanket over the top sheet. Remove the sheet without exposing the resident. Place the soiled sheet in the hamper, or dispose of it according to facility policy.

4 Help the resident to turn on the side away from you.

5 Loosen bottom linens.

6 Roll the soiled draw sheet and rubber sheet, and tuck along the resident's back.

Note: It is not necessary to wear gloves when handling dry, used linen. Wear gloves if the linen is known or suspected to be contaminated with blood or body fluids, secretions, or excretions. Remove gloves and wash hands (or use an alcohol-based hand cleaner) after handling soiled linen, before handling clean linen. If you are working alone, remove gloves and wash hands after applying the clean bottom sheet. Avoid contaminating environmental surfaces in the room with used gloves.

7 Place the clean sheet on the bed with the center fold at the center of the bed.

8 Unfold one-half of the sheet.

9 Place the bottom hem of the sheet even with the edge of the mattress, or fit the corner of the fitted sheet.

10 Tuck the top of the sheet under half of the head end of the mattress.

11 Miter the corner.

12 Tuck the sheet under the side of the entire mattress, working from the head to the foot of the bed.

13 Roll the remaining half sheet and tuck it under the soiled sheet.

14 Place the rubber draw sheet in the middle of the bed. Tuck in at the side.

15 Place a clean linen draw sheet over the rubber draw sheet. Tuck in at the side. If a bed protector is used, place it on top of the draw sheet and roll it inside the draw sheet.

16 Roll the remaining halves of draw sheets and tuck them along the resident's back under the soiled sheets.

17 Help the resident roll over the linen pile on the side facing you.

18 Raise the side rail.

19 Go to the other side of the bed.

20 Lower the side rail.

21 Loosen and remove soiled linens from under the mattress.

22 Raise the side rail if leaving the bedside.

(continues)

34 *continued*

23   Dispose of soiled linens according to facility policy. *Do not put soiled linen on the floor. Hold soiled linen away from your uniform.*

24   Remove gloves and dispose according to facility policy.

25   Wash your hands.

26   Return to the bedside and lower the side rail.

27   Pull the clean bottom sheet over the mattress.

28   Tuck the bottom sheet tightly under the head of the mattress.

29   Miter the corner of the sheet at the head of the bed, or fit the corner of the fitted sheet.

30   Pull the bottom sheet tight and tuck under the side of the mattress, working from head to foot.

31   Pull the rubber sheet tight and tuck over the bottom sheet at the side of the mattress.

32   Pull the draw sheet tight and tuck over the rubber sheet at the side of the mattress. If a bed protector is used, smooth and straighten it.

33   Help the resident to roll on her back. Cover the resident with the bath blanket.

34   Place the clean sheet over the bath blanket, centering the center fold of the sheet.

35   Pull the bath blanket from under the clean sheet.

36   Place the blanket and bedspread over the sheet.

37   Fold the top sheet over the edge of the blanket. Spread to make a cuff with the sheet.

38   Tuck the top linens under the foot of the mattress, allowing room for the resident's toes. Follow the care plan instructions for special devices, such as bed cradles and footboards.

39   Miter the corner of top linens at the foot of the bed.

40   Raise the side rail.

41   Go to the other side of the bed.

42   Lower the side rail.

43   Miter the corner of the top linens at the foot of the bed.

44   Remove the pillow and soiled pillowcase.

45   Place a clean pillowcase on the pillow.

46   Perform your procedure completion actions.

KEY POINTS IN THIS CHAPTER

▲ The skin of the elderly is fragile. It tears and breaks readily, and is much more easily damaged compared with younger adults.

▲ The skin in the elderly produces less oil, which causes dryness and flaking.

▲ Pressure ulcers are breaks in the skin caused by unrelieved pressure.

▲ Changing the resident's position is often the best prevention for pressure ulcers.

▲ Encourage residents to do as much of their personal care as possible.

▲ Allow the resident choices over routines and procedures.

▲ An important responsibility of the nursing assistant is observing and reporting any redness or other signs of skin irritation.

▲ The resident's self-esteem can be increased by appropriate clothing and attractive grooming.

▲ Anti-embolism stockings, which must be applied when the resident is lying down, must fit very well and smoothly to be effective.

REVIEW QUIZ

1. Which organ of the body provides it with a protective covering?
   a. skin
   b. hair
   c. nails
   d. heart

2. Age-related changes in the skin include:
   a. oily skin.
   b. brittle nails.
   c. fatty tissue increases.
   d. skin becomes more elastic.

3. All of the following are goals of skin care *except:*
   a. removal of bacteria on the skin.
   b. removal of perspiration and other body discharges.
   c. improving sensitivity to heat and cold.
   d. stimulating blood circulation.

4. Another term for pressure ulcers is:
   a. mucous membranes.
   b. decubiti.
   c. cyanosis.
   d. edema.

5. Which of the following help prevent pressure ulcers?
   a. changing the resident's position every shift
   b. giving adequate amounts of food and fluids
   c. using alcohol to toughen the resident's skin
   d. keeping the resident up in a chair all day

6. A sign of a pressure ulcer developing is:
   a. an area of redness on the skin.
   b. foul-smelling breath.
   c. change in bowel habits.
   d. pain in the chest.

7. What is included in oral hygiene?
   a. a complete bed bath and linen change
   b. cleaning of the mouth, teeth, and gums
   c. helping the resident ambulate
   d. cleansing the perineal area

8. Which of the following is true about dentures?
   a. Dentures should be cleaned while in the resident's mouth.
   b. Dentures should be removed when eating.
   c. Dentures are expensive and can break if dropped.
   d. Only the nurse should handle the resident's dentures.

9. You are assigned to care for Mrs. White. She cannot walk, spends most of her day in the wheelchair, and is able to use her hands and arms well. What is the best way for you to help her brush her teeth?

   a. Brush her teeth for her while she is in bed.
   b. Brush her teeth for her when she is up in the wheelchair.
   c. Get the nurse to help her brush her teeth.
   d. Help her brush her own teeth by taking her in the bathroom and getting the supplies she needs.

10. Which of the following should be done when giving a partial bath to Mrs. White?
    a. Take her to the shower room to give the partial bath.
    b. Let her do as much of the bath as possible.
    c. Wash Mrs. White's hands and feet as part of the procedure.
    d. Avoid giving pericare, as this is not part of the procedure.

11. What is perineal care?
    a. cleaning the genital area
    b. washing the resident's hair
    c. cleaning the tub and bathroom
    d. cleaning the fingernails and toenails

12. Anti-embolism stockings should be put on the resident:
    a. after the resident has been walking about.
    b. so the stockings fit loosely.
    c. when the resident is lying down.
    d. only at night when the feet are elevated.

13. When is an occupied bed made?
    a. whenever the resident is in the room
    b. when the resident is on bedrest
    c. when all the linens are changed
    d. when the resident has a complete bath

14. A prosthesis is:
    a. a part of your body.
    b. the medical term for a disease.
    c. an artificial body part.
    d. a self-help device.

15. When giving perineal care to a female resident, you should:
    a. wash from back to front.
    b. wash from front to back.
    c. wash back and forth vigorously.
    d. use plenty of soap.

16. When giving perineal care to a male, you should:
    a. wash the scrotum and anus only.
    b. wash from the anus toward the penis.
    c. wash from the penis to the anus.
    d. wash the scrotum and penis only.

17. You are assigned to care for Mr. Caldwell, a 71-year-old alert resident with Parkinson's disease.

Mr. Caldwell's hands shake because of his illness. He is able to wash his face and upper body. You finish the rest of his bath. It is time to shave the resident. He uses a safety razor and shaving cream. When Mr. Caldwell begins to shave his cheek, his hand is shaking badly. He seems embarrassed. You should:

a. leave the room so that the resident is not embarrassed.

b. ask Mr. Caldwell if he would like you to shave him.

c. tell Mr. Caldwell not to shave until he buys an electric razor.

d. tell the resident that he must grow a beard.

18. Mrs. Beverlin is a 57-year-old comatose resident. She is fed by tube because she cannot eat. You are assigned to do special oral hygiene for this resident. You should do all of the following *except:*

a. turn the resident's head to the side when doing mouth care.

b. explain what you are going to do even though you are not sure if the resident can hear you.

c. use a toothbrush and toothpaste, scrubbing well.

d. observe the resident's mouth for signs of irritation.

19. Mrs. Sinski is an 84-year-old resident being treated for pressure ulcers on her hips. The nurse tells you in report that Mrs. Sinski is at high risk for further skin breakdown, so you must give her good skin care. You should:

a. turn Mrs. Sinski at least every 2 hours.

b. bathe Mrs. Sinski with a large amount of soap to be sure she is clean.

c. massage her arms and legs well.

d. use plenty of powder in the skin folds and creases.

20. Mrs. Hyde is a 71-year-old alert resident who is on complete bedrest. You are assigned to give her a bed bath and oral hygiene. Mrs. Hyde wears dentures. She insists on removing them from her mouth herself. When she hands them to you, her hand bumps the overbed table and the dentures fall to the floor, breaking in half. Mrs. Hyde begins yelling that you are careless and that you broke her dentures. You should:

a. hide the dentures and tell everyone that the resident is confused.

b. explain what happened to your supervisor.

c. glue the dentures together.

d. tell the resident it was her fault.

CHAPTER 10
CROSSWORD PUZZLE

Directions: Complete the puzzle using these words found in Chapter 10.

abrasion
anus
axilla
decubitus

dentures
embolism
genital
incontinent

perineal
pressure
prosthesis
ulcer

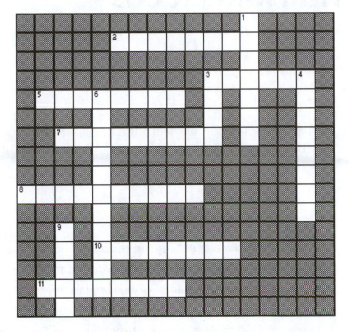

CHAPTER 10
PUZZLE CLUES

ACROSS

2. Bedsores are the direct result of _____.
3. The armpit
5. Cleansing the genital area is called _____ care.
7. A pressure sore or pressure ulcer may also be called a _____ ulcer.
8. An artificial body part is a _____.
10. Elastic stockings that improve circulation are called anti-_____ stockings.
11. Artificial teeth

DOWN

1. The area that includes the external sex organs and anus
3. The outlet for the rectum
4. A rubbing away or scraping of the skin
6. Unable to control the discharge of urine or stool
9. Pressure sore or pressure _____

Nutrition and Fluid Needs

OBJECTIVES

In this chapter, you will learn the importance of your role in helping residents with good nutrition and hydration. After reading this chapter, you will be able to:

- Spell and define key terms.
- Describe proper nutrition.
- Identify factors affecting the resident's nutrition.
- Describe special diets and alternative nutrition.
- Describe the importance of fluid balance.
- Demonstrate how to help with meals and feed a resident.
- Identify alternative means of meeting residents' nutritional needs.
- Record intake and output.

KEY TERMS

aspiration: breathing liquid or food into the air passages

constipation: difficult or infrequent bowel movements

cubic centimeter (cc): a metric unit of measurement; 30 cc equals one ounce

dehydration: a serious condition that develops as a result of inadequate water in the body

digestion: the process by which food is broken down in the body and changed into usable forms

emesis: vomiting or what is vomited

enteral feeding: feeding liquid nutrients through a tube; this procedure is done by the nurse

essential nutrients: substances in food that are necessary for good nutrition

food guide pyramid: a guide to proper nutrition that helps you select the foods you need in order to eat a well-balanced diet

force fluids: an order to encourage the resident to drink as much fluid as possible

gastrostomy (G) tube: a feeding tube that is surgically placed in the stomach to feed the resident a liquid formula diet

graduate: a pitcher used to measure liquids

infusion site: the location at which an intravenous needle or cannula is inserted

intake and output (I & O): recording of the amount of fluid taken in and fluid eliminated by a person

intravenous feeding: a liquid feeding given directly into a vein

lethargic: abnormally sleepy or drowsy

milliliter (mL): a metric unit of measurement; 30 mL equals one ounce

nasogastric (NG) tube: a method of feeding liquid nutrition to a resident in which a tube is passed through the nose into the stomach

nutrients: chemical substances necessary for life found in food

ounce: a unit of measurement equal to 30 cc or 30 mL

restrict fluids: an order to restrict the resident's fluid intake to a specific amount each shift because of a medical condition

therapeutic diet: a special or modified diet designed to meet the resident's medical needs

PROPER NUTRITION

Proper nutrition is important for everyone. An adequate intake of proper foods and fluids is necessary to live and grow. The **nutrients** in foods provide the elements we need for growth, energy, and repair of tissues. Nutrients essential for good nutrition include:

- proteins
- carbohydrates
- fats
- water
- vitamins
- minerals

Proper nutrition is when you take in an adequate amount of these nutrients. The **food guide pyramid** serves as a guide to proper nutrition (Figure 11-1).

The Food Guide Pyramid

A balanced diet contains the **essential nutrients.** Eating the right number of servings from each food group is a balanced diet. The following sections contain a listing of the food groups, number of servings per day, and why these nutrients are necessary. The amount of each serving is listed. People with lower calorie needs should select the lower number of servings from each group. People with higher calorie needs should select the higher number of servings. The food guide pyramid that was published in 2005 was designed to be individualized. It contains 12 intake levels, ranging from 1,000 calories per day to 3,200 calories per day. The pyramid should be individualized by each person to maintain a healthy weight. This can be easily done by visiting http://www.mypyramid.gov. The following examples are based on the average, 2,000-calorie-per-day diet.

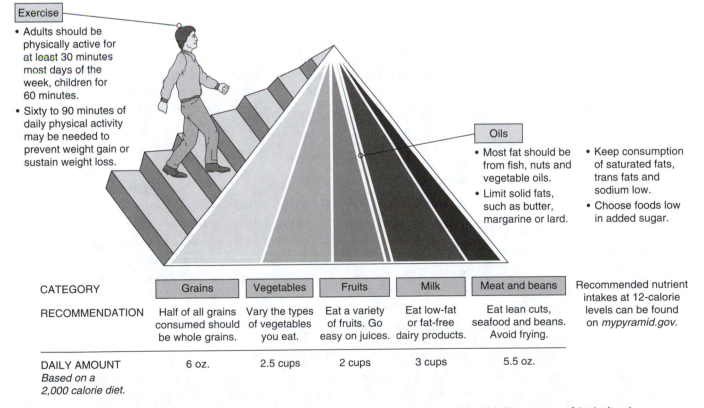

CATEGORY	Grains	Vegetables	Fruits	Milk	Meat and beans	Recommended nutrient intakes at 12-calorie levels can be found on *mypyramid.gov.*
RECOMMENDATION	Half of all grains consumed should be whole grains.	Vary the types of vegetables you eat.	Eat a variety of fruits. Go easy on juices.	Eat low-fat or fat-free dairy products.	Eat lean cuts, seafood and beans. Avoid frying.	
DAILY AMOUNT *Based on a 2,000 calorie diet.*	6 oz.	2.5 cups	2 cups	3 cups	5.5 oz.	

Exercise
- Adults should be physically active for at least 30 minutes most days of the week, children for 60 minutes.
- Sixty to 90 minutes of daily physical activity may be needed to prevent weight gain or sustain weight loss.

Oils
- Most fat should be from fish, nuts and vegetable oils.
- Limit solid fats, such as butter, margarine or lard.
- Keep consumption of saturated fats, trans fats and sodium low.
- Choose foods low in added sugar.

Figure 11-1 The USDA food guide pyramid serves as a guide for menu planning. (Courtesy of the U.S. Department of Agriculture)

- Grains group
  — Eat at least 6 ounces per day.
  — At least half the grains you eat each day should be whole grains (3 ounces per day; look for the name "whole" on the ingredients list). Whole grains contain the entire grain kernel.

- Vegetables group
  — Eat at least 2½ cups each day.
  — Vary your vegetables. Eat more dark green and orange vegetables. Eat dry beans and peas.
  — Vegetable juice is also a member of this group.
  — Vegetables may be raw, cooked, canned, frozen, dried, dehydrated, whole, cut up, or mashed.

- Fruits group
  — Eat at least 2 cups each day.
  — Eat a variety of fruits.
  — Choose fresh, frozen, canned, or dry fruit.
  — Go easy on fruit juices.

- Oils group
  — *Oils* are fats that are liquid at room temperature; they come from many different plants and fish. Some are used mainly as flavorings, such as walnut oil and sesame oil. Foods such as nuts, olives, and avocados are naturally high in oil.
  — Free oils, such as mayonnaise, butter, margarine, lard, and shortening, should be used sparingly.
  — Make the most of the fat sources in fish, nuts, and vegetable oils.
  — If solid fat is used in cooking (such as frying chicken), the extra oil consumed is part of the discretionary calorie allowance.

- Milk group
  — Consume 3 cups each day.
  — Use low-fat or fat-free products whenever possible.
  — Cheese, yogurt, and milk-based desserts are included in this group.
  — If you cannot consume milk because of lactose intolerance, choose lactose-free products and other sources that are rich in calcium.
  — Foods such as cream, butter, and cream cheese are low in calcium and are not considered part of this group.

- Meat and beans group
  — Eat 5½ ounces per day.
  — This group includes meat, fish, poultry, and eggs.
  — Dry beans and peas are part of this group as well as the vegetable group.
  — Choose lean and low-fat meats and poultry.
  — Meat may be baked, grilled, or broiled.
  — Vary your choices with more fish, beans, peas, nuts, and seeds.
  — Fish, nuts, and seeds contain healthy oils, so select these instead of meat and poultry when possible.
  — If high-fat meats are used, the extra oil consumed is part of the discretionary calorie allowance.

Discretionary calories. Each person needs a certain number of calories each day for proper body function and to provide energy for physical activities. The essential calories are the minimum calories required to meet your nutrient needs. By selecting food items that have low fat and low or no sugar content, you may be able to take in more calories than the amount required to meet your nutrient needs. These *discretionary calories* are extra calories that can be "spent" on solid fats, added sugars, alcohol, or extra food from any food group. For most people, the discretionary calorie allowance is very small (between 100 and 300 calories daily). Many people regularly use their discretionary calories by making unwise food choices, such as high-fat meats, cheeses, whole milk, or sweetened bakery products. You can use your discretionary calories to:

- Eat more foods from any food group than the food guide recommends.
- Eat higher-calorie forms of foods, such as those containing solid fats or added sugars, like whole milk, cheese, sausage, biscuits, sweetened cereal, and sweetened yogurt.
- Add fats or sweeteners to foods, such as sauces, salad dressings, sugar, syrup, and butter.
- Eat or drink items that are mostly fats, caloric sweeteners, and/or alcohol, such as candy, soda, wine, and beer.

Water

Water is an essential nutrient that is necessary to life. A person can live only a few days without water. Water is necessary for all cellular functions in the body. An adequate intake of fluids is required to replace fluids lost through urine, stool, sweat, and evaporation through skin. The normal adult intake of fluids should be two to three quarts a day.

Offering liquids to residents frequently is extremely important for the following reasons:

- Many residents are not able to drink liquids without your help.
- The sense of thirst is less in the elderly.
- An adequate fluid intake is necessary to prevent urinary problems and constipation.

Vitamins and Minerals

A person must have enough vitamins and minerals to stay healthy. Therefore, a regular diet should provide the necessary vitamins and minerals for a healthy adult. A balanced diet contains all of the vitamins and minerals needed to stay healthy. Some elderly and ill people also take vitamin pills to give them extra nutrients. Signs of good nutrition include:

- shiny hair
- bright, clear eyes
- alert mind
- healthy sleep patterns
- good appetite
- normal elimination
- healthy skin, nails, and teeth

FACTORS THAT AFFECT RESIDENT NUTRITION

Nutritional needs of the older person are the same as for younger adults. However, meeting these needs can be more difficult for the elderly person. Often the resident in the long-term care facility depends on your help to receive proper nutrition. Know these considerations for nutritional care:

- General factors
  - fatigue level
  - level of alertness
  - absence or presence of disease
  - medical conditions affecting the appetite
  - some medications affect the appetite
- Sensory loss
  - Sensory loss can mean decreased taste, smell, and vision. Meals may have to be enhanced with proper seasonings, unless this is against the diet ordered by the resident's physician.
  - Sight, smell, taste, and even the sound of food preparation affect appetite.
- Physical comfort
  - Assure the resident's comfort.
  - Position the resident properly to prevent **aspiration,** or choking, on food.
  - Position residents so they can reach their food.
- Dentures
  - Dentures that do not fit properly impair the resident's ability to enjoy mealtime.
  - Be sure the resident has dentures properly in place at mealtime.
- Ability to chew and swallow
  - Residents who cannot chew or swallow require special diets or procedures such as pureed foods or tube feeding.
  - Residents who cannot swallow easily have a hard time eating.
- Cultural influences. Culture may affect the resident's nutrition. The following are some common cultural influences that affect residents' food choices:
  - religion
  - national culture
  - family customs
  - economic background
  - personal tastes
- Emotional factors. These common emotional states can affect the resident's eating habits:
  - loneliness
  - depression
  - anger, frustration
  - eating disorders
- Environmental factors. The environment in which food is served can affect nutrition:
  - Mealtime is a source of social contact.
  - All staff members can make mealtime pleasant.
  - Pleasant table companions and conversation at mealtime are important.
  - Too much noise in the dining room can be a problem. Avoid shouting and clanging dishes.
  - Eliminate unpleasant odors, sights, and smells; these can cause the resident to lose his appetite quickly.
  - The food served should be attractive and appetizing in appearance.

— The food served should be the correct temperature. Hot foods should be served hot and cold foods served cold.

SPECIAL DIETS

Most residents will be on a general or regular diet. The dietitian in the long-term care facility plans meals for the residents. The dietitian makes menu changes for residents on special diets. Knowledge of various special and **therapeutic diets** will help you understand their effect on the disease process and know if the resident is allowed to have certain food items.

Common Therapeutic Diets

Clear liquids.   The clear liquid diet is used for persons who have stomach or intestinal distress or as first foods after surgery.

- Clear liquids include tea, broth, gelatin, some fruit juices, and some soft drinks (Figure 11–2).
- This diet is not generally used for residents who have swallowing problems.
- This diet is usually only served for short periods because it does not contain adequate nutrients.

Full liquid.   The full liquid diet is given to residents who have digestive disorders.

- Full liquid is clear liquid plus milk, custards and puddings, cream soups, ice cream and sherbet.
- This diet is usually only served for short periods because it does not contain adequate nutrients.

Mechanical soft.   This diet is used for residents who cannot chew well or those who have missing teeth.

- The diet is used for residents who have difficulty chewing or swallowing solid foods.
- The diet is the same as a regular diet, but the food has been ground in a blender or chopped finely. The food is not reduced to liquid in this diet. Items that are hard to chew, such as meats, are ground and finely chopped until they are about the consistency of hamburger. Some soft foods, such as bread and canned fruit, are not blended.

Diabetic, no concentrated sweets, or calorie-controlled diet.   These diets are ordered for residents who have diabetes or who must lose weight.

- No sugar is included on the tray.
- No foods with high sugar content:
  — honey
  — syrup
  — regular soft drinks
  — jelly, jams
  — candy
- Residents may have sugar-free substitutes, if indicated on the diet plan.
- Snacks are very important for some residents on this diet. If snacks are ordered, they are part of the calorie count upon which the resident's medication is based.

Low-sodium (low-salt) diet.   A low-sodium diet is ordered for persons with high blood pressure, heart, or kidney disease.

- No salt is included on the tray.
- Foods that are high in salt are limited (Figure 11-3):
  — bacon
  — ham

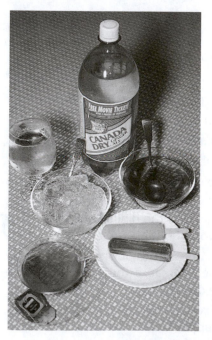

Figure 11-2 Items found on a tray for a clear liquid diet.

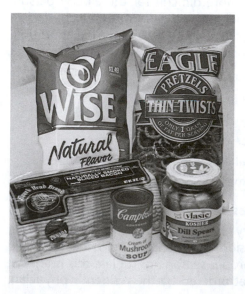

Figure 11-3 Foods that are high in sodium

— luncheon meats

— canned meats and fish

— some cheeses and soups

— some soft drinks

— many common snack food items

— pickles and olives

Pureed diets.   Pureed diets have been mechanically altered so they are the consistency of baby food. These diets contain the same foods as the diets listed, but they have been blended so they are easy to swallow. They are given to people who have problems chewing and swallowing regular foods. If a pureed food is the correct consistency, a plastic spoon will stand up in it. If the food will not support the spoon, it may be too watery to feed the resident.

FLUID BALANCE

Proper fluid balance occurs when the loss of body fluids is about the same as fluid taken in. The nursing assistant has an important role in helping the resident maintain proper fluid balance.

Reasons for Proper Fluid Balance

Water makes up more than one-half of body weight. Maintaining the proper fluid balance is important because it:

* helps proper blood flow
* helps food **digestion**
* improves removal of body waste
* protects cells by keeping:
  — skin moist
  — mouth and throat moist
  — eyeballs moist
* regulates body temperature

Dehydration

Dehydration occurs when there is not enough fluid in the body. This condition may cause serious harm to vital body organs. Death occurs when loss of body fluid is severe.

Signs of dehydration.   Be aware of these signs of dehydration:

* Mouth becomes dry. The resident may have trouble swallowing.
* Tongue becomes thick and coated.
* Skin becomes dry, itches, or cracks. It may tear easily and show evidence of "tenting" when it is pinched lightly. If the tent does not go away immediately, this should be reported to the nurse.

* Urine output decreases.
* Urine is darker and cloudy, and may have a strong odor.
* The resident may be tired or **lethargic.**
* Confusion and mental impairment may develop.
* The resident may show signs of **constipation.**

Edema

Edema may occur as the result of poor circulation, heart, or kidney disease. *Edema* is swelling or the retention of fluid in the tissues. The nursing assistant must be alert for signs of edema in the resident. Indications of edema are:

* swelling or puffiness, usually in feet, ankles, hands, eyes, face, and abdomen
* difficulty breathing, such as:
  — congestion or cough
  — wheezing when breathing
* quick weight gain
* decrease in urine output

Providing Adequate Hydration

Assist residents to take enough fluids in the following ways:

* Refer to the care plan. Know which fluids are restricted or encouraged. Some may be given between meals.
* Offer fluids every time you are in the room. Give the resident fluids that he likes, if allowed on his diet.
* Fluids are especially important in hot weather or when the resident has a fever.
* Help the resident drink properly. Hold the glass and straw if necessary.
* Encourage the resident to help himself. Use hand-over-hand technique or adaptive cups.
* Be sure that the resident always has fresh drinking water available in the room.
* Record all fluid intake and output accurately when ordered.
* Serve water with meals. Offer refills of coffee, tea, and other beverages at mealtime.

Special Situations

Sometimes the physician writes special fluid orders because of the resident's disease or condition. Special fluid orders are noted on the care plan. **Force fluids** is ordered for residents who do not take in an adequate amount of fluid each day. The term "force fluids" is deceiving. You do not really force the resident to drink. Rather, you must encourage the resident to drink as much as possible. Sometimes it helps if you offer the resident a variety of beverages. If you offer fluids frequently in small cups, the resident may drink more than if you give him a large glass and instruct him to drink it all. Getting to know the resident's patterns, likes, and dislikes is important. Give him fluids that he likes in quantities that he will drink. It may be necessary for you to stay in the room while the resident drinks the liquids. Residents who have orders to force fluids are often on intake and output. This means their fluid intake is measured to be certain that they drink enough.

An order to **restrict fluids** is sometimes written for residents with heart or kidney disease. Orders to restrict fluids are highly individualized. Instructions for the amount of fluids that the resident is allowed are written on the care plan. Often this amount is restricted to what is on the meal trays, with some additional liquids for the nurses to give with medications. Residents who have orders to restrict fluids are usually on intake and output so that their fluid intake can be measured. They often have orders for frequent weights. If they gain weight rapidly, this may be because they have consumed too much liquid. If you observe a resident with a fluid restriction order drinking extra liquids, notify the nurse.

HELPING WITH MEALS

You will be responsible for helping residents eat. This may include spoon-feeding some residents. You have already learned many factors that affect residents' overall nutrition. Making mealtime pleasant and enjoyable should be your goal. Encourage proper nutrition by helping residents as follows:

- Pleasant environment
  - Most residents eat their meals in the dining room.
  - If the resident stays in his room, be sure the room is clean and neat. Remove objectionable items such as commodes, bedpans, and urinals.
- Social concerns
  - Ask residents where and with whom they wish to eat, if consistent with the care plan.
  - If facility policy permits, encourage the resident's family to occasionally eat a meal with the resident.
  - Realize that the resident may feel resentment or be embarrassed if he is unable to feed himself.
  - Remember that eating is a social occasion. Residents usually eat better in a group than they do when they are alone.
  - If the resident must have his clothing protected because of spills, do not call the clothing protector a "bib." Some elderly residents feel that this is degrading and childlike. Call this garment an "adult clothing protector" or "apron."
- Resident comfort
  - Be sure the resident is clean and has recently toileted. Wash the residents' hands before meals.
  - Dress the resident in comfortable clothing.
  - Be sure the resident is wearing dentures, eyeglasses, and hearing aid, if used, at mealtime.
- Proper positioning
  - Be sure the resident is not too low to reach the table, or too far away because of the arms of a wheelchair.
  - It is the policy in many facilities to seat residents in regular dining room chairs instead of wheelchairs at mealtime.
- Adaptive equipment (Figure 11-4)
  - plate guards
  - adaptive silverware
  - special cups or glasses
- Serving trays
  - Wash your hands (or use an alcohol-based hand cleaner) before serving trays. If you must feed or physically assist a resident during the meal, wash your hands again when you have finished.
  - Be sure that the resident receives the right tray.
  - Keep food covered during transportation to maintain temperature and prevent contamination.
  - If a closed cart is used, shut the door to the food cart as soon as you remove each tray. This helps maintain food temperature and prevent contamination.
  - Serve one table at a time. Residents should not have to watch their tablemates eat while they are waiting for their own food. If possible, serve slow eaters first.
  - Leave trays on the food cart until you are ready to feed residents. Do not put a tray in front of a resident who must be spoon-fed until you are available to assist with the meal.

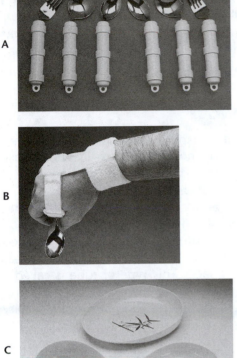

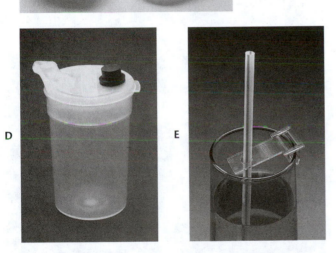

Figure 11-4 Adaptive devices that enable residents to eat and drink independently. (A) This flatware has built-up handles for easy gripping. Some pieces are angled, making it easier to move from the tray into the mouth without spilling. (B) The wrist cuff enables the resident to hold silverware and eat independently. (C) Adaptive plates and bowls have raised edges so residents can scoop food easily. (D) An adaptive cup. (E) The straw holder centers the straw and holds it in place. (Courtesy of Maddak, Inc.)

— Visually check the items on the tray to be sure that they are allowed on the resident's diet. Ask if you are unsure.

— Replace missing items, if needed.

— Make sure that residents have condiments and other seasonings of choice.

— Be sure food is served at the proper temperature. Hot foods should be served hot and cold foods cold.

— Offer to replace or reheat food that has become cold.

— Notice and report the resident's likes and dislikes, as well as techniques that do and do not help the resident meet nutritional needs.

— Offer substitutes if the resident does not eat. A substitute should always be available for the meat and vegetable. Follow your facility policy.

— Serve all clean trays before returning used trays to the food cart. Do not return used trays if unserved food remains on the cart.

— After all trays are served, check on residents. Honor resident requests for substitutes and extra portions, if allowed. Always offer beverage refills.

— Accurately record how much the resident eats, if this is the policy of your facility. Report any changes in appetite to the nurse.

— Record fluid intake if the resident is on intake and output.

— Be aware that residents with some medical conditions, such as a stroke, may not have a full field of vision. If the resident does not eat the food on a certain area of the tray, turn the tray around so the food is on the opposite side.

Feeding Techniques

Proper positioning. Various feeding techniques encourage optimal nutrition in residents. Position is important to prevent aspiration and choking.

• The resident's head should be elevated as much as possible.

• Feeding the resident with the head in a flat position creates a risk of choking. If the resident's head cannot be elevated, position the resident on his side.

Prepare the food. Cut food, open cartons, remove wrappers, and assist in other ways according to the resident's needs. In addition:

• Season food if the resident wishes.

• Tell the resident which items are hot.

• Use a clock description for the resident with a visual impairment. For example, the meat is on the plate at the six o'clock location.

• Remind and encourage residents to eat. Assist if they are unable to feed themselves.

Encourage self-care.

- Let the resident feed himself foods that can be handled easily.

- If the resident eats slowly, some food may have to be reheated. When the resident is eating independently, do not feed him even though he is slow. Assist only when he is unable to feed himself.

- Use adaptive equipment to enable the resident to be independent.

Feeding residents.

- Check the temperature of foods before feeding.

- Explain what foods are on the tray. Ask the resident what he would like to eat first.

- Do not mix foods together when feeding.

- Feed residents who are unable to feed themselves. Check the care plan goals.

Many residents who must be spoon-fed are encouraged to eat their own finger foods, such as bread.

- Check the temperature of a hot food by placing a drop on your wrist. If it feels too hot, wait a few minutes before feeding (Figure 11-5).

- Use hand-over-hand technique to help residents feed themselves.

- Offer liquids at intervals.

- Use a straw or spouted cup for liquids.

- Make pleasant conversation, but do not ask the resident questions that take a long time to answer.

- Never rush the resident.

- Sitting next to the resident conveys a relaxed feeling and is less intimidating than standing over the resident to feed him.

- Sit at or below eye level to prevent the resident from bending his head backward, which may cause choking.

TUBE FEEDING

Some residents are unable to eat solid food and are fed in different ways. The nursing assistant does not usually give these types of feedings, but an understanding of the techniques will help you care for the resident.

A feeding tube may be used for residents who have difficulty swallowing. Tube feeding may also be called **enteral feeding.** Some tubes are inserted through the nose and threaded through the throat and into the stomach. This type of tube is called a **nasogastric (NG) tube.** Most residents who receive tube feedings in the long-term care facility have permanent tubes surgically placed into the stomach. The most common type of permanent feeding tube is called a **gastrostomy (G) tube.** The resident is fed a liquid formula through the tube. The head of the bed should always be elevated when the tube feeding is running (Figure 11-6). The

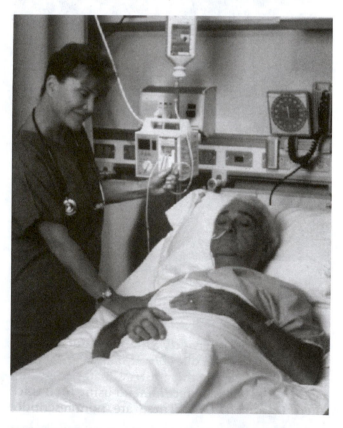

Figure 11-6 Always keep the head of the bed elevated during and after tube feeding.

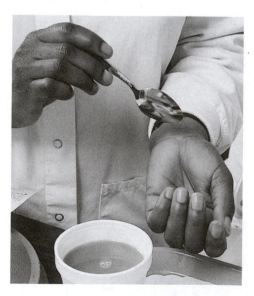

Figure 11-5 Test hot foods by placing a drop on your wrist.

PERFORMANCE PROCEDURE

35 Feeding the Resident

Supplies needed:
- adult clothing protector
- napkin or towel
- adaptive equipment as needed

1 Perform your beginning procedure actions.

2 Check the name on the tray and the diet served.

3 Check the meal tray for utensils and spilled foods.

4 Place the tray on the table. Remove food covers.

5 Sit near the resident.

6 Explain what is on the tray.

7 Ask the resident what foods he would like to eat first.

8 Encourage the resident to feed himself, if able, by using finger foods or adaptive equipment.

9 Use hand-over-hand technique to help the resident feed himself, if consistent with the care plan.

10 Fill the fork or spoon only half full or less, according to the resident's ability to swallow.

11 Use a straw for liquids.

12 Encourage the resident to eat. Talk pleasantly. Do not rush.

13 Wipe the resident's mouth.

14 Offer liquids between bites of solid food.

15 Remove the tray when the resident is finished.

16 Wash the resident's hands, if necessary.

17 Perform your procedure completion actions.

---

head should remain elevated for a specified period after the feeding stops. The care plan gives specific instructions. Residents who are tube-fed require frequent mouth care. Check your facility policy and the care plan for the type of solution to use and how often mouth care should be done.

When residents have feeding tubes in place, be very careful not to pull or tug on the tubing. Serious complications can occur if the tube becomes dislodged.

Safety Precautions

When caring for a resident who has a feeding tube, be sure to:

- keep the skin around the tube clean
- keep the head of the bed elevated

Oral Hygiene

Residents who use feeding tubes need frequent mouth care.

Nasogastric Tube

Follow these guidelines for a resident who has a nasogastric tube:

- Clean the nose around the tube.
- The tube is usually taped at the nose.
- The end of the tubing is pinned to the resident's clothing to prevent pulling.

Gastrostomy Tube

Follow these guidelines for a resident who has a gastrostomy tube:

- Clean the skin around the tube if it is open to the air.
- The nurse may place clean gauze around the wound opening. Do not remove gauze dressings.

Reporting

Report to the nurse immediately if the:

- alarm used to monitor the feeding solution sounds

- tube becomes dislodged
- resident begins to cough, choke, or vomit
- feeding solution is not flowing properly
- level of the formula in the bag is low or empty
- feeding is leaking around the gastrostomy tube
- skin appears irritated where the tube contacts the skin
- resident has loose stools

INTRAVENOUS FEEDINGS

Intravenous feedings, or IVs, are sometimes used to add to the resident's nutrition (Figure 11-7). Sometimes residents who receive intravenous feedings also receive a meal tray. Some residents receive only the intravenous solution. Check with the care plan and the nurse for instructions regarding a meal tray. The intravenous line can be placed in the veins of the arms or legs. Sometimes the intravenous line is in the neck or chest. When caring for the resident, be very careful not to dislodge the tubing. If you notice that the solution in the intravenous bag or bottle is running low, inform the nurse.

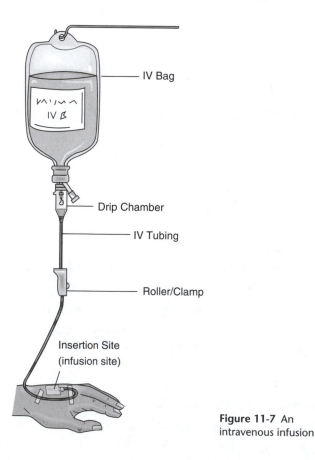

Figure 11-7 An intravenous infusion

IV Bag

IV B

Drip Chamber

IV Tubing

Roller/Clamp

Insertion Site (infusion site)

Safety Precautions

When caring for a resident who has an intravenous line, observe these precautions:

- Make sure the intravenous solution is flowing.
- Handle the **infusion site** carefully.
- Do not adjust the clamps on the tubing.
- Be careful when changing the resident's gown.

Reporting

Report to the nurse immediately if:

- the alarm used to monitor the intravenous solution sounds
- there is swelling, redness, pain, or bleeding at the site of needle insertion
- fluid is not dripping
- the level of the fluid in the bag is low or empty
- the needle or tubing becomes dislodged
- there is blood in the tubing

INTAKE AND OUTPUT

Intake and output (I & O) is a procedure in which all liquids taken in by the resident and all liquids put out by the resident are recorded. This procedure is done to monitor the resident's fluid balance. Recording intake and output is the nursing assistant's responsibility. Intake and output is abbreviated in most facilities as I & O. Note the following considerations for caring for a resident on I & O:

- Explain the procedure to the resident. Request the resident's cooperation if he is able.
- Record the information accurately.
- I & O worksheets are often kept at the bedside (Figure 11-8).
- Know your facility policy for I & O. Usually amounts taken by the resident are totaled at the end of shift and recorded on the medical record.

Note: Each facility has a listing of abbreviations that may be used in documentation in the facility. In 2004, an accreditation organization focused on eliminating certain abbreviations that often cause errors and are often misinterpreted because of sloppy or illegible handwriting. One such abbreviation is "cc," for cubic centimeter. Because of this, some facilities began documenting intake and output and other fluid measurements in milliliters (mL). However, many facilities continue to use "cc" for I & O

INTAKE – OUTPUT WORKSHEET

*INTAKE EQUIVALENTS

Medicine Cup – 30 cc
Water Pitcher – 800 cc/1,000 cc
Water Glass – 8 oz. – 240 cc
Styrofoam Cup (hot) – 6 oz./180 cc
Juice Glass – 4 oz./120 cc

Soup Bowl – 8 oz./240 cc
Ice Cream – 3 oz./90 cc
Carton Milk – 8 oz./240 cc

*Chart in CC's

TIME	INTAKE	OUTPUT	
	NOC	URINE	Emesis
0200	150cc	300 cc	
0600	200cc	300 cc	BM
			Drainage
	AM	URINE	Emesis
0730	525cc		
0900		350cc	
1000	100 cc		BM
1100		200cc	
			Drainage
	PM	URINE	Emesis
			BM
			Drainage

*These are guidelines only, verify containers used in your facility.

Figure 11-8 An intake and output worksheet. Although this example documents intake and output in cubic centimeters, some facilities document using millimeters (which are equivalent to cubic centimeters).

documentation. Misinterpreting handwritten abbreviations is a major cause of error in health care facilities. Know and follow your facility documentation policies and procedures.

Recording Intake

- Remember that I & O includes *all liquid* that the resident takes in, including fluid consumed in the dining room and during activities.

- Foods that are liquid at room temperature are recorded on the I & O sheets. For example, ice cream and Jell-O® are recorded.

- Fluids from any source are recorded. The nurse records intravenous and tube feedings.

- Record amounts in the intake column in **cubic centimeters (cc)** or in **milliliters (mL)** according to facility policy.

- Some measurements to know are:
  - 1 **ounce** (oz.) equals 30 cc (or mL)
  - 1 cup (8 oz.) equals 240 cc (or mL)
  - 1 teaspoon equals 5 cc (or mL)

- When measuring intake, remember that the measurements given are usually for containers filled to the top. Most glasses and cups are not filled completely full, so you should adjust how much fluid you record.

- The nursing assistant must learn the equivalents used in the facility. Most facilities provide conversion tables for recording intake.

- Record only the amount actually taken by the resident. For example, do not record a full glass of water if the resident drinks only half of the glass.

Recording Output

- Output includes all fluids lost from the body:
  - urine
  - blood or drainage
  - **emesis** (vomiting)
  - diarrhea
  - sweat

- Apply the principles of standard precautions when measuring output.

- Output is measured by pouring urine or other discharge into a **graduate** or measuring pitcher. Record the amount shown on the side of the pitcher.

- If the resident is incontinent, follow facility policy for recording urinary output. In some facilities, wet underpads are weighed on a scale. The weight is compared with the weight of a dry pad and the output is estimated.

- Report any blood or wound drainage to the nurse immediately.

- Report excessive perspiration.

PERFORMANCE PROCEDURE

36   Recording Intake and Output

Note: The guidelines for documenting intake and output vary slightly from one facility to the next. Some facilities document in cubic centimeters (cc), and others document in milliliters (mL). These measurements are equivalent. One cc equals one mL. Your instructor will inform you if the documentation in your facility differs from the examples shown here. Know and follow the required documentation procedure for your facility.

Supplies needed:
- paper towel
- graduate pitcher
- disinfectant used by facility
- pen and paper or I & O worksheet
- disposable exam gloves

1 Perform your beginning procedure actions.

2 Check to identify equivalents used in your facility.

3 Identify foods considered to be liquid as taken by the resident.

4 Estimate liquid food taken.

5 Record how much liquid is taken by the resident in cubic centimeters (cc) or milliliters (mL) according to facility policy.

6 Record amounts in the *intake* column.

7 Apply the principles of standard precautions when measuring output.

8 Measure output by pouring the contents of the bedpan, urinal, or emesis basin into the graduate. Remove one glove. Flush contents down the toilet after they are measured by holding graduate with gloved hand and pushing flush lever on toilet with ungloved hand.

9 Rinse and disinfect the graduate and bedpan, urinal, or emesis basin according to facility policy.

10 Record the elimination in the output column.

11 Perform your procedure completion actions.

KEY POINTS IN THIS CHAPTER

▲ A balanced diet containing the essential nutrients is necessary for good health.

▲ Some residents in the long-term care facility need help getting proper nutrition.

▲ Some residents are on special diets. Make sure the resident receives the right tray at mealtime.

▲ Fluid balance occurs when fluid intake and fluid output are about equal.

▲ Dehydration occurs when inadequate fluid is consumed and there is not enough liquid available in the body to perform essential functions.

▲ Making mealtime as pleasant as possible is important.

▲ Residents should feed themselves whenever possible.

▲ Be alert to safety when caring for residents who have feeding tubes.

▲ The head of the bed should always be elevated when the resident is receiving a tube feeding.

▲ When the resident is on I & O, all liquids taken in are recorded. Also, all liquid output must be measured and recorded.

REVIEW QUIZ

1. What is the purpose of the food pyramid?
   a. to provide a guide to eating a well-balanced diet
   b. to list foods that people on special diets should not eat
   c. to provide a plan for eating two meals a day for those who skip breakfast
   d. to provide a plan for those who plan school menus only

2. What is the normal daily fluid intake for an adult?
   a. 1 quart
   b. 1 to 2 quarts
   c. 2 to 3 quarts
   d. 6 to 8 quarts

3. Which of the following statements is true?
   a. Everyone should take a vitamin pill every day.
   b. Good nutrition can be obtained by eating proper amounts as listed on the food guide pyramid.
   c. The elderly should take extra vitamins once a week.
   d. Most foods do not contain vitamins or minerals.

4. If you feel that a food is too hot to feed to a dependent resident, you should:
   a. return the food to the tray cart uneaten.
   b. blow on the food to cool it.
   c. leave the food until it cools.
   d. put the food in the refrigerator.

5. Guidelines for passing trays to residents include all of the following except:
   a. handwashing and identifying the resident.
   b. placing the tray in front of residents who are spoon-fed; return later to feed the resident.
   c. checking the food on the tray to see if it is allowed and replacing missing food items.
   d. preparing the tray, seasoning food as requested, and providing adaptive devices.

6. Cultural influences that may affect eating habits are:
   a. religion and family customs.
   b. well-fitting dentures.
   c. the ability to chew or swallow.
   d. hereditary conditions and diseases.

7. Making mealtime a pleasant experience is the responsibility of the:
   a. nursing assistant only.
   b. dietary staff only.
   c. housekeeping staff.
   d. entire facility staff.

8. The person responsible for planning meals for residents is the:
   a. nursing assistant.
   b. dietitian.
   c. head nurse.
   d. administrator.

9. Which of the following would not be included on a clear liquid diet?
   a. tea
   b. milk
   c. broth
   d. gelatin (Jell-O®)

10. When serving a tray to a resident who is on a diabetic diet, you should make sure:
    a. there is no salt on the tray.
    b. the resident does not have coffee.
    c. there is no sugar on the tray.
    d. the tray has no fruit or vegetables on it.

11. Some residents must have a low-salt diet. A food that is high in salt content is:
    a. ham.
    b. milk.
    c. bread.
    d. fruit.

12. Dehydration occurs when:
    a. there is too much fat in the body.
    b. there is not enough fluid in the body.
    c. one has overeaten.
    d. the body is at rest.

13. When feeding a resident:
    a. turn on your favorite television program.
    b. feed the resident all solids before giving liquids.
    c. give all foods at room temperature.
    d. avoid rushing the resident.

14. A feeding tube may be inserted for residents who:
    a. are on a low-calorie diet.
    b. are on salt-restricted diets.
    c. have problems swallowing.
    d. have dentures that do not fit well.

15. When a resident is on intake and output, you must record:
    a. all the food eaten by the resident.
    b. the liquids the resident drinks.
    c. all liquids served to the resident.
    d. both liquids and solids taken by the resident.

16. You are assigned to work in the dining room. Mrs. Martinez is feeding herself very slowly. Several of the other residents have finished eating, and Mrs. Martinez is still eating. You should:
    a. feed Mrs. Martinez so that she gets done quickly.

   b. ask Mrs. Martinez if she would like any of the food heated again.

   c. leave Mrs. Martinez alone and check on her again later.

   d. remove Mrs. Martinez's tray.

17. Mr. Burns is an 83-year-old resident who has had a stroke and is not able to swallow. He is fed through a nasogastric tube. Mr. Burns's tube feeding is administered by a pump that runs all the time during your shift. When you go to Mr. Burns's room at 10:00, you notice that he is coughing and choking. You should:

   a. ask another nursing assistant what to do.

   b. leave the room and check on Mr. Burns later to see if he is still coughing.

   c. stay with Mr. Burns and call for the nurse immediately.

   d. pull the nasogastric tube out.

18. Mrs. Carroll has an order on her care plan to force fluids. Mrs. Carroll is on a regular diet. You know that she does not like to drink water. To be sure that she takes enough liquid on your shift, you should:

   a. ask Mrs. Carroll what kinds of fluids she likes and offer them.

   b. provide fluids that you like.

   c. offer Mrs. Carroll water each time you are in the room.

   d. force the resident to drink one pitcher of water during your shift.

19. Mrs. Carroll drinks 3 ounces of the beverage that you offer her. You should record her fluid intake as:

   a. 3 cc.

   b. 30 cc.

   c. 60 cc.

   d. 90 cc.

20. At the end of the day shift, Mrs. Carroll has consumed 1,500 cc of liquid. You know that this is:

   a. not enough liquid.

   b. an adequate amount of liquid.

   c. too much liquid.

   d. enough fluid to meet her needs for 24 hours.

CHAPTER 11
CROSSWORD PUZZLE

Directions: Complete the following puzzle using the following words found in Chapter 11.

aspiration
centimeter
dehydration
digestion
edema
emesis
force

gastrostomy
graduate
infusion
intake
intravenous
milliliter
nutrients

ounce
output
pyramid
restrict
therapeutic

CHAPTER 11
PUZZLE CLUES

ACROSS

6. "cc" is the abbreviation for cubic _____.
9. _____ and output
10. "mL" is the abbreviation for _____.
12. A special or modified diet used to treat a disease
14. A pitcher used for measuring drainage
15. Abnormal swelling
16. Chemical substances found in food that are necessary for life
17. Process by which food is broken down and changed into nutrients
19. Intake and _____

DOWN

1. The location where the intravenous tubing is inserted is the _____ site.
2. A unit of measurement equal to 30 cc
3. An order to _____ fluids means to encourage the resident to drink.
4. A resident whose doctor has ordered a limited amount of fluids has an order to _____ fluids.
5. Breathing liquid into the air passages
7. A feeding tube that is surgically placed in the stomach
8. The food guide _____ provides a guide to eating a balanced diet
11. Less than adequate amount of fluid
13. A liquid feeding given into a vein
18. Vomiting or what is vomited

Elimination Needs

OBJECTIVES

In this chapter, you will learn how to help residents with elimination needs. After reading this chapter, you will be able to:

- Spell and define key terms.
- Describe normal elimination.
- Describe factors that interfere with normal elimination.
- Describe bowel and bladder management guidelines.
- Position a resident on a bedpan.
- Assist a resident with the urinal.
- List observations of elimination that should be reported to the nurse.
- Perform catheter care.
- Empty a catheter bag.
- Describe ostomy care.
- List guidelines for enema administration.

KEY TERMS

bedpan: a container used by bedridden residents to discharge body waste

bladder: a hollow muscle that stores urine until it is eliminated from the body

bowel: the same as intestine; part of the digestive system extending from the stomach to the rectum

catheter: a tube inserted into a body cavity; often inserted into the bladder to drain urine

colon: the large bowel or the lower part of the intestine

colostomy: a surgical procedure in which the colon is attached to the outside of the body and waste is eliminated into a plastic bag attached to the skin

commode: a portable toilet

defecate: to have a bowel movement

diarrhea: multiple loose bowel movements

enema: administration of fluid into the rectum; usually done to cleanse the bowel

feces: waste products from the bowel; the same as stool or bowel movement

homeostasis: a constant state of balance within the body

impaction: mass of hard feces that cannot be passed from the rectum normally

incontinence: inability to control the passage of urine or stool

involuntary: done without choice; often refers to inability to control stool passage

kidneys: organs that filter the blood, removing waste products

ostomy: a surgically created opening through the abdominal wall into the intestines; body waste passes through this opening

stoma: the opening in the abdomen created by an ostomy

stool: feces or bowel movement

ureters: tubes that connect the kidneys to the urinary bladder

urethra: the body tube through which urine passes from the body

urinal: a container used by males for urination

urinate: to pass urine

void: to pass urine

NORMAL ELIMINATION

Elimination is the body's way of removing waste products and toxic substances through the digestive and urinary systems. A review of these systems follows.

Urinary System

The urinary system eliminates waste products from the blood, forms urine, and allows the discharge of urine. The urinary system is very important in maintaining **homeostasis,** or stable body function.

Organs in the Urinary system.

- **Kidneys**
  - filter the blood
  - return necessary water and chemicals to the blood after filtering out waste
  - form urine from waste products taken from the blood

- **Bladder**
  - stores urine in a hollow muscle until it is passed out of the body

- **Ureters**
  - tubes that connect the kidneys to the bladder

- **Urethra**
  - tube through which urine passes out of the body

Characteristics of normal urine.

- clear or yellow-golden color
- nearly odorless, but smells like ammonia if it stands over time
- free from sediment or mucus
- urge to **urinate** is usually felt when the bladder contains 150 to 200 mL

Digestive System

In the digestive system, food is chemically broken down so it can be absorbed by the blood as nutrients.

Main organs of the digestive system.

- Mouth
  - orifice where food is chewed and mixed with saliva causing the food to break down

- Esophagus
  - the tube connecting the mouth to the stomach

- Stomach
  - a muscular organ where food is churned and mixed with digestive juices

- Intestines
  - large and small tube-like canals that extend from the stomach to the rectum
  - nutrients are absorbed into the blood as food passes through the intestine
  - undigested food passed on as **stool (feces)** into the rectum

- Rectum
  - the last five to six inches of the **colon**
  - feces are stored in the rectum until the urge to move the **bowel** is felt
  - feces are eliminated from the anus, or outlet to the rectum

Characteristics of normal feces.

- light to dark brown color
- soft and formed
- frequency from daily bowel movement to every three days
- no difficulty in passing normal stool

INTERFERENCE WITH NORMAL ELIMINATION

When caring for the elderly, you must be aware of things that can cause elimination problems.

Aging

- Normal aging slows all body functions, including the digestive and urinary systems.
- Feelings of hunger and thirst decrease with age. Many elderly do not take enough food or liquids to allow for proper elimination.
- Blood flow to the kidneys is decreased. Urine, therefore, is not produced as often.
- Feeling of a full bladder and bowel is reduced. Elderly residents often feel urgency only when actually eliminating.
- Incontinence is not a part of normal aging.

Disease and Disability

- Many residents have chronic illnesses that affect elimination.
- Residents may have nerve damage. The nerve damage causes limited, reduced, or no feelings of urgency.

Inactivity

- The elimination systems rely on the stimulation from muscle movements to function effectively.

Medication

- Many residents take medications that affect the elimination systems. Medications may cause **diarrhea,** constipation, or urinary problems.
- Many elderly persons have a history of taking laxatives. Laxatives affect normal intestinal function.

Improper Diet

- Inadequate fluid intake can cause elimination problems.
- Food should have sufficient bulk or roughage.

Lack of Privacy

- Many persons need privacy to have normal elimination.

Stress

- This emotion may cause diarrhea, constipation, or urinary frequency.

Abnormal Body Position

- Using a **bedpan** is often difficult.
- When the resident remains in bed, urine pools, making voiding difficult. This often leads to urinary tract infections.

Time

- A sufficient amount of time is needed.

BOWEL AND BLADDER MANAGEMENT

Many residents who are incontinent or **involuntary** can relearn to control urine and stool passage. Bowel and bladder training plans take time and attention of the entire nursing staff. A plan to retrain may require scheduling changes and a lot of effort by the nursing assistant (Figure 12-1). Once the process is relearned, however, it will become part of the daily routine and will save you time and energy.

The resident, of course, benefits from any bowel and bladder plan. Control of one's body functions adds to self-esteem, dignity, happiness, and health.

Considerations for Care

- Apply the principles of standard precautions.
- Establish regularity and prevent **incontinence.**
- Set plans according to each resident's pattern. You will collect information about the resident's pattern of elimination. The nurse will use this information to write the toileting plan.
- Explain the procedure to the resident. This helps ensure resident cooperation.
- Refer to the care plan about:
  — fluid intake
  — recording fluid output
  — positioning the resident
  — the schedule of voiding intervals
- Reporting and recording your observations is very important.
- Treat incontinence in a matter-of-fact manner. Never scold, yell at, or ridicule the resident.

Special Guidelines for Toileting

- Some residents cannot tell you they need to use the toilet. They may become restless or irritable instead.
- Loss of appetite and small, watery rectal discharge may indicate a fecal **impaction.** Report this to the nurse immediately.
- Pressure or a full feeling in the lower abdomen may suggest a full bladder or a hard fecal mass. Report this to the nurse immediately.
- The urge to eliminate may occur quickly and suddenly. Respond promptly.
- Many residents must void more often at night.

INITIAL INCONTINENCE EVALUATION 2 DAY VOIDING PATTERN ASSESSMENT

N615

O O Ø ... incontinent SMALL amount
O Ø O ... incontinent MODERATE amount
Ø O O ... incontinent LARGE amount

● Dry When Checked
(/) Stool Present
(/) Resident Asked to Use Toilet

Day _Wed._   Date _9 / 2000_

AIDE	TIME	INCONTINENT	DRY	STOOL	PATIENT REQUESTED	TOILETED
Ellen Stacey	24 Midnite	Ø O O	●	( )	( )	cc
Ellen Stacey	1 AM	O O O	/	( )	( )	cc
Ellen Stacey	2 AM	O O O	/	( )	( )	cc
Ellen Stacey	3 AM	O O Ø	●	( )	( )	cc
Ellen Stacey	4 AM	O O O	/	( )	( )	cc
Ellen Stacey	5 AM	O O O	/	( )	( )	cc
Ellen Stacey	6 AM	O O O	/	( )	( )	cc
Ellen Stacey	7 AM	O O O	●	( )	(/)	cc 300
Audrey King	8 AM	O O O	/	( )	( )	cc
Audrey King	9 AM	O O O	/	( )	( )	cc
Audrey King	10 AM	O O Ø	●	( )	( )	cc
Audrey King	11 AM	O O O	●	( )	(/)	cc 200
Audrey King	12 PM	O O O	/	( )	( )	cc
Audrey King	13 PM	O O O	/	( )	( )	cc
Audrey King	14 PM	O O O	/	( )	( )	cc
Audrey King	15 PM	O Ø O	●	( )	( )	cc
Carlos Ramos	16 PM	O O O	/	( )	( )	cc
Carlos Ramos	17 PM	O O Ø	●	( )	( )	cc
Carlos Ramos	18 PM	O O O	/	( )	( )	cc
Carlos Ramos	19 PM	O O O	/	( )	( )	cc
Carlos Ramos	20 PM	O O O	/	( )	( )	cc
Carlos Ramos	21 PM	O O O	●	( )	(/)	cc 150
Carlos Ramos	22 PM	O O O	/	( )	( )	cc
Carlos Ramos	23 PM	O O O	/	( )	( )	cc
TOTALS						

RESIDENT NAME _Martin, Frank_   ROOM NO. _409_

Figure 12-1 Accurate recordkeeping is an important nursing assistant responsibility in a bowel and bladder management program. The nurse uses this information to develop a toileting schedule for the resident.

Help with Elimination Needs

Some ways you will help the resident with elimination needs include helping the resident to the bathroom or commode. A **commode** is a portable toilet. You will also be giving the resident the bedpan or **urinal.**

These are specially shaped containers designed to help the bedridden resident urinate (**void**) or **defecate.** Other duties you will perform are observing and reporting unusual output, providing catheter care, helping with care for an ostomy, and giving enemas.

PERFORMANCE PROCEDURE

37   Giving a Bedpan

Supplies needed:
- bedpan
- bedpan cover or disposable bed protector for cover
- bed protector
- toilet tissue
- washbasin
- soap
- washcloth
- towel
- disposable exam gloves

1 Perform your beginning procedure actions.

2 Ask the resident to flex the knees and rest weight on the heels, if able.

3 Help the resident to raise the buttocks:

   a Put one hand under the small of the resident's back, and gently lift while the resident pushes with his feet.

   b With the other hand, insert the bed protector under the resident.

4 If the resident is unable to lift his buttocks:

   a Help the resident to turn on his side, with his back toward you.

   b Place the bed protector on the bed.

   c Place the bedpan flat against the resident's buttocks (Figure 12-2).

   d Roll the resident on his back while holding the bedpan in place.

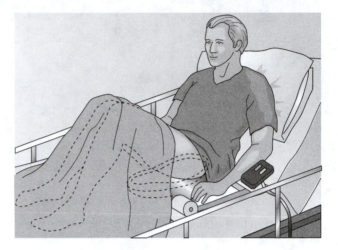

Figure 12-3 Elevate the head of the bed so that the resident is comfortable.

5 Cover the resident with the top sheet.

6 Raise the head of the bed slightly for comfort (Figure 12-3).

7 Remove the disposable gloves.

8 Raise the side rail.

9 Dispose of gloves according to facility policy.

10 Wash your hands.

11 Give the resident the call signal and toilet tissue. Instruct him to use the signal when he is done. Leave the room.

12 Return immediately when the resident calls.

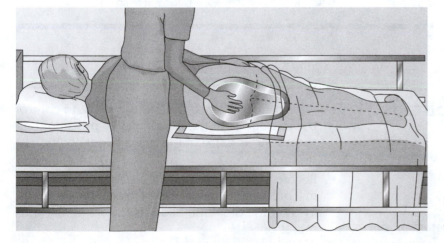

Figure 12-2 Position the bedpan flat against the resident's buttocks, then roll him back toward you while holding the pan in position.

(continues)

37 *continued*

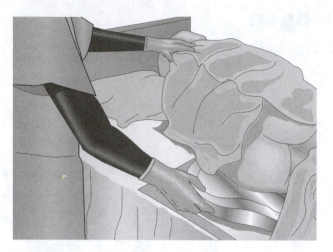

Figure 12-4 Hold the bedpan securely while the resident turns on his side.

13 Put on disposable gloves.

14 Lower the side rail.

15 Remove the bedpan by asking the resident to raise his hips.

16 If the resident is unable to raise his hips, hold the bedpan securely while the resident rolls to his side with back facing you (Figure 12-4). Remove the bedpan. Cover the pan with a bedpan cover or other cover according to facility policy (Figure 12-5).

17 Place the bedpan on a bed protector on the chair in the room, or according to facility policy. It is usually not placed on the overbed table or bedside stand.

18 Fill the washbasin with water (105°F). Help the resident to clean his perineal area, if necessary. Dispose of toilet tissue in the bedpan. Cover the bedpan.

19 Wash the resident's perineal area with soap and water. Rinse and dry.

20 Remove one glove and raise the side rail with the ungloved hand.

21 Take the covered bedpan to the bathroom. Empty and disinfect it according to facility policy. Use the ungloved hand to turn on faucets and flush the toilet. Store the bedpan in its proper location.

22 Remove the other glove and dispose according to facility policy.

23 Wash your hands.

24 Help the resident to wash his hands. Clean and return the basin to its proper location.

25 Perform your procedure completion actions.

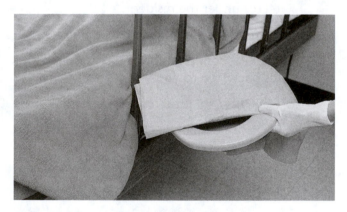

Figure 12-5 Cover the bedpan after you remove it.

OBSERVING AND MEASURING OUTPUT

Nursing Alert

Apply the principles of standard precautions when measuring residents' output.

Urine

- Measure and record in cubic centimeters or milliliters as indicated by facility policy.

- If the resident is incontinent, or unable to control the passage of urine, follow facility procedure by measuring the size of the urine puddle or weight of the pad.

- Record amounts in drainage bags by measuring in a graduate (Figure 12-6). Do not use the markings on the drainage bags, as the marks are estimates only.

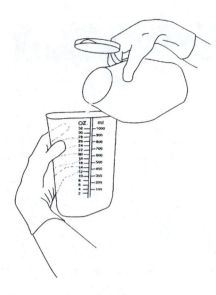

Figure 12-6 Pour the specimen into a graduate to measure the output. Read the numbers at eye level.

Feces (Bowel Movements)

- Recording bowel movements is very important to ensure that elimination is adequate.
- Most facilities use checklist charting for recording bowel movements.

Observe and Report Abnormalities

These abnormalities should be reported to the nurse immediately:

- blood
- mucus
- liquid stool
- very hard stool
- stool that is very dark in color
- undigested food or pills in the stool
- unusual color (clay color, black, etc.)

Record on I & O Sheet

Accurate reporting requires you to be observant. Be sure to record:

- amount of urine
- profuse perspiration or sweat
- time of output, if required
- amounts of emesis and liquid stools

PERFORMANCE PROCEDURE

38 Giving a Urinal

Supplies needed:
- urinal with cover
- washbasin
- soap
- washcloth
- towel
- disposable exam gloves

1 Perform your beginning procedure actions.

2 Lift the top covers and hand the resident the urinal under the covers. If the resident is unable to take the urinal, place the urinal in the bed and insert the resident's penis into the opening.

3 Remove the disposable gloves and dispose according to facility policy.

4 Raise the side rail.

5 Wash your hands.

6 Give the resident the call signal and instruct him to use it when he is done. Leave the room.

7 Return immediately when the resident calls.

8 Put on one disposable glove.

9 Ask the resident to hand you the urinal. Remove it if he is unable.

10 Take the urinal to the bathroom, and empty and disinfect it according to facility policy. Use the ungloved hand to turn on faucets and flush the toilet. Store the urinal in its proper location.

11 Remove the glove and dispose according to facility policy.

12 Wash your hands.

13 Fill the washbasin with water (105°F).

14 Lower the side rail.

15 Help the resident to wash his hands.

16 Raise the side rail.

17 Lower the height of the bed.

18 Clean and return the basin to its proper location.

19 Perform your procedure completion actions.

✔ GUIDELINES for Catheter Care

- ☐ Apply the principles of standard precautions when providing catheter care.
- ☐ Gently wash the genital area around the catheter with warm water.
- ☐ Wash the perineal area. Wash from front to back on females, and from the tip of the penis to the scrotum on males.
- ☐ Rinse and dry well.
- ☐ Some facilities include washing the catheter close to the body as part of this procedure. Follow your facility policy. If you are washing the catheter, always wash in the direction away from the body. Avoid rubbing back and forth.
- ☐ Make sure that the catheter tubing is without kinks.
- ☐ Make sure that all connections are tight.
- ☐ Make sure that the resident is not lying or sitting on the catheter tubing.
- ☐ Position the catheter to avoid pulling. Pulling the catheter is irritating to the resident. It is very painful for the resident if the catheter is accidentally dislodged. Use a Velcro strap or tape to secure the catheter to the leg to prevent pulling.
- ☐ Attach the drainage tubing to the sheet to allow the urine to drain well.
- ☐ The drainage bag should be below the level of the bladder at all times. If the bag is raised above the bladder, the urine will drain back into the body, causing the potential for an infection to develop.
- ☐ The catheter bag should never touch the floor.
- ☐ Attach the catheter bag to the bed frame, not the side rail.
- ☐ Take care when moving or transferring residents so that you do not pull on the catheter.

CATHETERS

A **catheter** is a tube inserted into a body cavity, usually for draining liquids. The most commonly used catheter is the indwelling urinary catheter, which is inserted by the nurse. You may hear this catheter called a "Foley." The catheter is usually left in the bladder, where it is held in place by a small, inflatable balloon (Figure 12-7). The catheter is attached to tubing that connects to the drainage bag that collects the urine.

Because the catheter opens into a body cavity, the resident is at high risk of infection. Many facilities have policies stating that the tubing and catheter are not to be disconnected. Some facilities use leg bags to collect the urine when the resident is out of bed during the day. The leg bag is worn under the clothing and is not as obvious as the regular catheter bag. Know and follow your facility policies and procedures for disconnecting the tubing and handling the catheter. This is a very important responsibility.

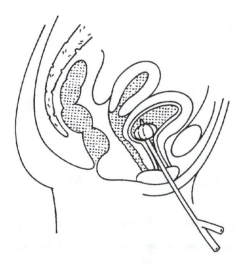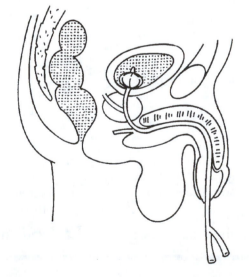

Figure 12-7 Placement of an indwelling catheter in the female and male resident

PERFORMANCE PROCEDURE

39   Giving Catheter Care

Note: The guidelines and sequence for this procedure vary slightly from state to state. Your instructor will inform you if the sequence in your state differs from the procedure listed here. Know and follow the required sequence for your state.

Supplies needed:
- bath blanket
- bed protector
- tape or catheter strap
- rubber band
- pin
- washbasin
- soap
- washcloth
- towel
- disposable exam gloves

1   Perform your beginning procedure actions.

2   Cover the resident with a bath blanket.

3   Fanfold the upper linen down to the foot of the bed.

4   Ask the resident to raise hips and place the bed protector under the resident.

5   Position the bath blanket to expose the resident's catheter.

6   Wash the urethra area around the catheter entrance.

7   Using a clean washcloth, wash the catheter for 3 inches from the insertion site into the body. Begin washing at the urinary meatus and wash downward. Avoid rubbing back and forth on the tubing.

8   Wash the genital area from front to back. Rinse well.

9   Dry the area well.

10 Secure the catheter with a catheter strap or tape.

11 Place the drainage tubing over the resident's leg.

12 Place the rubber band around the tubing and pin it to the sheet at the edge of the mattress to make sure that the tubing stays on the bed.

13 Cover the resident. Replace the bedding and remove the bath blanket.

14 Perform your procedure completion actions.

PERFORMANCE PROCEDURE

40   Emptying a Catheter Bag

Note: The guidelines and sequence for this procedure vary slightly from state to state. Your instructor will inform you if the sequence in your state differs from the procedure listed here. Know and follow the required sequence for your state.

Supplies needed:
- graduate pitcher
- paper towel
- alcohol sponge
- disposable exam gloves

1   Perform your beginning procedure actions.

2   Place a paper towel on the floor and place the graduate on top of it.

3   Remove the drainage spout from the bag and center it over the graduate (Figure 12-8). Be careful not to touch the tip of the drainage spout. Do not let the tip or the

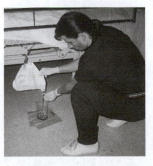

Figure 12-8 Place a paper towel on the floor. Center the tip of the tubing over the graduate. Avoid touching the tubing against the sides of the container. Keep the drain spout above the urine in the graduate.

(continues)

40 *continued*

sides of the drainage spout touch the graduate.

4 Open the clamp on the drainage spout and allow the urine to drain into the graduate.

5 After the urine has drained into the graduate, wipe the spout with the alcohol sponge, if this is your facility policy. Some facilities do not wipe the tip of the spout unless it has contacted your hands or the graduate.

6 Replace the drainage spout into the holder on the side of the catheter bag. Pick up the graduate. Dispose of the paper towel.

7 Note the amount, color, and character of urine.

8 Discard urine and disinfect the graduate according to facility policy. Store the graduate in its proper location. Record output.

9 Perform your procedure completion actions.

Catheter Care

This procedure may vary from one facility to another. Always refer to the care plan for specific instructions. Refer to the guidelines on page 210 for catheter care.

OSTOMIES

An **ostomy** is a surgical opening made through the abdomen for excretion of body waste (Figure 12-9). This procedure is done when disease or injury prevents normal elimination. An ostomy may be done to allow for urinary or fecal waste discharge. The opening of the ostomy is called the **stoma.** Ostomies may be temporary or permanent. The most common type of ostomy is the **colostomy,** an opening into the colon to allow for feces to be eliminated. Many people live well with ostomies. They work and are very active. Many people care for their own ostomy. The resident in a long-term care facility may need some assistance caring for

the ostomy. Procedures vary from one facility to another. However, some general guidelines apply.

Caring for the Resident with an Ostomy

Although policies vary, practice ostomy care carefully, and follow the guidelines on page 213.

ENEMAS

An **enema** is the injection of fluid into the rectum. This is usually done to empty the rectum of feces. You may be responsible for giving a resident an enema. In some facilities nursing assistants are not allowed to give enemas. Know and follow your facility policy.

There are two types of enemas: a cleansing enema and a retention enema. The cleansing enema is given to clean the rectum. The retention enema is given to soften the feces or to administer medication.

The type of enema nursing assistants usually administer is the cleansing enema. The solution for enemas may be plain water, a soap or salt solution, or a commercial preparation.

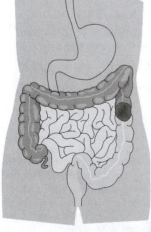 Colostomy

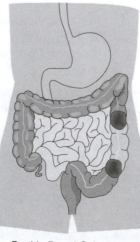 Double Barrel Colostomy

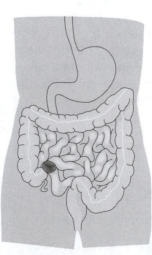 Ileostomy

Figure 12-9 The location of the ostomy determines the amount of water in the stool. The colostomy is the most common. The double-barrel colostomy is usually temporary. After the digestive system rests, the intestines are surgically reconnected.

✔ **GUIDELINES for Ostomy Care**

☐ Apply the principles of standard precautions when caring for an ostomy.

☐ Realize that the resident with an ostomy may feel a great loss of control and have a poor body image and low self-esteem. Be aware of your own body language during this procedure so that you do not further lower the resident's self-esteem.

☐ Be a good listener. Allow the resident to talk about her feelings.

☐ Report signs of depression to the nurse.

☐ Remove the soiled bag.

☐ Gently wash the area around the ostomy according to directions on the care plan.

☐ Observe and report any redness or irritation of the skin around the stoma.

☐ Apply protective cream around the stoma, if indicated on the care plan.

☐ Apply a clean bag.

☐ Change ostomy bags often to reduce odors. Some residents use deodorizer tablets or drops in the ostomy bag.

☐ Dispose of soiled bags according to facility policy.

✔ **GUIDELINES for Giving Enemas**

Policies of long-term care facilities vary regarding who is responsible for giving enemas. Check with the nurse before giving a resident an enema.

☐ Apply the principles of standard precautions when giving an enema.

☐ Check with the nurse about which solution to use.

☐ Enema solutions should be warm, about 105°F. Check the temperature with a bath thermometer.

☐ The amount of solution in a cleansing or tap water enema is usually 700 cc to 1,000 cc.

☐ Have the resident's bathrobe, slippers, bedpan, or commode nearby. The resident will feel urgency after the enema.

☐ When administering the enema solution, the resident should be lying on her left side in the Sims' position, with the right knee drawn toward the chest.

☐ Always lubricate the rectal tube of the enema.

☐ Before inserting the tubing into the rectum, clear air from the tubing by running water through the tubing. Clamp the tubing.

☐ Insert the tube about 2 to 3 inches.

☐ Raise the container of solution 12 to 18 inches above the rectum.

☐ Allow the solution to run in slowly.

☐ If the resident complains of cramping, clamp the tubing and instruct her to take deep breaths. Then open the tubing and continue the procedure.

☐ Give the amount of solution ordered by the physician and as tolerated by the resident.

☐ Ask the resident to hold the solution in the rectum for a few minutes, if possible.

☐ Help the resident to the bathroom, commode, or onto the bedpan.

☐ Make sure the resident's call light is in reach.

☐ Observe and report the results of the enema. Instruct the resident not to flush the toilet until results have been observed. If blood or other abnormalities are noted, do not flush the toilet until you have notified the nurse.

KEY POINTS IN CHAPTER

▲ Elimination of body waste is done through the body's digestive and urinary systems.

▲ Due to reduced sensitivity, the elderly person often feels urgency just when the elimination is felt.

▲ Some factors affecting normal elimination in the resident may be disease, inactivity, medications, and lack of privacy.

▲ Bowel and bladder management programs can help residents regain control over these body functions.

▲ Catheter care includes cleaning the genital area, and catheter, and watching for proper urine drainage.

▲ An enema involves the administration of fluid into the rectum, usually to remove feces.

▲ An ostomy is an opening into the abdomen to allow body waste to come out.

REVIEW QUIZ

1. The body's way of removing waste products is called:
   a. digestion.
   b. circulation.
   c. elimination.
   d. impaction.

2. The organs of the urinary system that filter the blood and form urine are the:
   a. bowels.
   b. kidneys.
   c. bladders.
   d. intestines.

3. Normal urine is:
   a. clear.
   b. dark yellow.
   c. foul-smelling.
   d. streaked with mucus.

4. What are the intestines?
   a. tubes connecting the kidneys and bladder
   b. tubelike canals extending from the stomach to the rectum
   c. a storage place for urine before discharge
   d. the tubes through which blood circulates throughout the body

5. In normal aging, the blood flow to the kidneys is:
   a. lessened.
   b. increased.
   c. stimulated.
   d. unchanged.

6. Incontinence:
   a. occurs naturally in aging.
   b. is always a psychological problem.
   c. is a medical problem.
   d. indicates behavior and adjustment problems.

7. Bowel and bladder training plans should include:
   a. the resident only.
   b. only the nursing staff on the night shift when the resident is incontinent.
   c. the entire nursing staff involved with the resident's care.
   d. facility administration.

8. All of the following statements are true *except*:
   a. Many residents will have the urge to urinate more frequently at night.
   b. The need to eliminate will occur quickly and urgently in many residents.
   c. Some residents may be restless and irritable, which may indicate a need to eliminate urine.
   d. Most residents are unable to control the passage of urine while sleeping.

9. What does the term *void* mean?
   a. to pass stool
   b. to urinate
   c. to insert a tube to drain urine
   d. to end the passage of urine or stool

10. A container that the male resident uses for urination in bed is the:
    a. urinal.
    b. regular bedpan.
    c. commode.
    d. indwelling catheter.

11. After removing a bedpan from a resident, you notice some blood in the urine. What is your best response?
    a. Empty the bedpan, and clean and replace equipment.
    b. Empty the bedpan into the toilet, then record the incident on the resident's chart.

c. Place the bedpan and contents in the bathroom. Report the appearance of blood in the urine to the nurse immediately.
d. Pour the urine into a cup and take it to the doctor's office for examination.

12. Caring for the resident who uses a urinary catheter includes:
a. securing the catheter to the resident's leg.
b. inserting the catheter into the resident.
c. removing the catheter at night.
d. changing the catheter every other day.

13. An opening made through the abdomen to allow for discharge of body waste is a/an:
a. enema.
b. ostomy.
c. catheter.
d. defecation.

14. When placing a resident on a commode to defecate, you are:
a. helping the resident to sit on a bedpan.
b. helping the resident to use a portable toilet to urinate.
c. placing the resident on a portable toilet to have a bowel movement.
d. placing the resident on a bedpan to have a bowel movement.

15. When giving a cleansing enema, you should insert the tubing into the rectum:
a. one inch.
b. two to three inches.
c. six to seven inches.
d. eight to nine inches.

16. You are caring for Mrs. Hunter, a 67-year-old resident who has had a stroke and is mentally confused. Mrs. Hunter has been having loose stools all morning that are watery in appearance. Her abdomen is hard to the touch. You know that:
a. Mrs. Hunter has had too much water to drink.
b. this is normal in residents who have had a stroke.
c. this could indicate a fecal impaction and should be reported to the nurse.
d. the loose stools will stop after the resident eats some solid food.

17. You are emptying catheter bags at the end of your shift. Mrs. McQueen's catheter bag only has 50 cc in it. You should:
a. record the output on the flow sheet and go home.
b. assume that another nursing assistant has emptied this catheter.
c. do nothing, as the bag does not have to be emptied.
d. report your observations to the nurse.

18. While you are emptying catheters, you accidentally touch the drain spout of Mr. Gates's catheter on the bed frame. You should:
a. insert the drain spout back in the catheter bag immediately.
b. wipe the drain spout with an alcohol sponge.
c. remove the catheter.
d. leave the drain spout exposed to the air after the bag is empty.

19. Miss Gunther is an 86-year-old resident who has Alzheimer's disease and is confused. This resident requires total care and is usually incontinent of urine. Miss Gunther urinates 10 times on your shift. The urine has a strong odor. You know that:
a. this may indicate a urinary tract infection and should be reported to the nurse.
b. Miss Gunther has had too much liquid to drink.
c. this is normal in Alzheimer's disease.
d. the resident is urinating frequently to get extra attention.

20. Mr. Haley is a 75-year-old resident with a colostomy. You are assigned to bathe him and do his colostomy care. The area around the stoma appears very red. You should:
a. wipe the area with an alcohol sponge.
b. remove the used colostomy bag and place a new one on the area immediately.
c. ask the nurse to look at the area before you reapply the bag.
d. apply moisturizing lotion to the area around the stoma.

CHAPTER 12
CROSSWORD PUZZLE

Directions: Complete the puzzle using these words found in Chapter 12.

anus
bedpan
bowel
catheter
colon
commode
colostomy

defecate
enema
feces
homeostasis
impaction
incontinent
involuntary

stoma
stool
urethra
urinal
void

CHAPTER 12
PUZZLE CLUES

ACROSS

3. A container that men use for urination
5. The lower part of the intestine
9. A tube inserted into a body cavity to drain liquid
10. The large bowel or lower part of the abdomen
12. Administration of fluid into the rectum to cleanse the bowel
13. A constant state of balance in the body
15. To have a bowel movement
17. The opening in the abdomen created by an ostomy
19. The tube through which the urine passes as it leaves the body

DOWN

1. A portable toilet
2. A surgically created opening into the abdominal wall to eliminate feces from the body
4. Unable to control the passage of urine
6. A mass of hard feces that the resident is unable to pass normally
7. Bowel movement
8. To urinate
11. Done without choice; usually refers to inability to control the passage of stool
14. Another word for stool
16. A special container that the resident uses to discharge body waste when in bed
18. The opening of the rectum

Vital Signs, Height, and Weight

OBJECTIVES

In this chapter, you will learn how to measure and record the vital signs of body temperature, pulse, respiration, and blood pressure. You will learn how to measure the resident's height and weight. After reading this chapter, you will be able to:

- Spell and define key terms.
- Describe vital signs.
- List four pulse sites.
- Measure the resident's temperature, pulse, and respirations.
- Measure the resident's blood pressure.
- Identify abnormal vital signs.
- Record the resident's vital signs.
- Measure and record the resident's height and weight.

KEY TERMS

apical pulse: the pulse heard through a stethoscope at the base of the heart

axillary: concerning the armpit area

blood pressure: the pressure of the blood against the walls of the arteries

body temperature: the amount of heat in the body measured by a thermometer

brachial pulse: the pulse felt on the inner side of the arm at the bend of the elbow

bradycardia: a pulse rate of less than 60 beats per minute

carotid pulse: the pulse felt on either side of the neck

Celsius: a metric unit of measuring temperature

cyanosis: a bluish color in the skin, lips, or fingertips due to lack of oxygen

diastolic pressure: the lower number of a blood pressure reading; the relaxing phase of the heartbeat cycle

dyspnea: difficult breathing; shortness of breath

exhalation: breathing air out

expiration: the same as exhalation; breathing air out

Fahrenheit: a scale for measuring temperature, commonly used in the United States

hypertension: abnormally high blood pressure

hypotension: abnormally low blood pressure

inhalation: breathing air in

inspiration: the same as inhalation; breathing air in

oral: concerning the mouth

palpated systolic pressure: systolic blood pressure determined by palpating the brachial or radial pulse while the sphygmomanometer is deflated; diastolic blood pressure cannot be determined by using this method

pulse: the beat of the heart that is felt when an artery is compressed against a bone

radial pulse: the pulse felt at the radial artery on the inner side of the wrist

rate: the number of pulse beats or respirations per minute

rectal: concerning the anus or rectum

respiration: the exchange of oxygen and carbon dioxide in the body

rhythm: the regularity of the pulse

sphygmomanometer: the piece of equipment used to take the blood pressure

stethoscope: the device used to listen to the resident's blood pressure, apical pulse, and other body sounds

systolic pressure: the top number of the blood pressure reading; the contraction phase of the heart cycle

tachycardia: a pulse rate of more than 100 beats per minute

temperature: measurement of heat in the body

tympanic: refers to the inner ear

vital signs: the temperature, pulse, respirations, and blood pressure

volume: the strength of the blood flow through the blood vessels

VITAL SIGNS

The **vital signs** measure the functions of vital organs of the body. These four functions are temperature, pulse, respiration, and blood pressure. All are necessary for life. When the body is not functioning normally, the rates and character of vital signs change. The resident's condition can be monitored and evaluated by measuring the vital signs.

It is important for you to learn how to correctly take and accurately record vital signs. Whenever you are not sure of the readings, tell the nurse immediately. Accurate measurement of vital signs takes learning and practice.

Abbreviations for Vital Signs, Height, and Weight

You must become familiar with the commonly used abbreviations for the vital signs, height, and weight. They are:

BP or B/P	blood pressure
V.S.	vital signs
TPR	temperature, pulse, and respiration
O or PO	oral temperature (taken in the mouth)
R	rectal temperature (taken in the anus)
A or AX	axillary temperature (taken in the axilla or armpit)
°	degrees
F	Fahrenheit measurement
C	Celsius measurement
Ht.	height
Wt.	weight
#	pounds

TEMPERATURE

The **temperature** measures body heat. Body heat is created by food changing into energy. Body heat is lost by perspiration, respiration, and excretion. The balance between heat produced by the body and the heat lost is the **body temperature.**

The normal aging process may interfere with the body's ability to regulate the temperature. Careful temperature monitoring is important for the resident in a long-term care facility. Other factors might affect the body temperature. Body temperature can be increased by:

- infection, illness, and disease
- dehydration
- physical exercise
- a very warm environment

Body temperature can be decreased by:

- shock
- a cold environment
- medications
- stress
- The oral temperature is increased or decreased by intake of hot or cold liquids, chewing gum, or smoking cigarettes

Thermometers

The temperature is taken using a thermometer. There are many types of thermometers, including:

- electronic (Figure 13-1)
- plastic or paper (Figure 13-2)
- glass (Figure 13-3)
- digital

The glass and electronic thermometers are most commonly used in long-term care facilities. Follow your facility's policy when using paper or plastic thermometers.

Thermometers measure body temperature using either the **Fahrenheit** or the **Celsius** (centigrade) scale. Both scales are divided into units called *degrees*. Check which type of thermometer your facility uses.

On glass thermometers, each long line on the thermometer equals one degree, and each short line

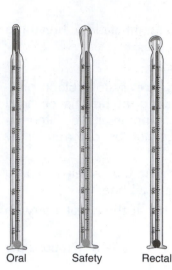

Figure 13-3 Three types of glass thermometers. The thermometer with a blue dot on the end is for both oral and axillary use. The thermometer with the red dot on the end is for rectal use.

equals two-tenths of a degree. The thermometer is read by noting the point at which the mercury column ends. The temperature is read to the nearest two-tenths of a degree.

Many facilities use disposable sheaths to cover the thermometer when taking the temperature. These sheaths protect the resident because they contain the glass if the thermometer is accidentally broken. Some types of sheaths used for rectal temperatures are prelubricated. The sheath on a glass thermometer is used once and discarded. Become familiar with the type of sheath your facility uses.

Mercury

Mercury is a neurotoxic, heavy metal that is linked to numerous health problems in wildlife and humans. A mercury thermometer is a small glass tube containing liquid mercury, a silvery-white substance that registers body heat. Mercury thermometers have been used for many years. However, in recent years the trend has been to avoid the use of products containing mercury because they can be very toxic to humans and wildlife, if broken.

Other products are being used in many glass thermometers because of the reduced potential for toxicity. Some thermometers contain a red or blue liquid. These are alcohol thermometers and contain no mercury. Other products may also be used. These thermometers are mercury-free, and are marked as such.

Mercury exposure can be toxic in small amounts, particularly if it vaporizes and is inhaled. Even small mercury spills must be cleaned up properly to prevent contamination and illness. If you accidentally break a mercury thermometer or other device containing mercury, inform the nurse promptly. Follow facility policies and procedures for picking up mercury. If no procedures are available, apply

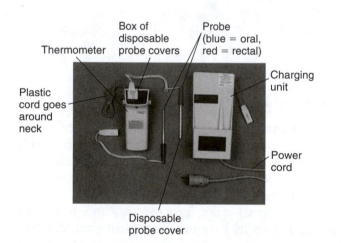

Figure 13-1 An electronic thermometer. Plastic probe covers are placed over the probe tip, then under the resident's tongue.

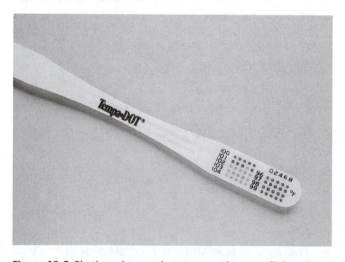

Figure 13-2 Plastic and paper thermometers have small dots that change color to record the temperature. They are used once and then discarded. Remove the thermometer slowly to prevent cutting under the resident's tongue.

gloves, face mask, and eye protection. Pick up broken glass and other debris and place in a puncture-resistant container. Use an index card to consolidate the droplets, then seal them in a plastic bag or covered container. Small droplets can be picked up with adhesive tape or wet paper towels. Seal the container and affix a label identifying the material as "mercury spill debris." Consult the nurse for information regarding where to discard this material.

Electronic thermometers. The electronic thermometer is a battery-operated unit that shows the temperature reading on a lighted display. This type of unit eliminates human error that may occur with other types of thermometers.

Two types of electronic thermometers are available. One type is used for oral, rectal, or axillary temperatures. This thermometer has a probe. A blue-colored probe is used for oral and axillary temperatures. A red-colored probe is used for the rectal temperature. This thermometer makes a "beep" sound when the temperature has been measured. The electronic thermometer usually has a cord to wear around your neck when you are walking down the hall or using the thermometer to take the temperature. Wear the thermometer like a necklace, and take care not to swing or drop it. The thermometer is very sensitive and will not work properly if it is banged or dropped.

Another type of electronic thermometer is used for taking the tympanic, or ear, temperature (Figure 13-4). This thermometer is inserted into the inner ear and records temperature very quickly. The display screen blinks when the temperature has been measured.

Disposable plastic sheaths, called *probe covers,* are inserted over the electronic probe of both types

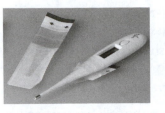

Figure 13-5 The handheld digital thermometer makes an audible sound when the temperature reading is ready. Always use a probe cover with this thermometer.

of electronic thermometers. A clean probe cover must be used for each resident's temperature. The batteries of electronic thermometers must be charged regularly to stay accurate. Follow facility policy when using electronic thermometers.

Digital thermometers. Some facilities use small, handheld digital thermometers (Figure 13-5). These thermometers are powered by a small battery, similar to a watch battery. A disposable probe cover must always be used with this thermometer. The guidelines for using this thermometer are the same as those for a glass thermometer. Follow your facility policies and procedures for disinfecting the thermometer between uses.

Methods of Measuring Body Temperature

There are four methods of measuring a resident's body temperature. The **oral** method is done by inserting the thermometer under the resident's tongue. The **rectal** method is done by inserting the thermometer one inch into the resident's rectum. The **axillary** method is done by placing the thermometer in the resident's armpit. The **tympanic** temperature is taken by inserting the thermometer into the resident's ear. Always refer to the care plan to learn which method must be used for each resident. Apply the principles of standard precautions when taking temperatures. A brief overview of each of these methods follows.

Oral temperature.   The oral temperature is taken by mouth. It is used when the resident is alert and cooperative.

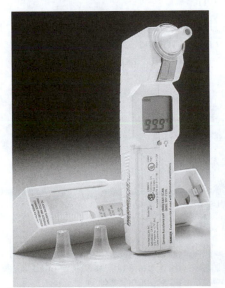

Figure 13-4 When positioned correctly, the tympanic thermometer is the fastest and most accurate method of taking the temperature.

- Do not take an oral temperature on residents with known seizure disorders.

- The oral thermometer may have a bulb or slender tip. Sometimes the end of the thermometer is blue or green.

- Do not take the temperature by mouth if the resident has just taken hot or cold liquids, smoked a cigarette, dipped tobacco, or chewed gum. Wait 15 minutes before taking the oral temperature.

- Do not take the temperature orally if the resident is using oxygen.

- Follow your facility policy for using a disposable sheath to cover the glass thermometer.
- The oral thermometer should remain in place for 3 minutes, or according to facility policy.
- The normal oral temperature is 98.6°F.

Rectal temperature. Note the following when using the rectal method.

- This thermometer has a shorter, rounded bulb tip that contains mercury or an alternative.
- The tip opposite the bulb end of the rectal thermometer is usually red.
- Follow your facility policy for using a disposable sheath to cover the glass thermometer.
- Use for residents receiving oxygen ("mouth breathers"), confused or disoriented residents, and others who cannot keep the thermometer in the mouth.
- Do not take a rectal temperature on residents who have hemorrhoids, diarrhea, fecal impaction, a colostomy, or recent prostate surgery.
- The thermometer must always be lubricated before it is inserted into the rectum. Some rectal thermometer sheaths are prelubricated.
- Insert the glass thermometer one inch into the rectum.
- Always hold the thermometer in place when taking rectal temperatures.
- This thermometer should remain in place for 3 minutes, or according to facility policy. Never leave the resident alone.
- The normal rectal temperature is 99.6°F.
- Record "R" if the temperature was taken rectally.

Axillary temperature. Take the axillary temperature using an oral thermometer.

- Follow your facility policy for using a disposable sheath to cover the glass thermometer.
- This is the *least accurate* method of taking the temperature and should not be used if you can take the temperature by using another method.
- An axillary temperature may not be accurate on residents who are underweight.
- Remove perspiration by wiping the axillary area before placing the thermometer.
- Some facilities require the nursing assistant to hold this thermometer in place. Know and follow the policy of your facility.
- This thermometer should remain in place for 10 minutes, or according to facility policy.
- The normal axillary temperature is 97.6°F.

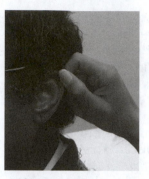

Figure 13-6 Gently pull the pinna up to straighten the ear canal.

- Record "AX" when the axillary temperature is taken, or follow your facility policy.

Tympanic temperature. This method of taking the temperature can be used for most residents.

- Use a special ear thermometer.
- Always use a disposable probe cover on the thermometer.
- Large amounts of ear wax may produce an inaccurate reading.
- Gently lift the top of the outer ear (Figure 13-6). This straightens the ear canal.
- Insert the end of the thermometer as far as it will go. For the temperature to be accurate, the detector at the end of the thermometer must be flat, facing the tympanic membrane. The reading will not be accurate if it is tipped to the side.
- Next, rotate the probe handle until it is aligned with the jaw, like speaking on the telephone (Figure 13-7). Quickly press the "scan" button. Hold the thermometer in place until the display flashes.
- Most ear thermometers can be set to give the equivalent of an oral or rectal reading.
- Follow your facility policy for recording the oral or rectal equivalent.

Some facilities use metric system measurements for temperatures. The formulas for converting temperatures between Fahrenheit and Centigrade are listed in Table 13-1.

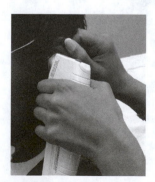

Figure 13-7 Insert the thermometer until it seals in the ear canal, then rotate until it is positioned like a telephone receiver.

✔ GUIDELINES for Taking Temperature

Some general rules are important when taking the resident's temperature:

☐ Apply the principles of standard precautions when taking temperatures.

☐ Check the thermometer for chips and cracks.

☐ Follow facility procedure for wiping up broken thermometers. The mercury in the glass is poisonous, and your facility will have special policies for cleanup.

☐ Be alert to thermometers with both Celsius and Fahrenheit scales. The markings on this type of thermometer are very small. Be sure to read accurately.

☐ Shake the column of liquid down below 96°F before inserting the thermometer.

☐ Use care when shaking down a thermometer. Stand away from the resident or surfaces that the thermometer may hit.

☐ Follow your facility policy for using disposable thermometer sheaths.

☐ Lubricate the rectal thermometer before inserting it.

☐ Hold the rectal thermometer in place with your gloved hand.

☐ Wipe the thermometer from the stem end to the bulb tip before inserting.

☐ Disinfect and store the thermometer according to facility policy.

☐ Never clean a glass thermometer with hot water. The thermometer may break.

☐ Use a clean probe cover for each resident when using an electronic thermometer or ear thermometer.

TABLE 13-1   Conversion Formulas

$F > C$ $C = 5/9 (F - 32)$
Example: To convert a Fahrenheit temperature of 212°F to Celsius, follow the procedure:
$5/9 = (212 - 32) = 5/9 \times 180 = 100°C$

$C > F$ $F = 9/5C + 32$
Example: To convert a Celsius temperature of 100°C to Fahrenheit, follow the procedure:
$100 \times 9/5 = 900/5 = 180 + 32 = 212°F$

PERFORMANCE PROCEDURE

41   Measuring an Oral Temperature

Note: The guidelines and sequence for this procedure vary slightly from state to state. Your instructor will inform you if the sequence in your state differs from the procedure listed here. Know and follow the required sequence for your state.

Supplies needed:
- thermometer
- disposable plastic sheath or probe cover
- pad and pen
- disposable gloves
- container for used thermometers

1 Perform your beginning procedure actions.

2 If using a glass thermometer, rinse the disinfectant off and dry the thermometer.

3 Shake the glass thermometer down to 96°.

4 Cover the thermometer with a plastic sheath or probe cover.

5 Apply gloves, if this is your facility policy.

(continued)

41   *continued*

(*Note:* Gloves are generally not necessary for taking oral temperatures unless there is a risk of contact with oral secretions, or unless wearing gloves is your facility policy.)

6 Place the bulb or tip of the probe under the resident's tongue and instruct the resident to close the lips.

7 Leave the thermometer in place for 3 minutes, or until the thermometer alarm sounds, according to facility policy and the type of thermometer used.

8 Remove the thermometer from the resident's mouth.

9 Discard the sheath or probe cover according to facility policy.

10 Hold the glass thermometer at eye level and read the mercury column.

OR

Read the digital display of the electronic thermometer.
Note the reading.

11 Shake the glass thermometer down to 96°. Place the thermometer in the container for used thermometers, or disinfect it according to facility policy.

OR

Place the probe for the electronic thermometer in the probe holder.

12 Remove your gloves and discard according to facility policy.

13 Record the temperature reading.

14 Perform your procedure completion actions.

PERFORMANCE PROCEDURE

42   Measuring a Rectal Temperature

Note: The guidelines and sequence for this procedure vary slightly from state to state. Your instructor will inform you if the sequence in your state differs from the procedure listed here. Know and follow the required sequence for your state.

Supplies needed:
- thermometer
- disposable plastic sheath or probe cover
- lubricant
- tissue or paper towel
- pad and pen
- disposable gloves
- container for used thermometers

1 Perform your beginning procedure actions.

2 If using a glass thermometer, rinse the disinfectant off and dry the thermometer. Shake the glass thermometer down to 96°.

3 Cover the thermometer with a plastic sheath or probe cover.

4 Position the resident in the Sims' position.

5 Apply gloves.

6 Place a small amount of lubricant on a tissue or paper towel. Use the tissue to lubricate the bulb of the thermometer. (*Note:* Some plastic sheaths are prelubricated.)

7 Separate the resident's buttocks with one hand.

8 Insert the bulb of the glass thermometer into the rectum one inch.

If using an electronic thermometer, insert the probe into the rectum half an inch, or according to facility policy.

9 Hold the thermometer in place for 3 minutes, or until the alarm sounds on the electronic thermometer.

10 Remove the thermometer from the resident's rectum.

11 Discard the sheath or probe cover according to facility policy.

(continued)

42 *continued*

12 Hold the glass thermometer at eye level and read the mercury column.

OR

Read the digital display of the electronic thermometer.

Note the reading.

13 Shake the glass thermometer down to 96°. Place the thermometer in the container for used thermometers or disinfect it according to facility policy.

OR

Place the probe for the electronic thermometer in the probe holder.

14 Remove your gloves and discard according to facility policy.

15 Record the temperature reading.

16 Perform your procedure completion actions.

PERFORMANCE PROCEDURE

43 Measuring an Axillary Temperature

Note: The guidelines and sequence for this procedure vary slightly from state to state. Your instructor will inform you if the sequence in your state differs from the procedure listed here. Know and follow the required sequence for your state.

Supplies needed:
- thermometer
- disposable plastic sheath or probe cover
- towel
- pad and pen
- disposable gloves
- container for used thermometers

1 Perform your beginning procedure actions.

2 If using a glass thermometer, rinse the disinfectant off and dry the thermometer. Shake the glass thermometer down to 96°.

3 Cover the thermometer with a plastic sheath or probe cover.

4 Apply gloves, if this is your facility policy.

5 Dry the axilla with a towel.

6 Insert the thermometer into the center of the axilla, then lower the resident's arm and bend it across the abdomen. Hold the thermometer in place, if this is your facility policy.

7 Leave the thermometer in place for 10 full minutes or until the thermometer alarm sounds.

8 Remove the thermometer from the resident's axilla.

9 Discard the sheath or probe cover according to facility policy.

10 Hold the glass thermometer at eye level and read the mercury column.

OR

Read the digital display of the electronic thermometer.

Note the reading.

11 Shake the glass thermometer down to 96°. Place the thermometer in the container for used thermometers or disinfect it according to facility policy.

OR

Place the probe for the electronic thermometer in the probe holder.

12 Remove your gloves and discard according to facility policy.

13 Record the temperature reading.

14 Perform your procedure completion actions.

PERFORMANCE PROCEDURE

44   Measuring a Tympanic Temperature

Note: The guidelines and sequence for this procedure vary slightly from state to state. Your instructor will inform you if the sequence in your state differs from the procedure listed here. Know and follow the required sequence for your state.

Supplies needed:
- tympanic thermometer
- probe cover
- pad and pen
- gloves if needed

1   Perform your beginning procedure actions.

2   Check the lens of the thermometer to make sure it is clean.

3   Cover the thermometer lens with a clean probe cover.

4   Select the appropriate mode (oral or rectal) on the thermometer.

5   Gently pull the ear up and back to straighten the ear canal.

6   Insert the thermometer, aiming it toward the tympanic membrane (eardrum). Insert until the tip seals in the ear canal. Rotate the probe handle slightly until it is aligned with the jaw, as if it were a telephone receiver.

7   Press the activation (scan) button. Hold the thermometer in place until the display flashes or the thermometer indicates that there is a reading.

8   Remove the thermometer from the resident's ear and discard the probe cover according to facility policy.

9   Record the temperature reading.

10 Perform your procedure completion actions.

PULSE

The **pulse** is the expansion and contraction of an artery. This rhythmic expansion and contraction in the artery indicates how fast or slow the heart is beating. It is felt in locations where an artery lies over a bone close to the surface of the skin (Figure 13-8). The pulse tells you how well the circulatory system is working. When you take the resident's pulse, be alert to the rate, rhythm, and volume of the pulse beat.

Pulse Rate

The pulse rate is the number of beats per minute. The pulse rate varies within individuals from time to time depending upon exercise or emotional state. The pulse should be counted while the resident is at rest. Characteristics for taking the pulse are as follows:

- The pulse rate varies. It depends on age, sex, body size, emotional state, and exercise.

- The pulse rate usually goes up as the body temperature increases.

- Pain usually increases the pulse rate.

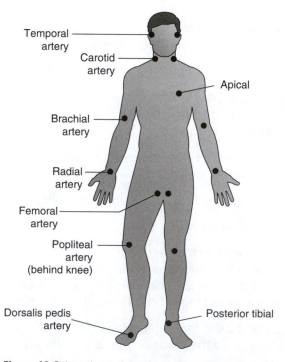

Figure 13-8 Locations where the pulse can be palpated

PERFORMANCE PROCEDURE

45   Taking the Radial Pulse

Note: The guidelines and sequence for this procedure vary slightly from state to state. Your instructor will inform you if the sequence in your state differs from the procedure listed here. Know and follow the required sequence for your state.

Supplies needed:
- watch with second hand
- pad and pen

1 Perform your beginning procedure actions.

2 Locate the radial pulse and place the first three fingers of your hand on it.

3 Look at your watch and begin counting.

4 Count the number of pulse beats for 60 seconds. (Count for 30 seconds and multiply by 2, if permitted by your state laws and facility policies.) Always count for one full minute if the pulse is irregular.

5 Record this figure.

6 If you are taking respirations, leave your fingers on the pulse.

7 If you are not counting respirations, perform your procedure completion actions.

- Medications may affect the pulse rate.
- The average adult pulse is 60 to 100 beats per minute.
- **Tachycardia** is a fast pulse rate of more than 100 beats per minute.
- **Bradycardia** is a slow pulse rate of less than 60 beats per minute.
- Report pulse rates of less than 60 or more than 100 to the nurse.

- The pulse is regular when the pulse beats are evenly spaced.
- The pulse is irregular when the beats are uneven or there are skipped beats.
- Report any irregular or unusual pulse beats.

Pulse Volume

The *pulse volume* is the forcefulness or degree of strength of the pulse. The volume of the pulse can be felt by noting how strong or weak the beat is

---

✔ GUIDELINES for Pulse Measurement

Several guidelines must be followed to measure the pulse properly:

☐ The resident should be at rest.

☐ The arm should rest comfortably on a surface.

☐ Use the tips of two or three fingers to take the pulse. Never use the thumb, because you may feel your own pulse in your thumb.

☐ Note the **rate,** or number of beats per minute.

☐ Note the **rhythm,** or regularity.

☐ Note the **volume**—weak, thready, or strong.

☐ Count the pulse for 60 seconds, or according to facility policy. In some facilities, counting for 30 seconds and multiplying by 2 is acceptable if the pulse is regular.

☐ The pulse is always recorded as the number of beats per minute.

☐ Report to the nurse immediately if the pulse is unusually fast, slow, or irregular.

when the artery is expanding and contracting. You will feel the pulse and note if it is:

- strong
- weak
- thready

Pulse Location

Learn these facts so you can record the pulse accurately.

- The **radial pulse** is felt at the wrist. It is the most common location for taking the pulse.
- The **carotid pulse** is felt on either side of the neck.
- The **apical pulse** is heard at the base of the heart. A **stethoscope** must be used to take the apical pulse.
- The **brachial pulse** is felt on the inner arm at the elbow. This is the pulse used to take the blood pressure.

RESPIRATION

Respiration is the process of breathing. It is this process that allows humans to take in oxygen and give off carbon dioxide. A single respiration or breath is one **inspiration** or **inhalation** (breathing air in) and one **expiration** or **exhalation** (breathing air out). As a nursing assistant you will be responsible for counting the resident's respirations.

Dyspnea is the medical term for shortness of breath. Shortness of breath always suggests a medical problem and should be reported to the nurse immediately. **Cyanosis** is a blue color of the skin, lips, or nailbeds caused by a lack of oxygen.

The process of breathing is both voluntary and involuntary. You breathe without thinking about it. However, you can control your respirations by holding your breath. This is the reason you do not explain to residents that you are counting the respirations. Counting respirations is usually done after counting the pulse. The resident will think you are taking the pulse while you are discreetly counting respirations.

Considerations for Care

Be aware of the following considerations regarding respiration:

- Normal respiration rate for adults is 12 to 20 per minute.
- Report respiratory rates below 12 or more than 20, or anything that differs from the normal range for that resident.
- Respirations increase with:
  — fever
  — infection
  — stress and emotional upsets
  — exercise

PERFORMANCE PROCEDURE

46 Counting Respirations

Note: The guidelines and sequence for this procedure vary slightly from state to state. Your instructor will inform you if the sequence in your state differs from the procedure listed here. Know and follow the required sequence for your state.

Supplies needed:
- watch with second hand
- pad and pen

1 Perform your beginning procedure actions.

2 Count the resident's pulse and remember the number.

3 After you have counted the pulse, glance at the resident's chest while continuing to look at your watch.

4 Count one inhalation and one exhalation as one respiration.

5 Count the number of respirations in one minute (60 seconds). (Count for 30 seconds and multiply by 2, if permitted by your state laws and facility policies. Always count for one full minute if the respirations are gasping or irregular.)

6 Record the respiration rate.

7 Record the resident's pulse and respirations on your note pad.

8 Perform your procedure completion actions.

✔ GUIDELINES for Counting Respirations

Know the following information so you will count respirations accurately:

☐ Breathing can be controlled, so avoid telling the resident when respirations are being counted.

☐ One inspiration and one expiration of breath are counted as one respiration. Watch the rise and fall of the resident's chest.

☐ Count respirations immediately after counting the pulse. Remember the pulse count as you count the rise and fall of the chest.

☐ Keep your fingers on the pulse while you are counting the respirations.

☐ Note if respirations are:

— regular

— shallow

— deep

— difficult or labored

☐ Count the respirations for one minute or as indicated by your facility policy.

☐ Record the respirations. Report any abnormalities to the nurse.

- Respirations decrease with:
  - some medications
  - some diseases
  - sleep

BLOOD PRESSURE

Measuring **blood pressure** gives valuable information about how the heart and blood vessels are working. The heart pumps the blood throughout the body through the arteries. The arteries carry blood away from the heart. When you take a resident's blood pressure, you are measuring how much pressure is exerted on the artery walls as the blood passes through. There is always some blood in the arteries, so there is always some pressure on the walls of the blood vessels. As the heart contracts to send out blood, a force is felt on the artery. This working phase of the heartbeat is called the **systolic pressure.** When the heart relaxes between beats, the pressure is lower. This is called the **diastolic pressure.** You will be reading both pressures when you take a blood pressure measurement.

The blood vessels of the older person are often thicker and less elastic, so the heart must work harder to push blood through the arteries. Therefore, the blood pressure in the older resident is often higher than a younger adult's blood pressure.

Equipment Used to Measure Blood Pressure

The equipment used in measuring blood pressure varies from one facility to another. In all cases you will be using something called a **sphygmomanometer,** commonly called a blood pressure cuff (Figure 13-9). Unless you use an electronic digital recording sphygmomanometer, you will also use a stethoscope to listen to the reading. Handle the sphygmomanometer carefully when you walk down the hall. Take care not to hit it against a wall or drop it. The sphygmomanometer may not provide an accurate reading if it is banged or dropped. Two types of sphygmomanometer are used:

- Mercury sphygmomanometer
  - A column of mercury is observed as you read the blood pressure.
  - This unit should be placed on a flat surface.
  - Read the mercury column at eye level.
  - No satisfactory alternative has been found for mercury in blood pressure devices, and many of these are still in use in health care facilities. Use mercury devices carefully to avoid breakage. Your facility will have policies and procedures for discarding mercury debris or intact mercury items, such as thermometers and blood pressure devices. Follow these procedures carefully.

- Aneroid sphygmomanometer. A pointer on a dial is observed as you read the blood pressure.

Accuracy is very important in taking the blood pressure. It takes skill and practice to learn to take accurate blood pressure readings. Ask the nurse to recheck a reading if you are not sure.

✓ GUIDELINES for Taking Blood Pressure

Follow these guidelines when taking blood pressure:

☐ Equipment should be in good working condition.

☐ Wipe the diaphragm or bell and earpieces of the stethoscope with an alcohol sponge before and after use.

☐ Use the proper size cuff.

☐ Read the gauge at eye level.

☐ The resident should be sitting or lying in a relaxed, comfortable position, with the arm resting on a solid surface.

☐ Do not take blood pressure in an arm:

— with an intravenous feeding

— with a dialysis access device

— weakened by a stroke

— on the side where a breast has been removed

☐ Do not reinflate the cuff immediately if you do not hear the blood pressure the first time. Let all of the air out, wait a minute, and take the blood pressure again.

☐ Record the blood pressure accurately in fraction form; for example, 120/80. Blood pressure is recorded as millimeters of mercury. For this reason, you may see the reading recorded as 120/80 mm Hg.

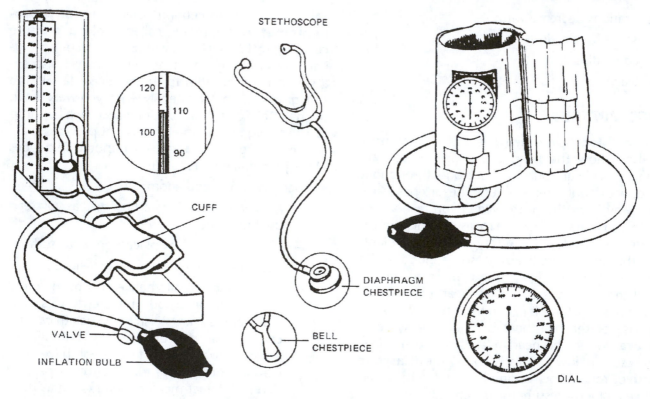

Figure 13-9 Equipment used to measure blood pressure

Terms Associated with Blood Pressure

Understand the terms **hypertension** and **hypotension**.

Hypertension. High blood pressure, usually 140/90 or higher, is considered hypertension. An elderly person's blood pressure may be higher than 140/90.

Hypotension. Low blood pressure, usually 100/60 or less, is considered hypotension.

Know and follow your facility policy for reporting blood pressure that is too high or too low.

47 Measuring the Blood Pressure (Two-Step Procedure)

Note: This is the "two-step" procedure recommended by the American Heart Association (AHA) beginning in 1993. The AHA considers the two-step procedure the most reliable for normal blood pressure measurement. (The most accurate values are obtained by internal monitoring, in which a catheter is placed in an artery. The internal method is not practical for most clinical situations.)

Note: The guidelines and reportable values for this procedure vary slightly from state to state, and from one facility to the next. Your instructor will inform you if the guidelines or reportable values in your state or facility differ from those listed here. Know and follow the required guidelines for your state.

Supplies needed:
- sphygmomanometer (blood pressure cuff)
- stethoscope
- alcohol sponges
- pad and pen

1 Perform your beginning procedure actions.

2 Wipe the earpieces and diaphragm of the stethoscope with the alcohol sponge.

3 Push the resident's sleeve up at least 5 inches above the elbow.

4 Extend the resident's arm and rest it on the arm of the chair, the bed, or the resident's lap, with the palm upward.

5 Unroll the cuff and open the valve on the bulb. Squeeze the cuff to deflate the cuff completely.

6 Locate the brachial artery, on the thumb side of the inner upper arm, by palpating with two or three fingers.

7 Wrap the cuff around the resident's arm, centering the bladder over the brachial artery. The cuff should be one inch above the artery in the antecubital space, in front of the elbow.

8 Locate the radial pulse on the thumb side of the wrist. Keep your fingers on it.

9 Close the screw on the handset and inflate the bulb until you can no longer feel the radial pulse. This is known as the **palpated systolic pressure.** Mentally add 30 to this number.

10 Open the screw and deflate the cuff.

11 Wait 30 seconds.

12 Place the stethoscope in your ears. Place the diaphragm of the stethoscope over the brachial artery.

13 Close the screw and inflate the cuff to 30 points higher than where the radial pulse was last palpated.

14 Slowly release the screw so the pressure in the cuff falls by increments of 2 mm Hg.

15 Listen for a sound. When you hear it, note the closest number on the gauge. This is the systolic pressure.

16 Continue to listen until the sound stops. Note the closest number on the gauge. This is the diastolic pressure. Continue to listen for 10 to 20 mm Hg below this sound.

17 Open the screw completely and deflate the cuff.

18 Remove the stethoscope from your ears.

19 Remove the cuff from the resident's arm.

20 Record the blood pressure on your note pad as a fraction, with the systolic reading first, followed by the diastolic reading.

21 If you are unsure of the blood pressure, wait one to two minutes, then check it again.

22 Wipe the earpieces and diaphragm of the stethoscope with the alcohol sponge.

23 Perform your procedure completion actions.

24 Report blood pressures over 140/90 or under 100/60 to the nurse immediately, or according to facility policy.

PERFORMANCE PROCEDURE

48   Measuring the Blood Pressure (One-Step Procedure)

Note: In some states, nursing assistants use a one-step procedure for measuring blood pressure. For your convenience, the one-step procedure is listed here.

Note: The guidelines and reportable values for this procedure vary slightly from state to state, and from one facility to the next. Your instructor will inform you if the guidelines or reportable values in your state or facility differ from those listed here. Know and follow the required guidelines for your state.

Supplies needed:
- sphygmomanometer (blood pressure cuff)
- stethoscope
- alcohol sponge
- pad and pen

1   Wipe the earpieces and diaphragm of the stethoscope with alcohol pads.

2   Perform your beginning procedure actions. The resident may be lying down or seated in a chair for this procedure.

3   Push the resident's sleeve up at least 5 inches above the elbow.

4   Extend the resident's arm and rest it on the arm of the chair, the bed, or the resident's lap, with the palm upward.

5   Unroll the cuff and open the valve on the bulb. Squeeze the cuff to deflate the cuff completely.

6   Locate the brachial artery, on the thumb side of the inner elbow, by palpating with two or three fingers.

7   Wrap the cuff snugly around the resident's arm, centering the bladder over the brachial artery. The cuff should be one inch above the artery in the antecubital space, in front of the elbow.

8   Position the gauge so you can see the numbers clearly.

9   Confirm the location of the brachial artery.

10   Place the earpieces of the stethoscope in your ears. Position the diaphragm to the stethoscope over the brachial artery. The diaphragm should not be touching the blood pressure cuff. Hold the diaphragm in place with the fingers of your nondominant hand.

11   With your dominant hand, tighten the thumbscrew on the valve (turn clockwise) to close it. Do not tighten it so much that you will have difficulty releasing it.

12   Pump the bulb to inflate the cuff until the gauge reaches 160, or according to facility policy.

13   Slowly open the valve by turning the thumbscrew counterclockwise. Allow the air to escape slowly.

14   Listen for the sound of the pulse in the stethoscope. A few seconds will pass without sound. If you hear pulse sounds immediately, deflate the cuff. Wait a minute, then repeat the procedure, this time inflating the cuff to 200.

15   Note the number on the gauge when you hear the first sound. This is the systolic blood pressure.

16   Continue listening as the air escapes slowly from the cuff. You will hear a continuous pulse sound. Note the number on the gauge when the sounds disappear completely. This is the diastolic blood pressure.

17   After the sounds disappear entirely, open the thumbscrew completely to deflate the cuff.

18   Remove the stethoscope from your ears.

19   Remove the cuff from the resident's arm.

20   Record the blood pressure on your note pad. Blood pressure is recorded as a fraction, with the systolic reading first, followed by the diastolic reading, such as 120/80.

21   Roll the blood pressure cuff over the gauge and return it to the case.

(continued)

48   *continued*

22   Wipe the earpieces and diaphragm of the stethoscope with an alcohol sponge. If the stethoscope tubing came in contact with the bed linen, wipe it as well.

23   Perform your procedure completion actions.

24   Report blood pressure over 140/90 or under 100/60 to the nurse immediately, or according to facility policy.

REPORTING AND RECORDING VITAL SIGNS

It is a good idea to check the vital signs a second time if you think the values are abnormal. Report to the nurse any vital signs that are outside the normal range. Recording vital signs you have measured is an important part of your role as a nursing assistant. Accuracy and writing clearly are necessary. Your facility may require you to record the vital signs on a graphic sheet or on a daily flow sheet. Ask for help if you are unsure of the method your facility uses. Remember these abbreviations for vital signs:

T	temperature
P	pulse
R	respiration
BP	blood pressure
V.S.	vital signs (includes all of the above)

Proper Way to Record Vital Signs

Be sure to go about recording vital signs in the manner you have been taught:

1. List temperature first.
2. List the pulse count second.
3. List the respirations third.
4. Example: 98.6(O)- 80-16
5. Always write "R" after the temperature reading when the temperature is taken rectally.
6. Always write "A" or "AX" after the temperature reading when the temperature is taken by the axillary method.
7. Follow your facility policy for recording tympanic temperature readings.
8. Some facilities assume that the temperature is oral if no letter is written behind the reading. Other facilities use "O" to denote an oral temperature.
9. Write the blood pressure as a fraction, such as 120/80.
10. Record vital signs accurately.

MEASURING AND RECORDING HEIGHT AND WEIGHT

Measuring the resident's height and weight is the responsibility of the nursing assistant in the long-term care facility. Knowing the height and weight is very important to members of the interdisciplinary team. The dietitian uses the information to plan the diet. The physician uses the information to calculate doses of medications. If the resident has a heart or kidney condition, having an accurate weight is important so that gains or losses of fluid can be detected readily. The following points are important to remember when recording height and weight:

*   Follow your facility policy to learn how often to weigh residents. Some residents are weighed daily or weekly. Most residents are weighed once a month.

*   Obtaining the height and weight on the day of admission of a new resident is very important. Many individuals use this information when doing admission assessments.

*   Refer to the care plan, or follow the nurse's instructions regarding the method and time.

*   When recording weight, compare it with the previous month. If the difference is five pounds or more, recheck the weight.

*   Follow facility policy for reporting changes in weight to the nurse. Usually, the nurse is notified if there is a difference of five pounds or more from the previous weight.

Methods of Weighing Residents

There are several ways to weigh residents.

*   Balance scale (Figure 13-10). The resident must be able to stand without help to use this type of scale.

*   Chair scale. The chair scale is manufactured with a chair permanently mounted on it. The resident sits in the chair while you obtain the weight.

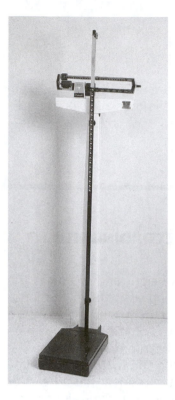

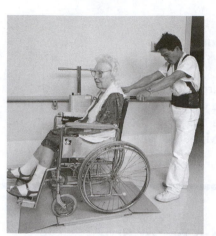

Figure 13-11 The wheelchair scale. Subtract the weight of the empty wheelchair from the total weight.

Figure 13-10 A balance scale may be used for residents who can stand independently.

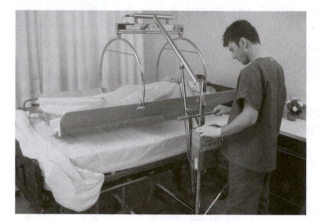

- Wheelchair scale (Figure 13-11). You must weigh the wheelchair without the resident before weighing him in the wheelchair. The weight of the chair is subtracted from the total weight.

- Bed scale (Figure 13-12). Bed scales are commonly attached to a mechanical lifting device. Make sure that the resident is not touching the bed when you obtain the weight.

Figure 13-12 The bed scale is used for nonambulatory residents who cannot sit in a chair. Make sure the sling is not touching the bed when you take the weight reading.

Methods of Measuring Height

- Balance scale. Most balance scales have a height bar that can be used for the resident who can stand. Follow your facility policy. In some facilities residents remove their shoes and stand on a paper towel.

- Tape measure. A tape measure is used to measure the resident who cannot stand. The resident lies in bed. Position the resident in the supine position. Straighten the resident's back, arms, and legs so that she is lying as straight as possible. Straighten and tighten the sheets. Place a pencil mark on the sheet even with the resident's head. Place another pencil mark at the level of the resident's heels. The distance between the two marks is measured with a tape measure to obtain the resident's height.

✓ GUIDELINES for Weight and Height Measurements

Follow these guidelines for taking accurate height and weight measurements:

- ☐ Weigh residents at the same time of day.
- ☐ Use the same scale each time the resident is weighed.
- ☐ Be certain scales are balanced before weighing the resident.
- ☐ Have the resident wear similar clothing each time he is weighed.

(continued)

✔ GUIDELINES for Weight and Height Measurements *(continued)*

❑ If you are taking a standing weight and height on a balance scale, have the resident remove his shoes and stand on a paper towel.

❑ Have the resident empty the bladder before being weighed.

❑ If the resident is wearing an incontinence brief, make sure it is dry before doing the weighing.

❑ If the resident has an indwelling catheter, make sure the bag is empty before doing the weighing.

❑ If the resident has a cast, has recently had a cast removed, or has new-onset edema, consult the nurse about possible weight discrepancies.

❑ If you are responsible for documenting the weight on the resident's chart, compare it with the previous month's weight. If there is a difference of 5 pounds or more (or according to facility policy), recheck the resident's weight. If, after rechecking the weight, there is still a difference, inform the nurse.

❑ There are electronic scales for standing weights, electronic chair scales, and electronic bed scales. Follow the manufacturer's directions for the type of scale you are using.

PERFORMANCE PROCEDURE

49   Measuring Weight and Height

Supplies needed:
- scale
- paper towels
- pad and pen

1 Perform your beginning procedure actions.

2 Standing scale:

a   Balance the scale.

b   Place a paper towel on the scale platform.

c   Assist the resident to remove shoes and stand on the platform.

d   Adjust the weights on the scale until the bar hangs freely on the end.

e   Add the weight on the two bars to determine the weight. Write this down on your note pad or remember it. (See Figure B-42 on page 298.)

f   Assist the resident to turn around, facing away from the scale.

g   Raise the height bar until it is level with the top of the head.

h   Record the measurement in the center of the height bar.

i   Help the resident down from the scale and assist to put on shoes, if necessary.

j   Remove and discard the paper towel.

3 Chair scale

a   Balance the scale.

b   Assist the resident to transfer from the wheelchair to the chair scale.

c   Place the resident's feet on the footrest of the chair.

d   Move the weights until the balance bar hangs freely, or read the electronic display screen. Remember this number or write it down on your note pad.

e   Transfer the resident back to the wheelchair.

4 Wheelchair scale

a   Balance the scale.

b   Obtain a wheelchair and take it to the scale and weigh it. Write down the weight.

- If the resident uses a lap tray on the wheelchair, remove the tray before weighing the resident. If the tray cannot be removed, weigh the tray and the wheelchair together during the first step of the procedure, then subtract the combined weight from the total. Lap trays can add as much as 8 pounds to the total weight.

c   Take the wheelchair to the resident's room and assist the resident to transfer into it.

d   Take the resident to the scale. Roll the wheelchair up the ramp and lock the brakes.

(continued)

49   *continued*

e   Adjust the weights until the balance bar hangs freely on the end. Write down this number on your note pad.

f   Unlock the brakes and slowly guide the wheelchair down the ramp.

g   Return to the resident's room and assist the resident to transfer out of the wheelchair.

h   Subtract the weight of the empty wheelchair from the total weight of the resident and chair and record this number.

5   Bed scale (follow the guidelines in Procedure 20 for assisting the resident into the lift seat or sling).

a   Balance the scale. The scale should be balanced with the canvas seat, chains, or straps attached.

b   Remove the sling from the scale and position the resident on the sling.

c   Connect the straps and elevate the lift above the level of the bed. Raise the sling so the resident's body and the sling hang freely over the bed.

d   Adjust the weights until the balance bar hangs freely on the end, or read the electronic display screen. Remember this number or write it on your note pad.

e   Lower the resident back into the bed and remove the sling.

6   Perform your procedure completion actions.

KEY POINTS IN THIS CHAPTER

▲ The vital signs tell you how well the body's vital organs are working.

▲ The body temperature can be measured using oral, rectal, axillary, or tympanic methods.

▲ The most commonly used site for taking the pulse is the radial artery in the wrist.

▲ When taking the respirations of a resident, hold the wrist as if taking the pulse.

▲ While measuring the blood pressure, note the systolic and diastolic pressure.

▲ Always report any unusual vital signs to the nurse immediately.

▲ Accuracy is very important when taking and recording vital signs.

▲ The nursing assistant is responsible for obtaining and accurately recording the residents' height and weight.

REVIEW QUIZ

1. Measuring the function of vital organs of the body is called taking:
   a. vital statistics.
   b. vital signs.
   c. blood pressure.
   d. pulse.

2. Which of the following may cause the body temperature to decrease?
   a. drinking coffee
   b. dehydration
   c. exercise
   d. shock

3. When reading the glass thermometer, each long line represents:
   a. one degree.
   b. one-tenth of a degree.
   c. two-tenths of a degree.
   d. five-tenths of a degree.

4. An oral temperature should *not* be used for the resident who:
   a. has dentures.
   b. is a mouth breather.
   c. has eaten in the past hour.
   d. used oxygen yesterday.

5. The thermometer must be lubricated before taking a/an:
   a. axillary temperature.
   b. oral temperature.
   c. rectal temperature.
   d. tympanic temperature.

6. The rhythmic expansion and contraction of an artery is called the:
   a. rate.
   b. pulse.
   c. volume.
   d. blood pressure.

7. What body system are you checking when you measure the pulse?
   a. respiratory
   b. digestive
   c. circulatory
   d. elimination

8. The pulse felt at the wrist is the:
   a. carotid.
   b. brachial.
   c. apical.
   d. radial.

9. Which of the following is *true* about counting the resident's respirations?
   a. Respirations are counted by watching the rise and fall of the chest.
   b. Counting of respirations is usually done simultaneously with counting the pulse.
   c. Always tell the resident when you begin counting the respirations.
   d. One rise and fall of the chest equals two respirations.

10. Measurement of the amount of force exerted on the walls of the arteries as blood flows through is:
    a. pulse.
    b. blood pressure.
    c. pressure factor.
    d. arterial pulse.

11. The resident's blood pressure reading is 130/84. The diastolic reading is:
    a. 214.
    b. 130.
    c. 84.
    d. 56.

12. What is hypertension?
    a. high blood pressure
    b. low blood pressure
    c. nervousness
    d. rapid pulse

13. What is your best action when you have taken the blood pressure of a resident and are not sure of the reading?
    a. Tell another nursing assistant.
    b. Look up the last reading and record the same numbers.
    c. Tell the nurse about your uncertainty and ask her what to do.
    d. Forget the reading and try to take the resident's blood pressure the next day.

14. What should you do when the measurements of any vital sign are abnormally high or low?
    a. Record the measurements on the chart at the end of your shift.
    b. Alert the nurse immediately to the abnormal measurements.
    c. Tell the resident and ask what he would like you to do.
    d. Report to the nurse at the end of your shift.

15. The proper way to record the temperature, pulse, and respirations is to write the:
    a. temperature first, pulse second, respirations third.
    b. respirations first, pulse second, temperature third.
    c. temperature first, respirations second, pulse last.
    d. respirations first, temperature second, pulse last.

16. You have just taken Mrs. Heinrich's weight. Last month she weighed 120 pounds. This month her weight has dropped to 80 pounds. You should:
    a. notify the nurse immediately.
    b. record the 80-pound weight on the flow sheet.
    c. recheck the weight.
    d. order a high-calorie food for the resident from the kitchen.

17. You were assigned to take the TPR and B/P on Mrs. James, an 84-year-old resident who recently was admitted after a stroke. The readings were B/P 132/82, T 98.8, P 96, R 42. Which of these readings is *not* in the normal range?
    a. blood pressure
    b. temperature
    c. pulse
    d. respirations

18. Ramona Kelley is a 72-year-old resident with kidney disease. She is on a fluid restriction. She goes to the dialysis center three times a week. You must take her vital signs when she returns from dialysis. The care plan states that you are to weigh her daily. Her weight on Monday is 133 pounds. On Tuesday, her weight is 140. You should:
    a. inform the nurse.
    b. record the weight on the flow sheet at the end of your shift.

c. call the dialysis center and ask their advice.
d. tell the resident she is drinking too many fluids.

19. Mrs. Springer is a 92-year-old resident with a diagnosis of chronic obstructive pulmonary disease. When you enter her room to give her breakfast, you find her sitting up in bed. She has a blue color around her lips. You count her respirations and find that they are 40 and appear shallow. You should:
a. feed Mrs. Springer breakfast.
b. leave the breakfast tray in the room and continue your assignment.

c. give the resident oxygen at 8 liters per minute.
d. advise the nurse of Mrs. Springer's condition immediately.

20. You take Bill Walker's blood pressure and find that it is 220/160. Mr. Walker has hypertension and previously had a stroke. You know that the blood pressure reading is:
a. too high.
b. normal for a resident with hypertension.
c. hypotensive.
d. too low.

CHAPTER 13
CROSSWORD PUZZLE

Directions: Complete the puzzle using these words found in Chapter 13.

aural
axillary
brachial
bradycardia
cyanosis
diastolic
dyspnea
exhalation
expiration
height
hypertension

hypotension
inhalation
inspiration
oral
oxygen
palpated
pressure
pulse
radial
rate
rectal

respiration
rhythm
sphygmomanometer
systolic
tachycardia
temperature
vital
volume
weight

CHAPTER 13
PUZZLE CLUES

ACROSS

1. The top number of the blood pressure that is recorded when the heart is working
6. High blood pressure above 140/90
7. _____ can be taken on a standing scale or a chair scale.
8. The pressure indicated on the blood pressure gauge when the radial pulse can no longer be felt is the _____ systolic pressure.
9. A colorless, odorless, tasteless gas necessary for human life
10. The pulse at the wrist is the _____ pulse.
11. Having to do with the armpit
14. Having to do with the mouth
16. Bluish color
17. Pulse more than 100 beats per minute
21. The exchange of oxygen and carbon dioxide in the body
24. The pulse felt on the inner side of the elbow
25. Measurement of how tall the resident is
28. Measurement of heat in the body
29. Shortness of breath
30. The number of pulse beats or respirations in a minute

DOWN

1. The blood pressure cuff
2. Temperature, pulse, respirations, and blood pressure are known as _____ signs.
3. The lower number of the blood pressure taken when the heart is resting
4. Another word for inhalation
5. Temperature taken in the anus
12. Blood _____
13. The beat of the heart that is felt when an artery is compressed against a bone
15. Breathing air out
18. Low blood pressure below 100/60
19. A pulse rate less than 60 beats per minute
20. The force of the blood moving through the blood vessels
22. Another word for exhalation
23. Breathing in
26. The regularity of the pulse
27. Having to do with the ear

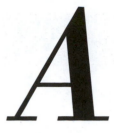

Anatomy Diagrams

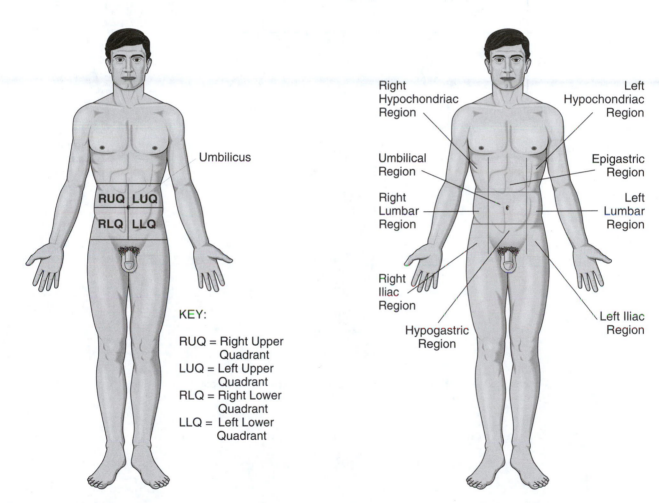

Umbilicus

| RUQ | LUQ |
| RLQ | LLQ |

KEY:

RUQ = Right Upper
        Quadrant
LUQ = Left Upper
        Quadrant
RLQ = Right Lower
        Quadrant
LLQ = Left Lower
        Quadrant

Right
Hypochondriac
Region

Left
Hypochondriac
Region

Umbilical
Region

Epigastric
Region

Right
Lumbar
Region

Left
Lumbar
Region

Right
Iliac
Region

Left Iliac
Region

Hypogastric
Region

A-1A The four abdominal quadrants

A-1B The abdomen can be divided into nine regions.

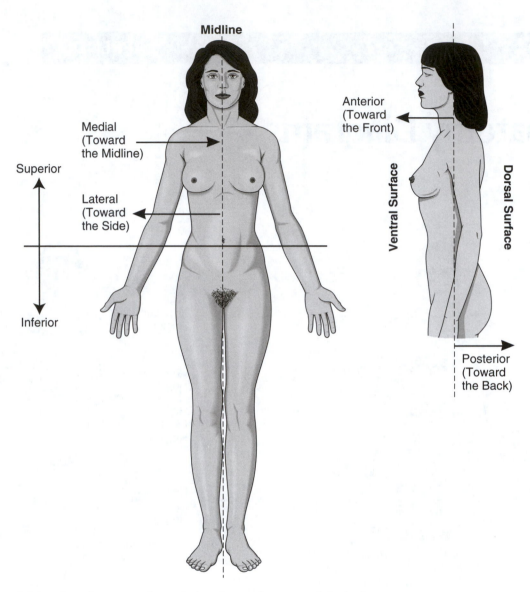

A-2 Imaginary lines are used to make it easier to refer to parts of the body.

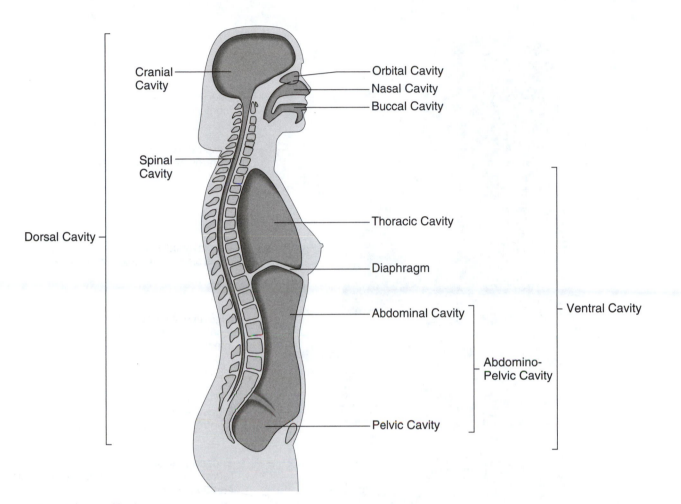

Cranial Cavity

Orbital Cavity

Nasal Cavity

Buccal Cavity

Spinal Cavity

Thoracic Cavity

Diaphragm

Dorsal Cavity

Abdominal Cavity

Ventral Cavity

Abdomino-Pelvic Cavity

Pelvic Cavity

A-3 Lateral view of body cavities

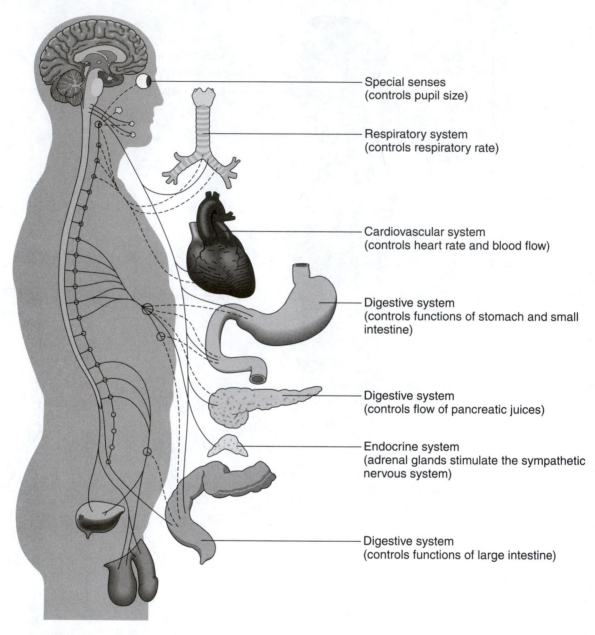

Special senses
(controls pupil size)

Respiratory system
(controls respiratory rate)

Cardiovascular system
(controls heart rate and blood flow)

Digestive system
(controls functions of stomach and small intestine)

Digestive system
(controls flow of pancreatic juices)

Endocrine system
(adrenal glands stimulate the sympathetic nervous system)

Digestive system
(controls functions of large intestine)

A-4 The autonomic nervous system

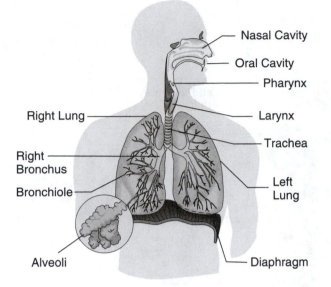

Nasal Cavity

Oral Cavity

Pharynx

Right Lung

Larynx

Trachea

Right Bronchus

Bronchiole

Left Lung

Alveoli

Diaphragm

A-5 The respiratory system

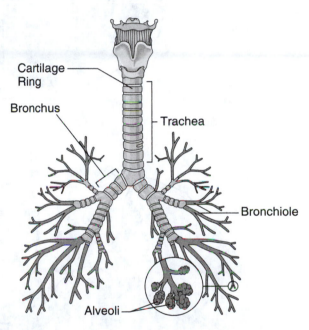

Cartilage Ring

Bronchus

Trachea

Bronchiole

Alveoli

A-6 Structures of the lower respiratory tract

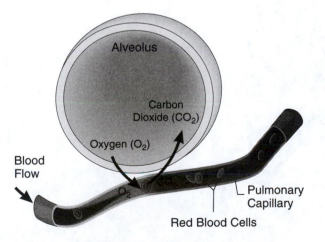

Alveolus

Carbon Dioxide (CO_2)

Oxygen (O_2)

Blood Flow

O_2

Pulmonary Capillary

Red Blood Cells

A-7 Oxygen and carbon dioxide exchange in the capillaries of the alveoli

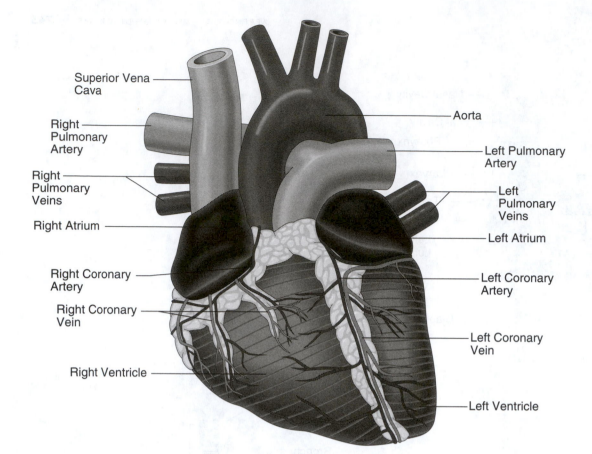

Superior Vena Cava

Right Pulmonary Artery

Right Pulmonary Veins

Right Atrium

Right Coronary Artery

Right Coronary Vein

Right Ventricle

Aorta

Left Pulmonary Artery

Left Pulmonary Veins

Left Atrium

Left Coronary Artery

Left Coronary Vein

Left Ventricle

A-8 The heart and blood vessels

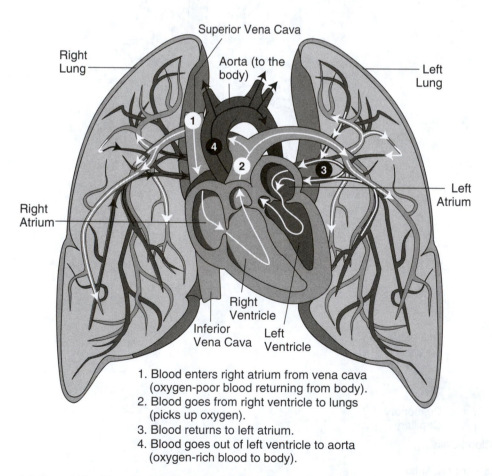

Superior Vena Cava

Right Lung

Aorta (to the body)

Left Lung

Left Atrium

Right Atrium

Inferior Vena Cava

Right Ventricle

Left Ventricle

1. Blood enters right atrium from vena cava (oxygen-poor blood returning from body).
2. Blood goes from right ventricle to lungs (picks up oxygen).
3. Blood returns to left atrium.
4. Blood goes out of left ventricle to aorta (oxygen-rich blood to body).

A-9 Flow of blood from the heart to the lungs, to the body, and back to the heart, where the cycle begins again.

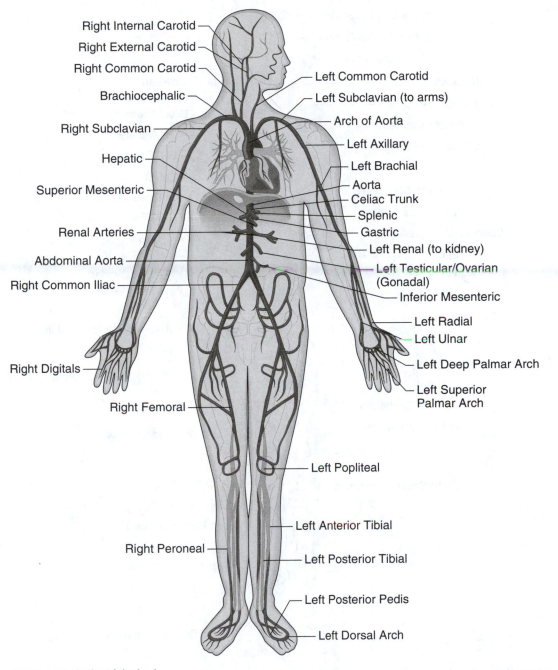

Right Internal Carotid

Right External Carotid

Right Common Carotid

Brachiocephalic

Right Subclavian

Hepatic

Superior Mesenteric

Renal Arteries

Abdominal Aorta

Right Common Iliac

Right Digitals

Right Femoral

Right Peroneal

Left Common Carotid

Left Subclavian (to arms)

Arch of Aorta

Left Axillary

Left Brachial

Aorta

Celiac Trunk

Splenic

Gastric

Left Renal (to kidney)

Left Testicular/Ovarian (Gonadal)

Inferior Mesenteric

Left Radial

Left Ulnar

Left Deep Palmar Arch

Left Superior Palmar Arch

Left Popliteal

Left Anterior Tibial

Left Posterior Tibial

Left Posterior Pedis

Left Dorsal Arch

A-10 Major arteries of the body

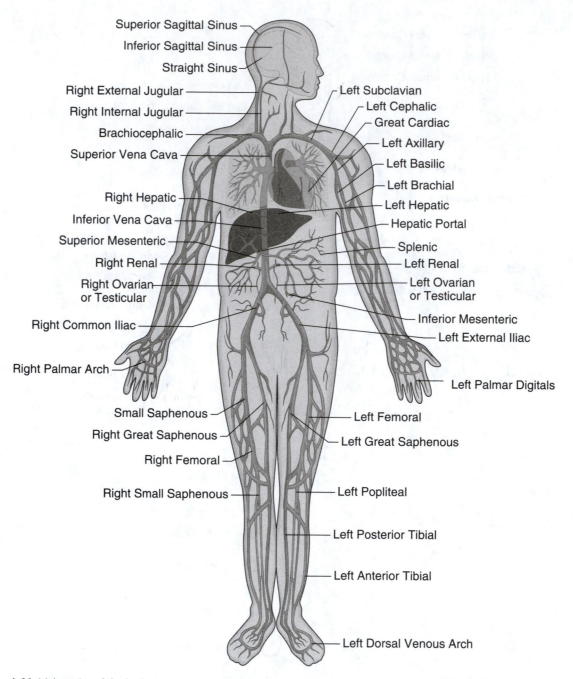

Superior Sagittal Sinus
Inferior Sagittal Sinus
Straight Sinus
Right External Jugular
Right Internal Jugular
Brachiocephalic
Superior Vena Cava
Right Hepatic
Inferior Vena Cava
Superior Mesenteric
Right Renal
Right Ovarian or Testicular
Right Common Iliac
Right Palmar Arch
Small Saphenous
Right Great Saphenous
Right Femoral
Right Small Saphenous

Left Subclavian
Left Cephalic
Great Cardiac
Left Axillary
Left Basilic
Left Brachial
Left Hepatic
Hepatic Portal
Splenic
Left Renal
Left Ovarian or Testicular
Inferior Mesenteric
Left External Iliac
Left Palmar Digitals
Left Femoral
Left Great Saphenous
Left Popliteal
Left Posterior Tibial
Left Anterior Tibial
Left Dorsal Venous Arch

A-11 Major veins of the body

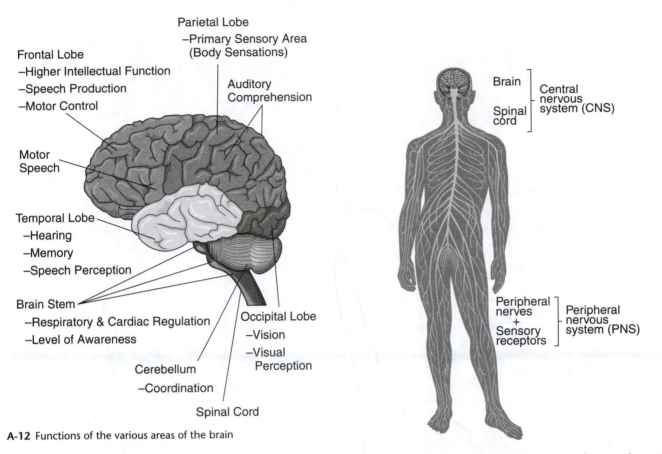

Frontal Lobe
–Higher Intellectual Function
–Speech Production
–Motor Control

Parietal Lobe
–Primary Sensory Area
(Body Sensations)

Auditory
Comprehension

Motor
Speech

Temporal Lobe
–Hearing
–Memory
–Speech Perception

Brain Stem
–Respiratory & Cardiac Regulation
–Level of Awareness

Occipital Lobe
–Vision
–Visual
Perception

Cerebellum
–Coordination

Spinal Cord

Brain
Spinal
cord
Central
nervous
system (CNS)

Peripheral
nerves
+
Sensory
receptors
Peripheral
nervous
system (PNS)

A-12 Functions of the various areas of the brain

A-14 The peripheral nervous system connects the central nervous system to the various parts of the body. Messages are relayed to these structures through the brain and spinal cord.

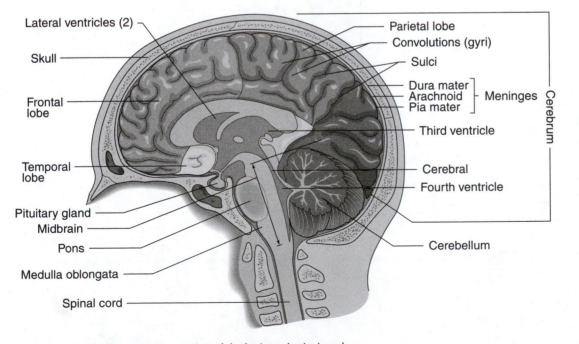

Lateral ventricles (2)

Skull

Frontal
lobe

Temporal
lobe

Pituitary gland

Midbrain

Pons

Medulla oblongata

Spinal cord

Parietal lobe
Convolutions (gyri)
Sulci
Dura mater
Arachnoid
Pia mater
Meninges
Cerebrum
Third ventricle
Cerebral
Fourth ventricle
Cerebellum

A-13 The central nervous system consists of the brain and spinal cord.

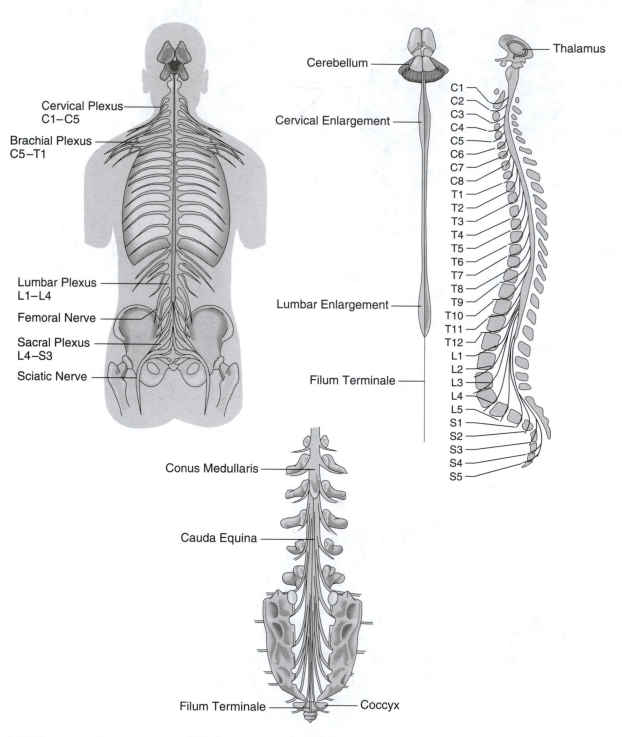

A-15 Nerves controlling various parts of the body

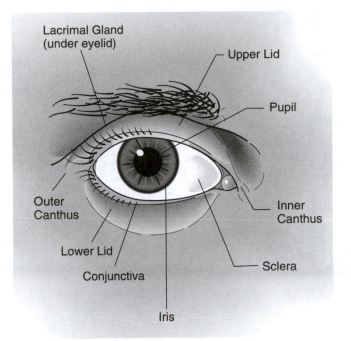

Lacrimal Gland
(under eyelid)

Upper Lid

Pupil

Outer
Canthus

Inner
Canthus

Lower Lid

Sclera

Conjunctiva

Iris

A-16 Structures of the external eye

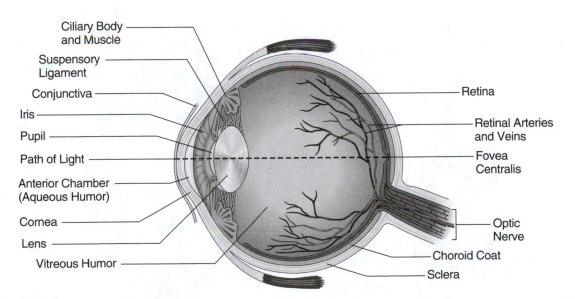

Ciliary Body
and Muscle

Suspensory
Ligament

Conjunctiva

Iris

Pupil

Path of Light

Anterior Chamber
(Aqueous Humor)

Cornea

Lens

Vitreous Humor

Retina

Retinal Arteries
and Veins

Fovea
Centralis

Optic
Nerve

Choroid Coat

Sclera

A-17 Internal structures of the eye

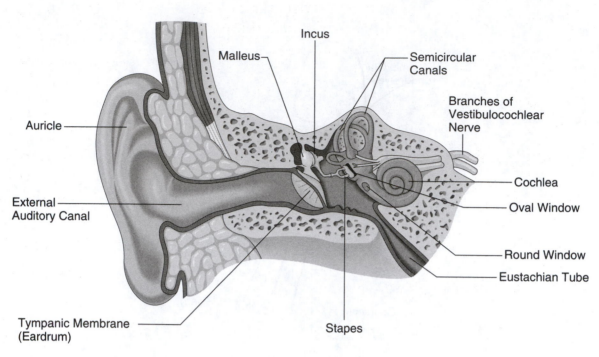

Incus

Malleus

Semicircular
Canals

Branches of
Vestibulocochlear
Nerve

Auricle

External
Auditory Canal

Cochlea

Oval Window

Round Window

Eustachian Tube

Tympanic Membrane
(Eardrum)

Stapes

A-18 Internal structures of the ear

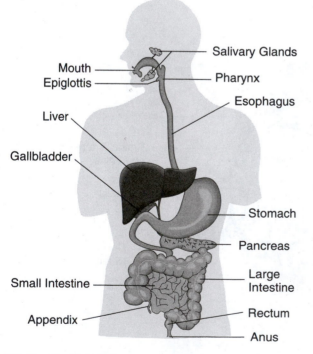

Salivary Glands

Mouth

Pharynx

Epiglottis

Esophagus

Liver

Gallbladder

Stomach

Pancreas

Small Intestine

Large
Intestine

Appendix

Rectum

Anus

A-19A The digestive system

Upper Lip

Incisors

Hard Palate

Soft Palate

Uvula

Posterior
Pharynx

Tonsil

Molars

Papillae
(Taste Buds)

Gingiva (Gums)

Lower Lip

A-19B Structures of the mouth

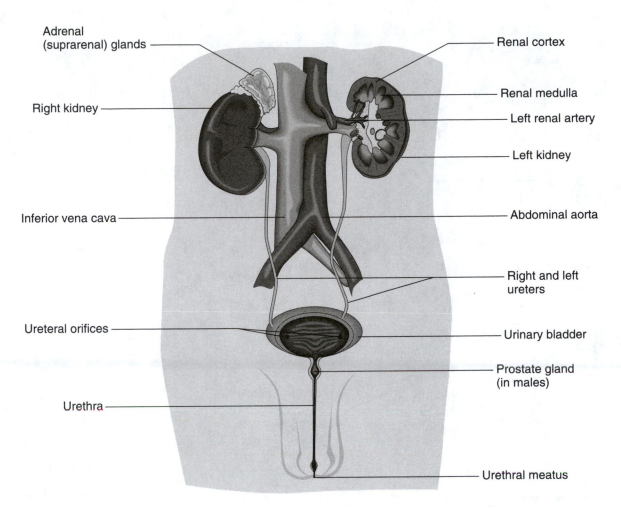

Adrenal (suprarenal) glands

Right kidney

Inferior vena cava

Ureteral orifices

Urethra

Renal cortex

Renal medulla

Left renal artery

Left kidney

Abdominal aorta

Right and left ureters

Urinary bladder

Prostate gland (in males)

Urethral meatus

A-20 The urinary system

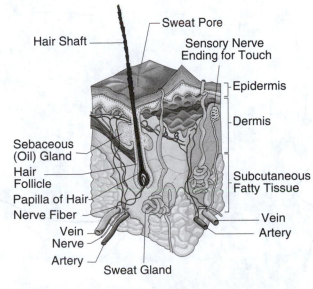

Hair Shaft

Sweat Pore

Sensory Nerve Ending for Touch

Epidermis

Dermis

Sebaceous (Oil) Gland

Hair Follicle

Papilla of Hair

Nerve Fiber

Vein
Nerve

Artery

Sweat Gland

Subcutaneous Fatty Tissue

Vein

Artery

A-21 Cross-section of the skin

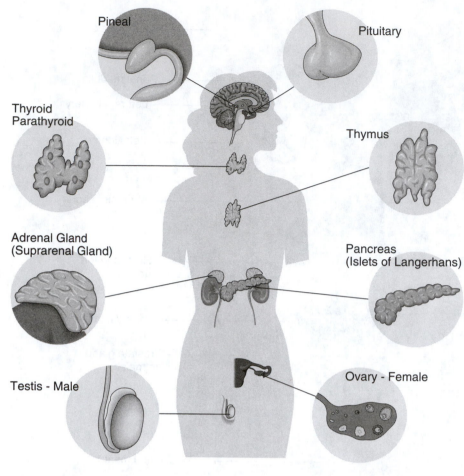

Pineal

Pituitary

Thyroid
Parathyroid

Thymus

Adrenal Gland
(Suprarenal Gland)

Pancreas
(Islets of Langerhans)

Testis - Male

Ovary - Female

A-22 The endocrine system

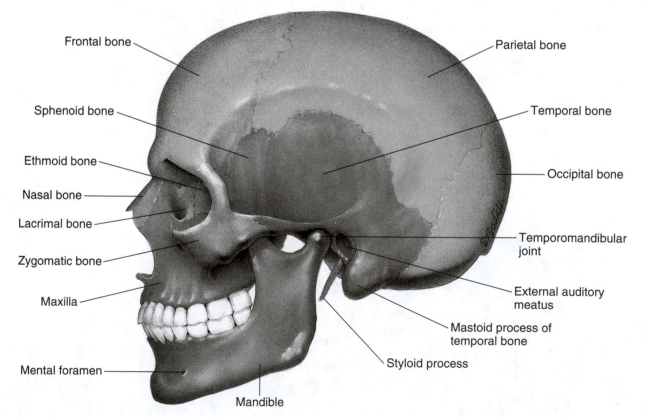

Frontal bone

Parietal bone

Sphenoid bone

Temporal bone

Ethmoid bone

Nasal bone

Lacrimal bone

Occipital bone

Zygomatic bone

Temporomandibular
joint

Maxilla

External auditory
meatus

Mental foramen

Mastoid process of
temporal bone

Styloid process

Mandible

A-23 Bones of the skull

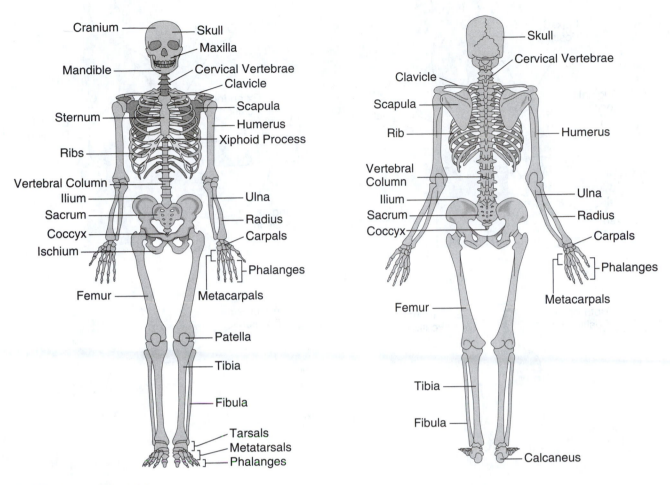

A-24 Major bones of the skeleton

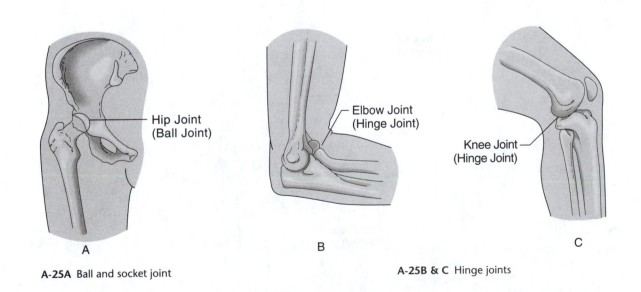

A-25A Ball and socket joint

A-25B & C Hinge joints

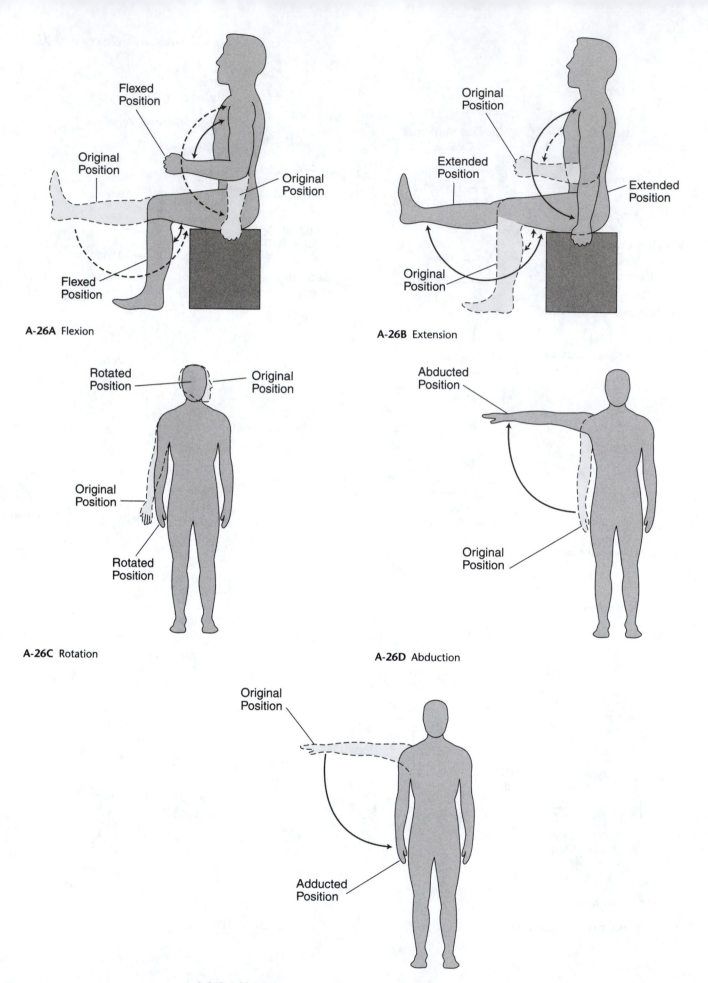

A-26A Flexion

Flexed Position

Original Position

Original Position

Flexed Position

A-26B Extension

Original Position

Extended Position

Extended Position

Original Position

A-26C Rotation

Rotated Position

Original Position

Original Position

Rotated Position

A-26D Abduction

Abducted Position

Original Position

A-26E Adduction

Original Position

Adducted Position

256

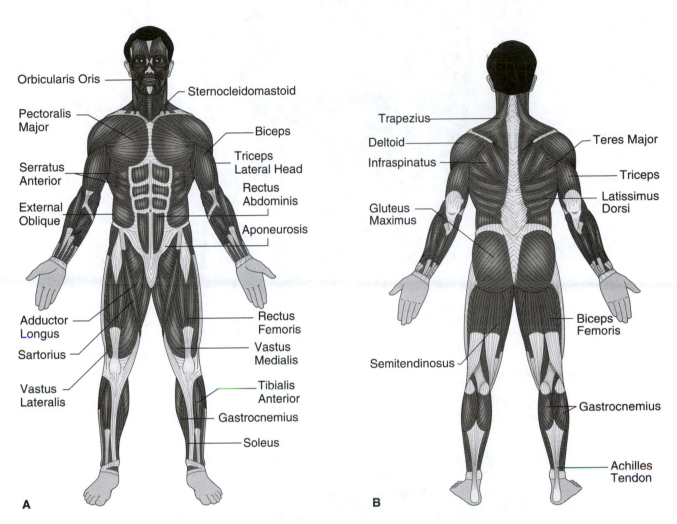

A-27A & B Major muscles of the body

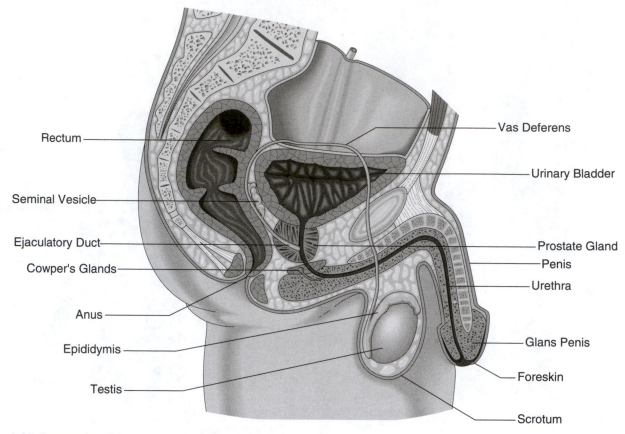

Rectum

Seminal Vesicle

Ejaculatory Duct

Cowper's Glands

Anus

Epididymis

Testis

Vas Deferens

Urinary Bladder

Prostate Gland

Penis

Urethra

Glans Penis

Foreskin

Scrotum

A-28 Cross-section of the male reproductive system and genitalia

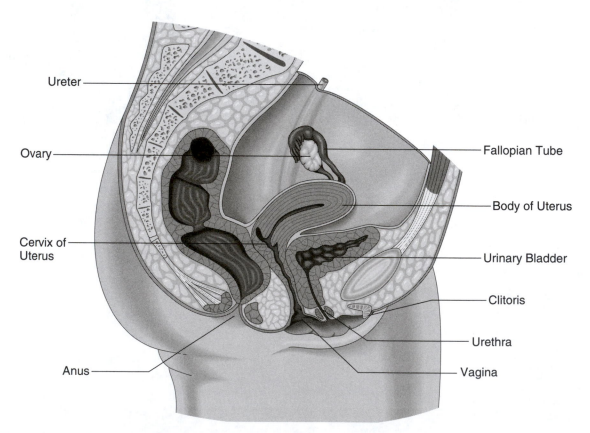

Ureter

Ovary

Cervix of
Uterus

Anus

Fallopian Tube

Body of Uterus

Urinary Bladder

Clitoris

Urethra

Vagina

A-29 Cross-section of the female reproductive system and genitalia

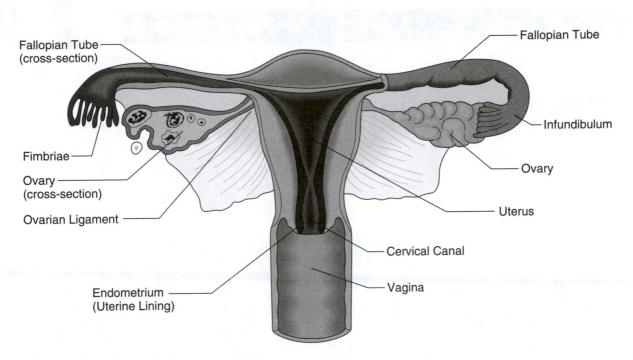

Fallopian Tube
(cross-section)

Fallopian Tube

Infundibulum

Fimbriae

Ovary
(cross-section)

Ovary

Ovarian Ligament

Uterus

Cervical Canal

Endometrium
(Uterine Lining)

Vagina

A-30 Internal female reproductive organs

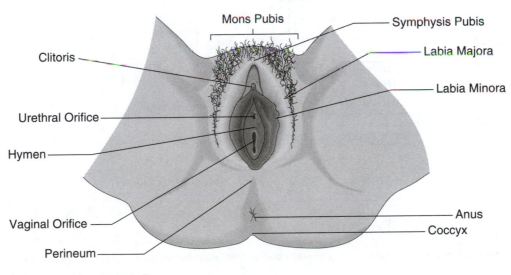

Mons Pubis

Symphysis Pubis

Clitoris

Labia Majora

Labia Minora

Urethral Orifice

Hymen

Vaginal Orifice

Anus

Coccyx

Perineum

A-31 External female genitalia

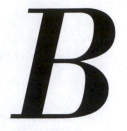

Useful Information

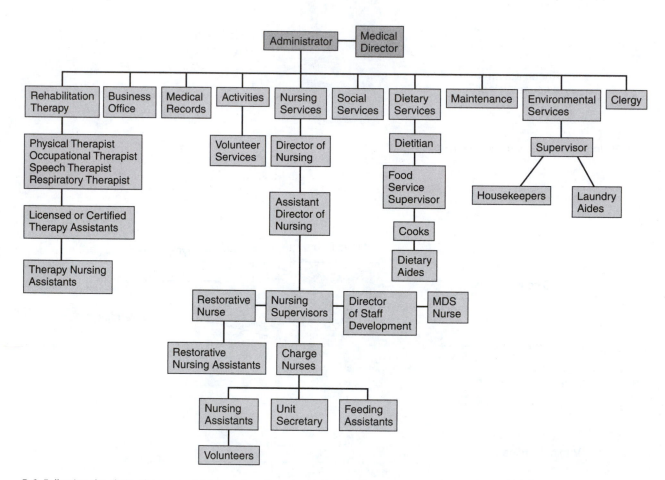

B-1 Following the chain of command for reporting shows respect and enhances communication in the long-term care facility.

Interdisciplinary Health Care Team Members

Team Member	Responsibilities
Provide Most of the Direct Care Services to Residents	
Licensed Nurse (licensed nurses may be either RNs or LPN/LVNs)	Directs the care of residents, administers medications, and performs treatments. Supervises and directs nursing assistant staff.
Nursing Assistant (NA, CNA, or STNA)	Provides most of the personal care to residents under the supervision of the licensed nurse. The nursing assistant spends more time with the residents than other team members.
Medication Aide (MA) (Certified Medication Assistant [CMA]) (Medication Technician [MT])	A certified nursing assistant who has met certain criteria, taken additional classes in medication administration methods, and completed a state certification examination. Allowed to pass medications in skilled nursing facilities, assisted living facilities, and home health care in 25 states.
Restorative Nursing Assistant (RNA)	A certified nursing assistant who has additional education and experience in restorative nursing care. Delivers care designed to assist the resident to attain and maintain his or her highest level of function, and prevent physical deformities.
Dining Assistant (Feeding Assistant, Nutrition Assistant)	A single-task worker with at least 8 hours education in nutrition and hydration. Assists stable residents with eating and drinking. May not assist residents with complex feeding problems.
Dietary Staff Member	Prepares meals and is responsible for ordering groceries, washing dishes, and other kitchen duties.
Registered Dietitian (RD)	Writes the menus for meals prepared by the dietary department. Responsible for seeing that residents on special diets receive the right food in the proper amounts. Assesses each resident's individual dietary needs; calculates individual calorie, fluid, and other requirements; and makes recommendations for care of chronic illnesses and complications.
Activities	Provides activities for resident enjoyment. Some activities are done to provide exercise for residents. Other types of activities are designed to provide positive self-esteem. Activities also provide opportunities for residents to socialize with others.
Social Service Worker (LSW or SSD)	Helps meet residents' mental and emotional needs. Coordinates functions with personnel and agencies inside and outside the facility to see that resident needs are met. When it is time for the resident to be discharged home or to another health care agency, the social worker coordinates the resources the resident will need and makes the transition as smooth as possible. An LSW is a licensed social worker. The SSD is a social services designee.
Physical Therapist (PT, LPT)	Helps residents regain strength and physical function lost because of illness or injury. The goal of the therapist is to help the resident achieve the highest possible level of physical function. The physical therapist also teaches residents and staff how to perform physical activities in a safe manner. A physical therapy assistant (PTA) may assist with physical therapy services.

Continues

B-2 Interdisciplinary team members

Interdisciplinary Health Care Team Members, *Continued*

Team Member	Responsibilities
Occupational Therapist (OT, OTR/L)	Helps residents regain strength and physical function lost because of illness or injury. This therapist helps residents to relearn self-care skills, such as feeding, bathing, grooming, and dressing. The goal of care is to help the resident become as independent as possible. Residents who have lost physical function may be able to use adaptive or self-help devices to be independent. The occupational therapist helps residents obtain these devices and learn how to use them. The OT may also fabricate or order splints and other equipment to prevent deformities. An occupational therapy assistant (OTA) may assist in providing occupational therapy services.
Respiratory Care Practitioner (RCP)	Works with residents who have breathing problems and those who need oxygen and other special treatments for their lungs. The goal of the treatment is to see that residents receive enough oxygen to meet their needs.
Speech Language Pathologist (SLP)	Works with residents who have diseases or injuries that have affected their ability to speak properly. This therapist also helps residents who have swallowing problems to learn to eat and drink without choking.
Physician (MD or DO)	Orders the resident's medical plan of care. Medications, diagnostic tests, and treatments must be ordered by the physician.
Clinical Nurse Specialist (CNS)	An advanced-practice registered nurse with a master's degree who focuses on a very specific resident population (e.g., medical, surgical, diabetic, cardiovascular, operating room, emergency room, critical care, geriatric, neonatal, etc.).
Nurse Practitioner (NP)	A registered nurse with advanced academic and clinical experience, which enables him or her to diagnose and manage common acute and chronic illnesses, either independently or as part of a health care team. A nurse practitioner provides some care previously offered only by physicians and in most states is legally permitted to prescribe medications.
Physician Assistant (PA)	A health care professional licensed to practice medicine with physician supervision. PAs conduct physical examinations, diagnose and treat illnesses, order and interpret tests, counsel on preventive health care, assist in surgery, and in most states are permitted to write prescriptions. Because of the close working relationship the PA has with the physician, PAs are educated in the medical model designed to complement physician training.
Provide Less Direct Resident Care	
Clergy	Members of the clergy are pastors of religious institutions or other religious workers who help residents meet their spiritual needs.
Bookkeeping or Office Worker	Responsible for answering the telephone, recordkeeping, and taking care of business and financial functions.
Medical Records Worker	Keeps permanent records of residents' care and treatment. Records are an important tool for communication with other members of the health care team. They are legal documents that may be used in court.
Maintenance Worker*	Responsible for seeing that the building and equipment are safe and in good repair at all times.
Laundry Worker*	Washes facility linen and keeps the nursing units supplied with sheets, towels, and other items needed to care for residents. The laundry worker in most long-term care facilities also washes residents' personal clothing.
Housekeeping Personnel*	Keeps the facility clean and sanitary.
Beautician/Barber	Provides haircuts and other services needed to care for residents' hair.

*These departments may be combined into one environmental service department.

Types of Abuse

Type of abuse	Description
Physical abuse	Willful, nonaccidental injury, such as handling a resident roughly or striking, slapping, or hitting a resident
Verbal abuse	Swearing, using demeaning terms to talk to a resident, or embarrassing a resident
Mental abuse	Threatening to harm a resident or threatening to withhold food, fluid, or care as a form of punishment
Sexual abuse	• Physical force or verbal threats are used to force a resident to perform a sexual act • Touching or fondling a resident inappropriately • Any behavior that is seductive, sexually demeaning, harassing, or reasonably interpreted as sexual by the resident

B-3 Examples of various types of abuse

Stages of Grief

Stages of Grief	Response of the Nursing Assistant
Denial	Reflect the resident's statements, but try not to confirm or deny the fact that the resident is dying. *Example: "The lab tests can't be right. I don't have cancer."* *"It must have been difficult for you to learn the results of your tests."*
Anger	Understand the source of the resident's anger. Provide understanding and support. Listen. Try to meet reasonable needs and demands quickly. *Example: "This food is terrible—not fit to eat."* *"Let me see if I can find something that would appeal to you more."*
Bargaining	If it is possible to meet the resident's requests, do so. Listen attentively. *Example: "If only God will spare me this, I'll go to church every week."* *"Would you like a visit from your clergy person?"*
Depression	Avoid clichés that dismiss the resident's depression ("It could be worse. You could be in more pain"). Be caring and supportive. Let the resident know that it is okay to be depressed. *Example: "There just isn't any sense in going on."* *"I understand you are feeling very depressed."*
Acceptance	Do not assume that, because the resident has accepted death, she or he is unafraid, or that she or he does not need emotional support. Listen attentively and be supportive and caring. *Example: "I feel so alone."* *"I am here with you. Would you like to talk?"*

B-4 Nursing assistant responses during the phases of the grieving process

Behavior Observations to Make and Report
Always report abnormal behavior to the nurse, even if you believe the behavior is "normal for the resident."
Who? Does the behavior involve another person or specific types of people? How are these individuals alike?
What? Describe the behavior. What were the circumstances in which the behavior occurred?
Where? Did the behavior occur in one specific location?
When? What is the time of day? Does the behavior occur at predictable times or in predictable situations, such as during bathing? When the resident is tired, when the resident awakens, or other times?
What were the environmental conditions? Was it light, dark, hot, cold, noisy, quiet?
How do others respond to the resident's behavior? Is there anyone who is never approached by the resident? If so, how does he or she manage or prevent the behavior?
Is there a pattern or clues to the behavior? Can you identify clues or signals that the behavior is about to begin?

B-5 Become familiar with the behavior care plan and implement it before the resident loses control. Your objective observations of the resident's behavior and response to the plan are important and should be reported to the nurse. Reinforce or reward appropriate resident behavior. Residents tend to repeat behavior that is rewarded.

Wanderers

Type of Wanderer	Characteristics	Approaches
Exit seeker/escapist wanderer	• Very high risk for leaving the facility. • The resident may not know where he or she is, but knows that he or she does not want to be there. • May be ambulatory or in a wheelchair. • Resident looks for opportunities to exit and leaves very quickly if presented with an opportunity. • Completely unaware of personal safety. • May not be properly dressed for the outside climate. • Uses very poor judgment. • Probably has a destination in mind.	• Try to determine the resident's intended location in advance. • Avoid arguing or using reality orientation, which agitate the resident. • Use distraction. • This wanderer is usually not looking for a physical location, but instead a state of mind. Try to provide it. If the resident says he or she must go to work, provide the state of mind by talking about the job, responsibilities, and so forth. • Make the resident feel good about himself or herself. • Remove hats, coats, coat rack, purses, shoes, and other items associated with going outside.
Critical/self-stimulation wanderer	• Completely disoriented. • Unaware of safety. • At very high risk of serious injury outside the facility. • Not deliberately trying to leave the facility. • If resident turns a doorknob or pushes the panic bar on the door for stimulation, he or she will exit.	• Close monitoring and supervision. • Diversional activity. • Exercise. • Walking in a small group inside the facility. • Responds well to repetition, structure, predictability, and familiar routines.
Akathisia wanderer	• Resident who has taken psychiatric drugs (chemical restraints) for many years. • Wandering is a side effect of years of drug therapy. • Very restless. • Wanders aimlessly with no apparent purpose. • May cross arms in front of the chest or abdomen when wandering. • Usually does not try to leave the facility.	• Close monitoring and supervision. • Diversional activity. • Exercise. • Walking in a small group inside the facility. • Responds well to repetition, structure, predictability, and familiar routines.
Purposeful wanderer	• Has a specific agenda, but is unable to communicate what it is. • May be looking for the bathroom. • May be bored. • May be overstimulated by noise and other factors in the environment. • May be in pain. • May be hungry or thirsty. • May be stressed and feeling overwhelmed. • May be dehydrated.	• Through trial and error, attempt to learn the resident's agenda and meet it.

Continues

B-6 A key to understanding wandering behavior is to realize that there are different types of wanderers. If the type of wandering behavior can be identified, approaches can be planned to keep the resident safe.

Wanderers, *Continued*

Type of Wanderer	Characteristics	Approaches
Aimless wanderer	• Totally disoriented. May think he or she is in own residence. • Frequently wanders into others' rooms. • May rummage through others' belongings. • Will enter housekeeping closets and unlocked service areas. • Totally unaware of personal safety. • Usually very upsetting to other residents and stressful for facility staff.	• Place cloth shields over doorknobs to change the texture. • Tape paper streamers across doorways. • Post signs that say "Stop," "Do Not Enter," or "Construction Zone." • Provide a dresser or nightstand of items to rummage through in the hallways. • Give the resident a repetitious task, such as folding towels or sorting coins.
Modeling wanderer	• Wander in pairs, usually for stimulation and companionship. • If the first resident exits the facility, the second resident will follow. • Usually completely unaware of safety.	• Provide diversional activities. • Determine the leader's agenda and keep him or her in the facility. • Place dark tile or construction paper on the floor by the doorway. It appears to be a hole, and residents usually will not attempt to cross it.

B-6

Managing Inappropriate Sexual Behavior

Behavior	Possible Trigger (Antecedent)	Approaches
Sexually suggestive comments, inappropriate sexual behavior	• Needs more affection, sense of belonging, need to be touched • As dementia progresses, the need for human contact is often expressed more physically • Environment reminds resident of sex • Fatigue, sensory overload, discomfort, boredom	• Focus on the person, not the behavior • Remain calm, do not overreact • Inform the resident that the behavior is not appropriate • Redirect the resident calmly and firmly • Involve the resident in an activities program • Do something the resident likes, such as listening to music, taking a walk, or having a snack • Give the resident something else to do • Leave and return later • Change your behavior • Change your physical position or approach • Touch the resident in an appropriate manner, such as by putting lotion on arms and hands • Find ways of incorporating appropriate touch into daily routine • Offer soothing objects to touch, fondle, and hold, such as stuffed animals or dolls • Assist in making the resident look good and feel physically attractive • If the behavior occurs at a certain time of day, keep the resident involved in a purposeful activity during this time • Do an environmental audit. Hot? Cold? Too much stimulation? Too little stimulation? • Offer to take the resident to the bathroom • Move the resident to another location • Encourage and reward appropriate behavior • Be aware of cues indicating unmet intimacy needs
Sexual gestures with staff or inappropriate touching during personal care or ADLs	• Misinterprets caregiver's intention • Resident misinterprets cues, perceives another's touch as sexual, such as touching or sitting next to the resident and touching his or her body with yours • Environment reminds resident of sex • Mistakes caregiver for his or her partner	• Distract during personal care • Avoid sending the resident mixed sexual messages, even in a joking manner • Ask a caregiver of the same sex (as the resident) to provide personal care • Remain calm, do not overreact • Inform the resident that the behavior is not appropriate • Respond to the resident in a matter-of-fact manner • Be aware that the behavior is a symptom of the resident's illness • Be aware of your own behavior, body language, and the message you send • Decide ahead of time how you will react if a resident makes inappropriate sexual advances. Advance planning will help you react appropriately when confronted with the situation

Continues

B-7 Types of inappropriate sexual behavior, potential triggers, and ways of managing the behavior

Managing Inappropriate Sexual Behavior, *Continued*		
Behavior	**Possible Trigger (Antecedent)**	**Approaches**
Removing clothes Exposing self Undressing in public Wearing only a shirt	• Too hot in environment • Need to use the bathroom • Clothing uncomfortable • Memory loss, forgets to put on clothes • Unaware of environment; may think he is in his bedroom or getting ready to bathe • Tired, wants to go to bed • Does not remember rules of social behavior	• Check and modify room temperature • Take to bathroom • Make sure clothing fits properly, is comfortable and not too tight • Allow resident to rest in bed • Dress in clothing that opens in back or is difficult to remove (do not put clothing on inside out or backward, use clothing designed to open in back)
Public masturbation or fondling self	• Genital irritation • Reacts to what feels good • No longer has judgment, awareness of appropriate behavior	• Check for irritation at an appropriate time • Remove from public area and provide privacy • Give resident repetitive manual activities to do, such as folding towels
Inappropriate advances toward other residents Sexual behavior with another resident Touching someone else in an inappropriate way	• Other person may remind the resident of a former partner • Other resident may be giving cues that are perceived as sexual advances, such as a woman lifting her skirt • Mistakes other resident for a former partner	• Calmly and firmly inform resident that the behavior is not appropriate • Keep residents separated as much as possible • Monitor helpless residents carefully; protect helpless residents • Seat away from residents of the opposite sex • Have care provided by staff member of same sex as the resident

B-7

Nursing Assistant Observations

Activity	Observations
Activities of daily living	• What the resident can do independently • The resident's need for assistance, how much assistance, type of assistance needed • The resident's ability to tolerate activity (does he become fatigued, short of breath, etc.) • The resident's motivation, preferences, abilities
Dressing and grooming	• Overall appearance—tidy, untidy, neat, clean
Walking	• Difficulty getting up and down • Need for an assistive device, such as a cane or walker • Safety awareness • Gait steady, unsteady, shuffling, rigid, etc. • Posture • Sudden onset of falls, difficulty balancing
Position, movement	• Ability to position/reposition self • Need for staff to reposition • Special positioning aids • Ability to move unassisted • Presence of contractures • Able/unable to move • Movements shaky, jerking, tremors, muscle spasms, etc. • Presence or absence of pain upon movement • Deformity, edema • Normal or abnormal range of motion • Ability to sit, stand, move, or walk
Eating	• Food likes and dislikes, refusals • Feeding ability, need for assistance, how much assistance, type of assistance needed • Percentage of meal consumed • Difficulty chewing or swallowing, coughing, choking
Drinking	• Ability to take a drink at will without assistance • Ability to drink from straw, cup, or need for special device • Need for assistance, how much assistance, type of assistance needed • Beverage preferences • Accepts or refuses water, if offered • Fluid intake • Difficulty swallowing liquids, coughing, choking
Urinary elimination	• Frequency of elimination • Inability to urinate, or voiding frequently in small amounts • Will the resident use the bathroom if given the opportunity? • Is the resident incontinent? • Color, clarity, odor, amount of urine • Presence of mucus, sediment, or other abnormalities in urine • Pain, burning, frequency of urination • Does the resident have a urinary catheter; if so, is it draining properly, leaking, etc.?
Bowel elimination	• Frequency of elimination • Will the resident use the bathroom if given the opportunity? • Is the resident incontinent? • Appearance of stool, presence of blood, mucus, parasites, or foreign matter; liquid or solid stool • Abnormal color stool (black, clay color, etc.) • Small or extremely large stool • Loose, watery stool • Complaints of pain, constipation, diarrhea, bleeding • Excessive gas (flatus)

Continues

B-8 Making observations, communicating with residents and other staff, reporting, and recording are important skills to master.

Nursing Assistant Observations, *Continued*	
Gastrointestinal system	• Frequent belching • Fruity smell to breath • Complaints of indigestion, gas (flatus), nausea, vomiting • Choking • Abdominal pain • Abdominal distention (swelling) • Oral or rectal bleeding • Vomitus, stool, or drainage from a nasogastric tube that looks like coffee grounds • Condition of mouth and teeth; report ulcerations, pain, drainage, obvious cavities, lesions on lips or inside mouth, abscesses, cracked or broken teeth, loose teeth, abnormalities such as grinding teeth • Dentures fit properly and do not cause pain or pressure • Dentures in good repair and marked with name or initials according to facility policy • Teeth/dentures clean, breath is fresh • Moisture of lips and mucous membranes inside mouth versus dry, chapped lips or dry mucous membranes (report)
Level of consciousness	• Conscious • Unconscious • Change in consciousness, awareness, or alertness • Ability to respond verbally or nonverbally • Sleepiness for no apparent reason
Sleeping	• Ability to sleep, or can't sleep • Sleeps constantly • Awakens easily • Difficult to awaken • Moves about in sleep • Need to be awakened for toileting • Repositions self or needs to be repositioned by staff
Skin	• Skin dry, oily, normal • Redness, unusual skin color, such as blue or gray color of the skin, lips, nailbeds, roof of mouth, or mucous membranes • Redness in the skin that does not go away within 30 minutes after pressure is relieved from a bony prominence or pressure area • In dark or yellow-skinned residents, spots or areas that are darker in appearance than normal skin tone • Pressure ulcers, open areas/skin breakdown, skin tears, abrasions, lacerations • Irritation, rash, bruises, skin discoloration, swelling, lumps, abnormal skin growths, change in color of a wart or mole, hives • Abnormal sweating, excessive heat or coolness to touch • Drainage • Foul odor
	• Complaints such as numbness, burning, tingling, itching • Signs of infection • Skin growths • Poor skin turgor/tenting of skin on forehead or over sternum • Edema, swelling • Moisture of lips and mucous membranes inside mouth
Cardiovascular system	• Pulse rate, regularity, strength • Blood pressure • Presence or absence of chest pain • Color, appearance of skin, nailbeds, mucous membranes

Continues

Nursing Assistant Observations, *Continued*	
Respiratory system	• Respiratory rate, rhythm, regularity • Respirations noisy, labored, quiet • Shortness of breath, gasping for breath, Cheyne-Stokes respirations • Wheezing • Presence or absence of coughing (dry or moist/productive) • Retractions • Skin color, color of lips, nailbeds, mucous membranes
Nervous system	• Weakness • Sensation, ability to feel touch, absence of sensation • Presence or absence of pain • Numbness, tingling • Normal, abnormal or involuntary motor function, spasticity • Ability or inability to move a body part • Coordination, lack of coordination

B-8

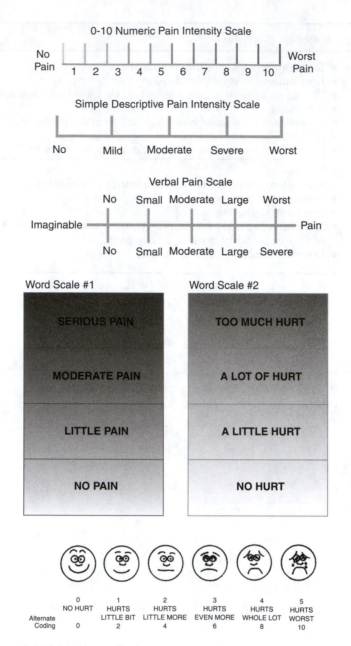

0-10 Numeric Pain Intensity Scale

No Pain | 1 2 3 4 5 6 7 8 9 10 | Worst Pain

Simple Descriptive Pain Intensity Scale

No   Mild   Moderate   Severe   Worst

Verbal Pain Scale

No Small Moderate Large Worst

Imaginable ——————————— Pain

No Small Moderate Large Severe

Word Scale #1

SERIOUS PAIN

MODERATE PAIN

LITTLE PAIN

NO PAIN

Word Scale #2

TOO MUCH HURT

A LOT OF HURT

A LITTLE HURT

NO HURT

| 0 | 1 | 2 | 3 | 4 | 5 |
| NO HURT | HURTS LITTLE BIT | HURTS LITTLE MORE | HURTS EVEN MORE | HURTS WHOLE LOT | HURTS WORST |

Alternate Coding   0   2   4   6   8   10

B-9 The resident will select the pain scale that best helps her communicate the level and intensity of her pain. (FACES pain scale from Wong D.L., Hockenberry-Eaton M., Wilson D., Winkelstein M.L., Schwartz P.: Wong's Essentials of Pediatric Nursing, ed. 7, St. Louis, 2005, p. 1259. Copyrighted by Mosby, Inc. Used with permission.)

The 24-Hour Clock

Standard Clock	24-Hour Clock	Standard Clock	24-Hour Clock
12:00 midnight	2400 or 0000	12:00 noon	1200
1:00 a.m.	0100	1:00 p.m.	1300
2:00 a.m.	0200	2:00 p.m.	1400
3:00 a.m.	0300	3:00 p.m.	1500
4:00 a.m.	0400	4:00 p.m.	1600
5:00 a.m.	0500	5:00 p.m.	1700
6:00 a.m.	0600	6:00 p.m.	1800
7:00 a.m.	0700	7:00 p.m.	1900
8:00 a.m.	0800	8:00 p.m.	2000
9:00 a.m.	0900	9:00 p.m.	2100
10:00 a.m.	1000	10:00 p.m.	2200
11:00 a.m.	1100	11:00 p.m.	2300

B-10 Entries in the chart are made in chronological order, by date and time. Some facilities use the 24-hour clock to document the time. When this system is used, indicating times by noting a.m. or p.m. is not necessary.

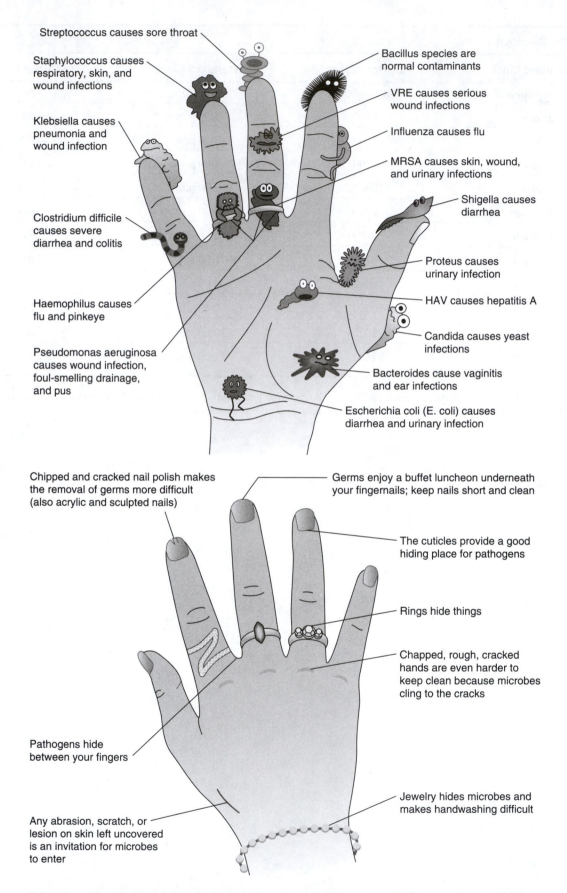

Streptococcus causes sore throat

Staphylococcus causes respiratory, skin, and wound infections

Klebsiella causes pneumonia and wound infection

Clostridium difficile causes severe diarrhea and colitis

Haemophilus causes flu and pinkeye

Pseudomonas aeruginosa causes wound infection, foul-smelling drainage, and pus

Bacillus species are normal contaminants

VRE causes serious wound infections

Influenza causes flu

MRSA causes skin, wound, and urinary infections

Shigella causes diarrhea

Proteus causes urinary infection

HAV causes hepatitis A

Candida causes yeast infections

Bacteroides cause vaginitis and ear infections

Escherichia coli (E. coli) causes diarrhea and urinary infection

Chipped and cracked nail polish makes the removal of germs more difficult (also acrylic and sculpted nails)

Pathogens hide between your fingers

Any abrasion, scratch, or lesion on skin left uncovered is an invitation for microbes to enter

Germs enjoy a buffet luncheon underneath your fingernails; keep nails short and clean

The cuticles provide a good hiding place for pathogens

Rings hide things

Chapped, rough, cracked hands are even harder to keep clean because microbes cling to the cracks

Jewelry hides microbes and makes handwashing difficult

B-11 Many infections are spread on the hands, so health care workers must pay close attention to good hand hygiene and eliminating areas where pathogens can hide. Jewelry with many stones or complicated settings provides a hiding place for pathogens. Long fingernails, chipped nail polish, and acrylic nails also provide hiding places for microbes. Chapped, cut, cracked hands increase the risk of contracting an infection.

Elements in the Chain of Infection

Causative Agent	Source or Reservoir	Portal of Exit	Mode of Transmission	Portal of Entry	Susceptible Host
Bacteria	People	Blood	Direct contact	Mucous membranes	Chronic diseases
Fungi	Medicine	Moist body fluid	Indirect contact	Nonintact skin	Immuno-suppression
Viruses	Food	Droplets	Airborne	Urinary tract	Surgery
Parasites	Water	Secretions	Droplet	GI tract	Diabetes
	Equipment	Excretions	Fomites	Respiratory tract	Elderly residents
		Skin	Common vehicle	Blood	Burns
			Vectors	Body fluid	Cardiopulmonary disease

B-12 Elements of the chain of infection

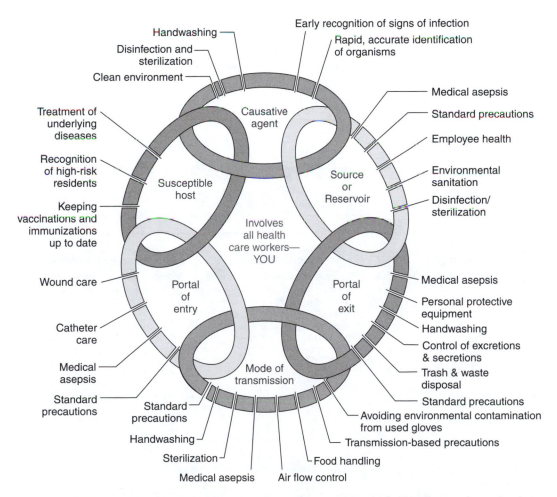

B-13 If one link in the chain is broken, the infection cannot be spread to others. This diagram shows the chain of infection, with examples of how health care workers can break each link of the chain.

Modes of Transmission of Microbes

Airborne	Tiny microbes are carried by moisture or dust particles in air and are inhaled
Droplet	Droplets spread within approximately three feet (no personal contact). Droplets are larger and heavier than airborne microbes, so they cannot travel as far. Droplet nuclei are inhaled: • Coughing • Laughing • Sneezing • Singing • Talking
Contact	Direct contact of health care provider with resident: • Touching • Rubbing • Toileting (urine and feces) • Blood, body fluid, mucous membranes, or nonintact skin • Bathing • Secretions or excretions from patient
	Indirect contact of health care provider with objects used by residents: • Clothing • Dressings • Bed linens • Diagnostic equipment • Personal belongings • Permanent or disposable health care equipment • Personal care equipment • Instruments and supplies used in treatments • Environmental surfaces such as counters, faucets, and doorknobs
Common Vehicle	Spread to many people through contact with items such as: • Food • Medication • Water • Contaminated blood products
Vector-Borne	Intermediate hosts such as: • Flies • Rats • Fleas • Mice • Ticks • Roaches

B-14 Examples of various methods of microbe transmission

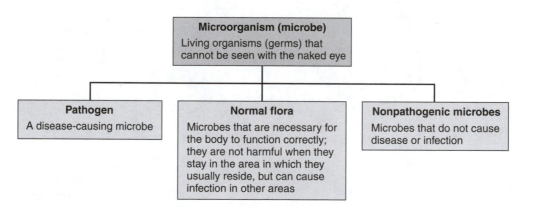

B-15 Various types of microbes

Examples of Personal Protective Equipment in Basic Resident Care

Resident Care Task	Gloves	Gown	Goggles/ Face Sheild	Surgical Mask
Controlling bleeding when blood is squirting	Yes	Yes	Yes	Yes
Wiping a wheelchair, shower chair, or bathtub with disinfectant solution	Yes	No	No	No
Emptying a catheter bag	Yes	Yes, if facility policy	Yes, if facility policy	Yes, if facility policy
Serving a meal tray	No	No	No	No
Giving a backrub to a resident who has intact skin	No	No	No	No
Brushing a resident's teeth	Yes	No	No	No
Helping the dentist with a procedure	Yes	Yes, if facility policy	Yes	Yes
Cleaning a resident and changing the bed after an episode of diarrhea	Yes	Yes	No	No
Changing a bed in which the linen is not visibly soiled	No, or follow facility policy. If gloves are worn for removing soiled linen, remove and wash hands before handling clean linen	No	No	No
Taking an oral temperature with a glass thermometer (gloves are not necessary with an electronic thermometer)	Yes	No	No	No
Taking a rectal temperature	Yes	No	No	No
Taking blood pressure	No	No	No	No
Cleaning soiled utensils, such as bedpans	Yes	Yes, if splashing is likely	Yes, if splashing is likely	Yes, if splashing is likely
Shaving a resident with a disposable razor	Yes, because of the high risk of this procedure for contact with blood	No	No	No
Giving eye care	Yes	No	No	No
Giving special mouth care to an unconscious resident	Yes	No, unless coughing is likely	No, unless coughing is likely	No, unless coughing is likely
Washing the resident's genital area	Yes	No	No	No
Washing the resident's arms and legs when the skin is not broken	No	No	No	No

B-16 There are exceptions to every rule. Use this chart as a general guideline only. Add personal protective equipment if special situations, such as likely splashing, exist. Follow your facility policies and procedures for the selection and use of protective apparel.

Material Safety Data Sheet

PRODUCT CODE NUMBERS:
MSC5300

SECTION 1

ISSUE DATE: 9-21-96
IDENTITY: **Exuderm Hydrocolloid Ultra Dressing**

MARKETED OR DISTRIBUTED BY:
Medline Industries, Inc.
One Medline Place
Mundelein, IL 60060
1.800.MEDLINE

Emergency Telephone Number:
Contact Your Regional Poison Control Center

SECTION 2 - HAZARDOUS INGREDIENTS/IDENTITY INFORMATION

HAZARDOUS COMPONENTS (SPECIFIC CHEMICAL IDENTITY, COMMON NAME(S)	CAS#	OSHA PEL	ACGIH TLV	OTHER LIMITS RECOMMENDED	% (OPTIONAL)
None					

SECTION 3 - PHYSICAL/CHEMICAL CHARACTERISTICS

BOILING POINT: N/A	SP GRAVITY (WATER=1): N/A
VAPOR PRESSURE (MM HG): N/A	MELTING POINT: N/A
VAPOR DENSITY (AIR=1): N/A	EVAPORATION RATE(BUTYL ACETATE=1): N/A
SOLUBILITY IN WATER: N/A	
APPEARANCE AND ODOR: Light caramel in color and no odor	

SECTION 4 - FIRE AND EXPLOSION HAZARD DATA

FLASH POINT (METHOD USED): N/A		
FLAMMABLE LIMITS: N/A	LEL: N/A	UEL: N/A
EXTINGUISHING MEDIA: Water, dry chemical or foam		
SPECIAL FIRE FIGHTING PROCEDURES: None		
UNUSUAL FIRE AND EXPLOSIVE HAZARDS: None		

SECTION 5 - REACTIVITY DATA

STABILITY: Stable
CONDITIONS TO AVOID: Avoid overheating and freezing.
INCOMPATIBILITY (MATERIALS TO AVOID): N/A
HAZARDOUS DECOMPOSITION OR BYPRODUCTS: N/A
HAZARDOUS POLYMERIZATION: Will not Occur
CONDITIONS TO AVOID: N/A

SECTION 6 - HEALTH HAZARD DATA

ROUTE(S) OF ENTRY: INHALATION: N/A	SKIN: N/A		INGESTION: N/A
HEALTH HAZARDS (ACUTE AND CHRONIC): None			
CARCINOGENICITY? N/A	NTP? N/A	IARC? N/A	OSHA REGULATED? N/A
SIGNS AND SYMPTOMS OF EXPOSURE: May cause moderate irritation in eyes			
MEDICAL CONDITIONS GENERALLY AGGRAVATED BY EXPOSURE: N/A			
EMERGENCY AND FIRST AID PROCEDURES: Eye contact: Flush. Excessive Ingestion: Induce vomiting and consult physician.			

SECTION 7 - SPILL, LEAK, AND WASTE DISPOSAL PROCEDURES

STEPS TO BE TAKEN IN CASE MATERIAL IS RELEASED OR SPILLED: N/A
WASTE DISPOSAL METHOD: In accordance with all local, state and federal regulations.
PRECAUTIONS TO BE TAKEN IN HANDLING AND STORING: N/A
OTHER PRECAUTIONS: N/A

SECTION 8 - CONTROL MEASURES

RESPIRATORY PROTECTION (SPECIFY TYPE): N/A		
VENTILATION:	LOCAL EXHAUST: N.A.	SPECIAL: N/A
	MECHANICAL (GENERAL): N/A	OTHER: N/A
PROTECTIVE GLOVES: N/A		EYE PROTECTION: N/A
SPECIAL CLOTHING: N/A		
WORK/HYGIENIC PRACTICES: None		

SECTION 9 - SPECIAL PRECAUTIONS

None

SECTION 10 - ADDITIONAL INFORMATION

Exuderm Hydrocolloid Dressing has passed all testing required for medical devices as outlined in the FDA Biocompatibility Guidelines for short term devices in contact with breached or compromised skin.

The information provided in this Material Safety Data Sheet has been obtained from sources believed to be reliable.

Medline Industries, Inc. provides no warranties, either expressed or implied and assumes no responsibility for the accuracy or completeness of the data contained herein.

ISSUE DATE: 9-21-96
Revised: 10/31/01 Updated telephone information

B-17 Material Safety Data Sheets provide important information and instructions on product use, health risks, first aid, and safety precautions. (Courtesy of Medline Industries, Inc.; (800) MEDLINE)

Bomb Threat Checklist

Questions to ask the caller:

• Where is the bomb right now? _____

• Did you place the bomb? _____

• Why did you place the bomb? _____

• When is the bomb going to explode? _____

• What will cause the bomb to explode? _____

• What kind of bomb is it? _____

• Where are you? _____

• What is your name? _____

Exact wording of the call:

_____

_____

_____

Date and time of the call: _____

Length of the call: _____

Caller's gender (sex): _____ Approximate age: _____ Accent: _____

Caller's Voice; Circle all that apply

calm	nasal	loud	distinct	lisp	clearing throat
angry	slow	laughing	slurred	raspy	coughing
agitated	rapid	crying	ethnic	deep	deep breathing
excited	soft	normal	stutter	ragged	cracking
disguised	foreign	accent	familiar		

If the voice sounded familiar, whose voice did it sound like? _____

Language; Circle all that apply

Well-spoken (educated)	Irrational	Message read by caller
Foul	Incoherent	Accent or dialect (specify) _____
	Taped message	

Background Sounds

Street (cars, buses, etc.)	Motor (fan, air conditioning)	Local call	Other (specify)
Airplanes	Church bells	Phone booth	_____
PA system	Animal noises	Office machinery	_____
Music	Clear	Video games, pinball, bowling, etc.	
House (dishes, TV, radio)	Static	Factory machinery	
Construction			

B-18 A bomb threat checklist is available in some facilities. Obtaining this information will help locate the bomb (if any), and will help identify the caller.

Complications of Restraints

Potential Physical Problems	Potential Psychosocial Problems	Potential Physical Problems	Potential Psychosocial Problems
Decreased independence	Worsening of behavior problems	Urge to void frequently, dribbling	Sense of abandonment
Increased dependence on staff		Incontinence	Loss of self-esteem
Pressure ulcers	Withdrawal, loss of social contact	Urinary tract infection	Crying
Weakness	Depression	Constipation	Screaming, yelling, calling out
Decreased range of motion	Forgetfulness	Fecal impaction	
Muscle wasting	Fear	Lethargy	Loss of dignity
Contractures (frozen, deformed joints)	Anger	Shortness of breath	Boredom
Pain from immobility Loss of ability to ambulate	Shame	Pneumonia	Feelings of hopelessness
	Agitation	Bruising, redness, cuts	
Edema of ankles, lower legs, feet, fingers	Mental confusion	Falls	Feelings of helplessness
		Impaired circulation	
Decreased appetite, weight loss	Combativeness	Blood clots	Irritability
Dehydration	Restlessness	Choking	Ritualistic behavior
Acute mental confusion		Death	
Distended abdomen			

B-19 Complications of restraints

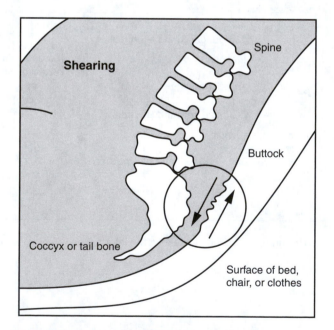

B-20 Shearing occurs when the skin is pulled in one direction while the underlying bone moves in the opposite direction. Many pressure ulcers develop and worsen because of shearing. The friction rubs the top layer of skin off, exposing nerve endings and increasing pain.

Stage I: Nonblanchable erythema of intact skin, the heralding lesion of skin ulceration. In individuals with darker skin, discoloration of the skin, warmth, edema, induration, or hardness may also be indicators.

Stage II: Partial-thickness skin loss involving epidermis, dermis, or both. The ulcer is superficial and presents clinically as an abrasion, blister, or shallow crater.

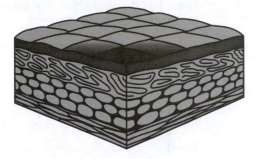
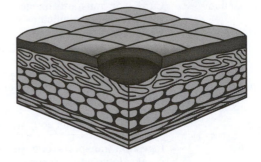

Stage III: Full-thickness skin loss involving damage to or necrosis of subcutaneous tissue that may extend down to, but not through, underlying fascia. The ulcer presents clinically as a deep crater with or without undermining of adjacent tissue.

Stage IV: Full-thickness skin loss with extensive destruction, tissue necrosis, or damage to muscle, bone, or supporting structures (e.g., tendon, joint capsule). Undermining and sinus tracts also may be associated with Stage IV pressure ulcers.

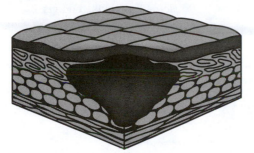
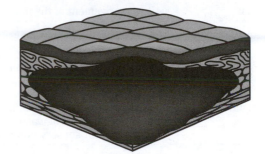

Avoidable and Unavoidable Pressure Ulcers [State Operations Manual. §483.25(c)]

- *Avoidable* means that the resident developed a pressure ulcer and that the facility did not do one or more of the following: evaluate the resident's clinical condition and pressure ulcer risk factors; define and implement interventions that are consistent with resident needs, resident goals, and recognized standards of practice; monitor and evaluate that impact of the interventions; or revise the interventions as appropriate.

- *Unavoidable* means that the resident developed a pressure ulcer even though the facility had evaluated the resident's clinical condition and pressure ulcer risk factors; defined and implemented interventions that are consistent with resident needs, goals, and recognized standards of practice; monitored and evaluated the impact of the interventions; and revised the approaches as appropriate.

B-21 The pressure ulcer stages reflect the amount of tissue destruction.

Body Systems: Components and Functions

System	Function	Organs
Cardiovascular	Carries or transports oxygen and water to the body and eliminates some forms of wast materials.	Heart, blood, arteries, veins, capillaries, spleen, lymph vessels and nodes.
Note: The cardiovascular system may also be called the circulatory system. The "immune system" is part of the cardiovascular system.		
Respiratory	Supplies oxygen to the body and eliminates carbon dioxide.	Lungs, nose, larynx, pharynx, trachea, bronchi.
Urinary	Elimination of liquid body wastes.	Kidneys, ureters, bladder, urethra.
Digestive	Ingestion transports food. Digestion breaks down and absorbs nutrients, and eliminates wastes.	Mouth, teeth, tongue, salivary glands, pharynx, esophagus, liver, gallbladder, stomach, small intestine, appendix, rectum, anus.
Nervous	Regulates body movement and functions. Controls all mental processes.	Brain, spinal cord, nerves.
Muscular	Allows movement of the body.	Muscles, ligaments, tendons.
Skeletal	Protects vital organs and gives shape and support to the body.	Bones, joints.
Note: Sometimes called the "musculoskeletal system." When used in this context, it refers to the combined structures and functions of the muscular and skeletal systems.		
Integumentary	Provides protection against infection, aids in the removal of waste, and serves as a vehicle for sensory perception.	Skin, hair, nails, sweat and oil glands.
Endocrine	Produces hormones to regulate body functions (metabolic processes).	Pituitary gland, pineal gland, parathyroid gland, thyroid gland, adrenal glands, thymus glands, testes, ovaries.
Reproductive	Reproduction of the species.	Female: ovaries, uterus, fallopian tubes, vagina. Male: testes, scrotum, penis, prostate gland.
Note: Sometimes called the "genitouyrinary system." When used in this context, it refers to the combined structures and functions of the urinary and reproductive systems.		

B-22 Structure and function of the body systems

Major Complications of Immobility

System	Complication
Respiratory	The resident has more difficulty expanding the lungs. Fluid and secretions collect in the lungs. This increases the risk of pneumonia and other lung infections.
Cardiovascular	Blood clots are caused by pooling of blood and pressure on the legs. Edema may be caused by lack of movement. The heart must work harder to pump blood through the body. Changes in the blood vessels may cause dizziness and fainting when the resident is placed in an upright position.
Integumentary (skin)	Pressure sores may develop in a short time from lack of oxygen to the tissues. Pressure ulcers may worsen quickly and be difficult or impossible to reverse.
Muscular	Weakness and atrophy develop from lack of use. Contractures (deformities) develop because of the resident's position. Contractures may be painful and are difficult or impossible to reverse. Contractures also promote pressure ulcer development, and make treating pressure ulcers more difficult. The contractures cause reduced capillary blood flow to bony prominences, and estimates are that up to 60% of all pressure ulcers involve some sort of unattended contracture. Voluntary movement of the contracted joint becomes difficult or impossible as the contracture worsens.
Skeletal	Calcium drains from the bones when they are inactive. This contributes to fractures, non-healing, osteoporosis, and other complications.
Urinary	The extra calcium in the system from the bones promotes the development of kidney stones. Retention of urine is common, and is often caused by the resident's position in bed. Overflow of a full bladder leads to incontinence. The resident is at high risk of urinary tract infection.
Gastrointestinal	Indigestion and heartburn may result if the resident is not positioned properly for meals. The resident is at risk for choking unless positioned upright during and after meals. Loss of appetite may occur from lack of activity, illness, and boredom. Constipation and fecal impaction result from immobility.
Nervous	Weakness and limited mobility develop. Insomnia may result from sleeping too much during the day, then being unable to sleep at night.
Mental changes	Irritability, boredom, lethargy, and depression result from the resident's frustration and feelings of helplessness.

B-23 Years ago, people who were sick stayed in bed for long periods. After childbirth, women were kept on bedrest for at least seven days. We now know that early activity is best for the resident. Bedrest, inactivity, and immobility negatively affect every system in the body. Bedrest is a medically prescribed treatment in which the resident cannot get out of bed. All residents should be up each day unless they have a specific doctors' order for bedrest. This table summarizes the major complications of immobility on each body system.

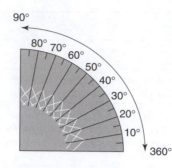

B-24 The nursing assistant must be familiar with degrees to use for resident positioning.

Range-of-Motion Terminology

- **Abduction** is moving an extremity *away from* the body.

- **Adduction** is moving an extremity *toward* the body.

- **Circumduction** is a circular movement of a joint, such as the thumb or wrist.

- **Dorsal flexion,** or **dorsiflexion,** is pulling the foot upward toward the head.

- **Eversion** is turning a joint outward.

- **Extension** is straightening a joint.

- **External rotation** is turning a joint outward *away from* the median line.

- **Flexion** is bending a joint.

- **Hyperextension** is gentle, excessive extension of a joint, slightly past the point of resistance.

- **Internal rotation** is turning a joint *inward toward* the median line.

- **Inversion** is turning a joint inward.

- **Medial** pertains to or is situated toward the midline of the body.

- **Median** means situated in the median plane or in the midline of the body.

- **Opposition** is touching each of the fingers against the thumb.

- **Palmar flexion** is the act of bending the hand down toward the palm.

- **Plantar flexion** is bending the foot downward, away from the body.

- **Pronation** is moving a joint to face downward.

- **Radial deviation** is turning the forearm toward the radius.

- **Retraction** is drawing back, away from the body.

- **Rotation** means moving a joint in, out, and around.

- **Supination** is moving a joint so it faces upward.

- **Ulnar deviation** is turning the forearm toward the ulna.

B-25 Terminology used for range-of-motion exercises

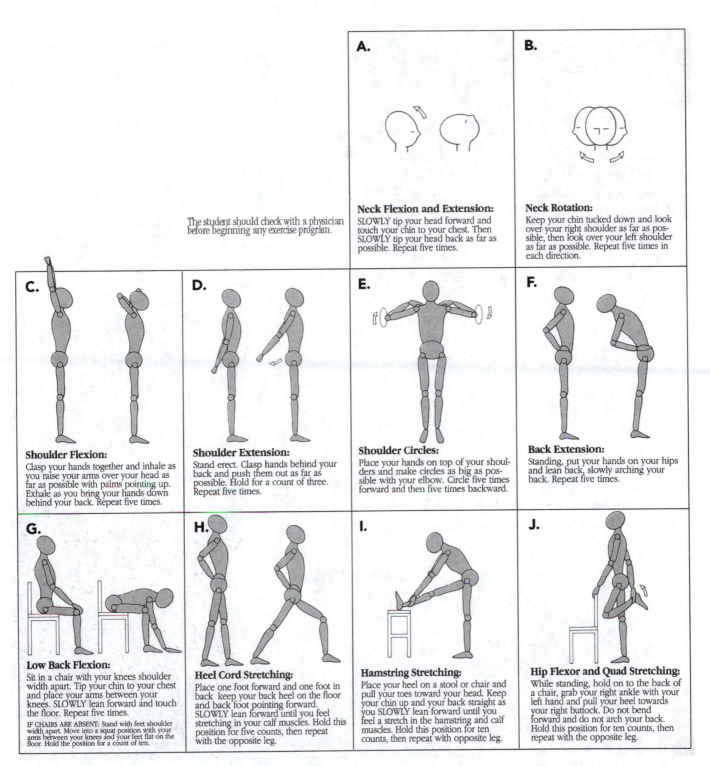

The student should check with a physician before beginning any exercise program.

A.

Neck Flexion and Extension:
SLOWLY tip your head forward and touch your chin to your chest. Then SLOWLY tip your head back as far as possible. Repeat five times.

B.

Neck Rotation:
Keep your chin tucked down and look over your right shoulder as far as possible, then look over your left shoulder as far as possible. Repeat five times in each direction.

C.

Shoulder Flexion:
Clasp your hands together and inhale as you raise your arms over your head as far as possible with palms pointing up. Exhale as you bring your hands down behind your back. Repeat five times.

D.

Shoulder Extension:
Stand erect. Clasp hands behind your back and push them out as far as possible. Hold for a count of three. Repeat five times.

E.

Shoulder Circles:
Place your hands on top of your shoulders and make circles as big as possible with your elbow. Circle five times forward and then five times backward.

F.

Back Extension:
Standing, put your hands on your hips and lean back, slowly arching your back. Repeat five times.

G.

Low Back Flexion:
Sit in a chair with your knees shoulder width apart. Tip your chin to your chest and place your arms between your knees. SLOWLY lean forward and touch the floor. Repeat five times.

IF CHAIRS ARE ABSENT: Stand with feet shoulder width apart. Move into a squat position with your arms between your knees and your feet flat on the floor. Hold the position for a count of ten.

H.

Heel Cord Stretching:
Place one foot forward and one foot in back keep your back heel on the floor and back foot pointing forward. SLOWLY lean forward until you feel stretching in your calf muscles. Hold this position for five counts, then repeat with the opposite leg.

I.

Hamstring Stretching:
Place your heel on a stool or chair and pull your toes toward your head. Keep your chin up and your back straight as you SLOWLY lean forward until you feel a stretch in the hamstring and calf muscles. Hold this position for ten counts, then repeat with opposite leg.

J.

Hip Flexor and Quad Stretching:
While standing, hold on to the back of a chair, grab your right ankle with your left hand and pull your heel towards your right buttock. Do not bend forward and do not arch your back. Hold this position for ten counts, then repeat with the opposite leg.

B-26 Warming up before work can help prevent injuries. (Reprinted with permission from Ergodyne Corporation, St. Paul, MN)

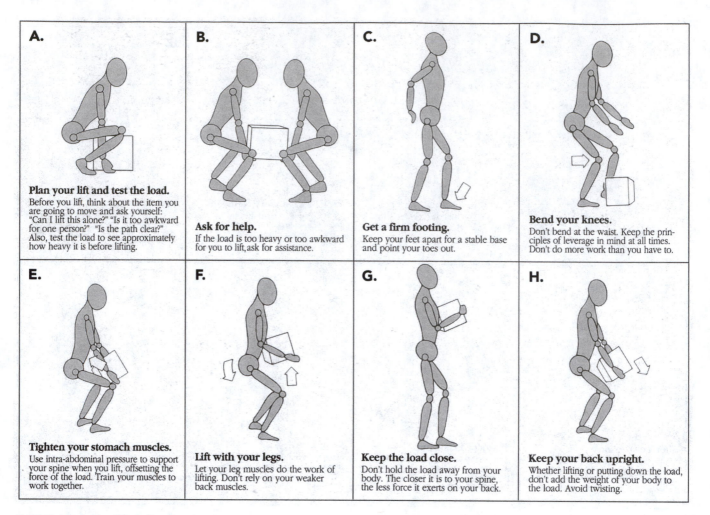

A.

Plan your lift and test the load.
Before you lift, think about the item you are going to move and ask yourself: "Can I lift this alone?" "Is it too awkward for one person?" "Is the path clear?" Also, test the load to see approximately how heavy it is before lifting.

B.

Ask for help.
If the load is too heavy or too awkward for you to lift, ask for assistance.

C.

Get a firm footing.
Keep your feet apart for a stable base and point your toes out.

D.

Bend your knees.
Don't bend at the waist. Keep the principles of leverage in mind at all times. Don't do more work than you have to.

E.

Tighten your stomach muscles.
Use intra-abdominal pressure to support your spine when you lift, offsetting the force of the load. Train your muscles to work together.

F.

Lift with your legs.
Let your leg muscles do the work of lifting. Don't rely on your weaker back muscles.

G.

Keep the load close.
Don't hold the load away from your body. The closer it is to your spine, the less force it exerts on your back.

H.

Keep your back upright.
Whether lifting or putting down the load, don't add the weight of your body to the load. Avoid twisting.

B-27 Eight rules for lifting. (Reprinted with permission from Ergodyne Corporation, St. Paul, MN)

Common Diseases/Conditions in Elderly Long-Term Care Residents

Disease or Condition	Description
Alzheimer's Disease	A progressive disease of brain cells in which the resident loses mental and physical ability. The disease is incurable and ends in death.
Amputation	Removal of an extremity. Amputation is usually performed because of diabetes, vascular disease, trauma, or gangrene.
Arteriosclerosis	A narrowing of the inside walls of the arteries that makes them rigid and thick. Adequate blood flow cannot pass through the vessel walls to nourish the body. High blood pressure is common because the heart has to work harder to force blood through the blocked vessels. Residents are at high risk of stroke and heart attack.
Arthritis	A painful inflammation of joints that results in limited movement, swelling, and deformities.
Atherosclerosis	A buildup of plaque, calcium, and fat on the walls of the arteries, which makes them rigid and thick. Adequate blood flow cannot pass through the vessel walls to nourish the body. High blood pressure is common because the heart has to work harder to force blood through the narrow vessels. Residents are at high risk of stroke and heart attack.
Cancer	A malignant tumor or new growth anywhere in the body. Cancer may spread slowly or rapidly.
Cerebrovascular Accident (CVA, Brain Attack, or Stroke)	An incident in the brain caused by a blood clot or bursting of blood vessels, allowing blood to spill out into the brain cavity. Common effects of a stroke are paralysis on one side of the body, loss of bowel and bladder control, and speech impairments. The effects may be temporary or permanent.
Congestive Heart Failure	A condition in which the heart is unable to pump sufficient blood to meet the needs of the body. Characterized by high blood pressure and fluid retention.
Diabetes Mellitus	A disorder of the endocrine system in which the body cannot metabolize carbohydrates, proteins, and fat properly.
Emphysema	A disorder in which the air sacs of the lungs have stretched and lost their elasticity, causing them to be unable to contract to remove excess air.
Head Injury	An injury to the brain that results from falls or trauma. Head injuries may affect mental function, physical function, or both. In the elderly, the effects are often permanent because of brain damage.
Hearing Impairment	Difficulty hearing from a number of causes. Impairment may range from being hard of hearing to complete deafness. Some residents may benefit from use of a hearing aid.
Heart Attack (Myocardial Infarction)	A serious medical emergency in which the blood vessels that nourish the heart muscle are blocked or burst, disrupting the normal flow of blood through the heart.
Heart Block	A condition that may require a pacemaker for treatment. Caused by a disruption in the electrical conduction of the heart in which the heart's own internal pacemaker does not beat regularly.
Hip Fracture	A broken hip that is usually the result of a fall but can result from trauma (such as an auto accident) or osteoporosis. The term "hip fracture" really is not accurate. This term refers to a fracture anywhere in the upper third or head of the femur. This is a serious injury, and there is a known relationship between hip fracture and mortality in the elderly.
Hip Replacement	*Total Hip Arthroplasty (THA)* involves removal of a portion of the pelvic bone and femur, and insertion of a prosthesis (artificial body part). This procedure may be done because the patient has fractured a hip, and it cannot be repaired by other methods, or for treatment of degenerative arthritis, when the hip joint has deteriorated and is very painful.

Continues

B-28 Because of aging changes, persons who are elderly are at greater risk of developing chronic diseases. These diseases require a change in lifestyle and a period of time to mentally adjust. This table summarizes common diseases and conditions in elderly long-term care residents.

Common Diseases/Conditions in Elderly Long-Term Care Residents, *Continued*

Disease or Condition	Description
Huntington's Disease	A progressive, hereditary disease that results in rapid, involuntary movements and progressive dementia.
Hypertension	High blood pressure. The resident may have no symptoms, or may develop dizziness, headaches, and fatigue. Serious complications can result if hypertension is not treated.
Multiple Sclerosis	A chronic, progressive disease marked by intermittent periods of remission. The resident has loss of muscle control, weakness, incoordination, and speech, visual, and sensory disturbances.
Paraplegia	Paralysis below the waist. The condition is usually caused by trauma, but can be caused by tumors and other conditions.
Parkinson's Disease	A neurological disorder that results in tremors, muscular rigidity, and a shuffling gait.
Peripheral Artery Disease	A condition caused by atherosclerosis that results in insufficient blood flow to the legs. It may result in leg ulcers or necessitate amputation.
Peripheral Vascular Disease	A disorder that is frequently the result of varicose veins. Blood return from the legs is not adequate. The condition commonly results in blood clots and leg ulcers.
Pneumonia and Influenza	Serious infections of the lungs contracted by the droplet method of transmission.
Post Polio Syndrome	Post polio syndrome is a neurologic disorder identified by increased weakness and/or abnormal muscle fatigue in persons who had paralytic polio many years earlier. Signs and symptoms are divided into two subgroups. Neuromuscular symptoms are believed to be caused by a progressive decline in motor neurons, resulting in new weakness and muscle fatigue. Musculoskeletal symptoms are probably caused by years of abnormal use and wear.
Tetraplegia	Paralysis below the neck. The usual cause is trauma, but can result from tumors, infection, and other conditions.
Transient Ischemic Attack (TIA)	A temporary period of diminished blood flow to the brain. An attack occurs suddenly and usually lasts from 2 to 15 minutes, although it may last longer. Signs and symptoms are similar to those of a stroke but are reversible and temporary. Persons who experience TIAs are at high risk for strokes.
Vision Impairment	Difficulty seeing, caused by any one of a number of causes. Sometimes vision can be improved with glasses or surgery. In some disorders, vision cannot be restored.

B-28

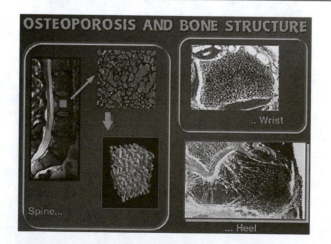

B-29 Bone loss from osteoporosis causes painful, disabling fractures in both men and women. About 40 percent of women and 13 percent of men will suffer a bone fracture due to osteoporosis in their lifetime. (Courtesy of Sharmila Majumdar, Ph.D., Professor, University of California, San Francisco)

GUIDELINES FOR

Resident Care and Compliance with Accepted Practice Standards

- Follow all facility policies and procedures for resident care.
- Know the care plan for the residents you are assigned to care for, including the major diagnosis, approaches to problems, and expected outcomes.
- Perform procedures in the way you were taught. Do not perform procedures for which you have not been trained.
- Practice safety in everything you do.
- All residents should have the call signal within reach at all times. Answer call signals promptly.
- Be polite and treat all residents with dignity and respect.
- Always close the door to the room when providing care. Pull the privacy curtain and close the window curtain. This should be done in the care of all residents, whether alert or confused.
- Cover residents completely in bed, chair, or hallways so they are not exposed.
- Always knock on the door before entering a room and wait for a response. If you do not get a response, open the door slightly and announce your presence.

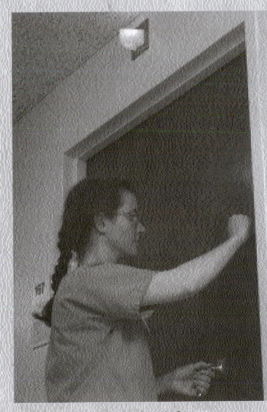

Knock on the door and wait for response before entering.

- If the resident's door is open, knock on the door frame or other surface and wait for permission to enter the room.
- Communicate with residents during care and explain procedures before you perform them.
- Know your responsibility for residents who use permanent equipment, such as oxygen, tube feeding, or IV pumps. The flow rate of the pump should match the ordered rate on the care plan. If it does not, notify the nurse. If an alarm sounds on a piece of medical equipment, notify the nurse immediately.
- Comb the resident's hair and tend to grooming needs early in the day so the resident is presentable in appearance for visitors. Assist with grooming needs throughout the day, if necessary.
- Check the resident's fingernails to be sure they are clean and neatly trimmed.
- Use handrolls or other props in the hands of dependent residents, to prevent contractures. Remove the handrolls and clean the palm of the hand daily, or according to facility policy.
- Shave male residents daily. Follow your facility policy for removing facial hair on female residents.
- Give residents oral care three times a day, or according to individual needs.
- Check residents frequently to be sure they are clean and dry. Give incontinent care as necessary.
- All residents should be clean and odor-free.
- Make sure the resident's appearance is presentable at all times. Remove spilled food from clothing, and change the clothing or gown if necessary. Make sure the resident is clean after meals. If food is spilled on bed linen or the floor, replace the linen or remove the food from the floor. When residents are up and dressed during the day, the clothing should be clean, in good repair, color-coordinated, and appropriate for age and season.
- Residents should have footwear appropriate to the floor surface on their feet during transfers. Feet should be covered when a resident is up in the chair so that bare feet are not resting on the floor.
- Pay attention to resident positioning in bed and chair. Preventive mattresses, heel and elbow protectors, and other devices are used if the resident is at risk of skin breakdown. Padding should be used for positioning residents if bony areas will rub against each other or against a firm surface.
- Footboards should be in place for bedfast residents.
- The feet should be supported when residents are up in the chair.
- Residents in wheelchairs should be positioned so that their hips are at the rear of the seat. They should be seated upright and not lean to the side. If you are responsible for residents who move about the facility in wheelchairs, find them and check on them periodically to be sure their needs are met.

Continues

B-30

GUIDELINES FOR

Resident Care and Compliance with Accepted Practice Standards, *Continued*

- When feeding residents, sit at eye level and maintain a conversation, even if the resident is confused.
- Alternate liquids with solids when feeding.
- Change incontinent residents promptly. Provide perineal care after each incontinent episode.
- Always notify the nurse of a change in the resident's condition, even if it seems insignificant.
- Notify the nurse immediately of red or open areas on a resident's skin.
- Document your care completely and accurately. Do not leave blank spaces in flow sheets. Read what you are signing on flow sheets before signing your initials to them. Surveyors review what you have documented. Inadequate documentation can adversely affect the survey. Your documentation is a permanent, legal record of the care provided, and you may have to defend it in court.

B-30

Survey Issues

Quality of Resident Life

- Residents are dressed appropriately
- Residents have appropriate footwear
- The way staff talk to and interact with residents
- How staff respond to resident requests
- Availability and receptiveness of staff to meet resident needs
- Scheduled activities and appropriateness of activities in meeting resident needs
- Adequate, timely mealtime assistance given

Emotional and Behavioral Conduct of Residents

- How staff respond and react to residents
- How staff meet resident needs
- Resident behavior problems and how these behaviors are addressed by staff
- How promptly staff respond to resident needs

Quality of Resident Care

- Skin condition, including pressure ulcers, rashes, excessive wetness, dry skin
- Skin tears, bruises, or injuries
- Availability of fresh drinking water and assistance with drinking given residents
- Signs and symptoms of dehydration, including dry skin, appearance of urine in drainage bags, dry mucous membranes and lips
- Clinical problems such as edema, contractures, underweight or emaciated appearance, significant weight loss
- Resident positioning, use of pillows, props, handrolls, footboards, and other devices
- Presence and prevalence of all types of infections
- Proper use of standard precautions and good handwashing
- Use of feeding tubes and position of residents when feeding is infusing
- Special care issues, such as ventilators, IV therapy, use of oxygen
- Amputations

Facility Environment and Safety

- Infection control
- Functional, clean, sanitary
- Free from hazards
- Homelike and clean
- Effectiveness of environment in meeting resident needs

B-31 Surveyors will focus on issues listed here. They will identify residents for closer evaluation.

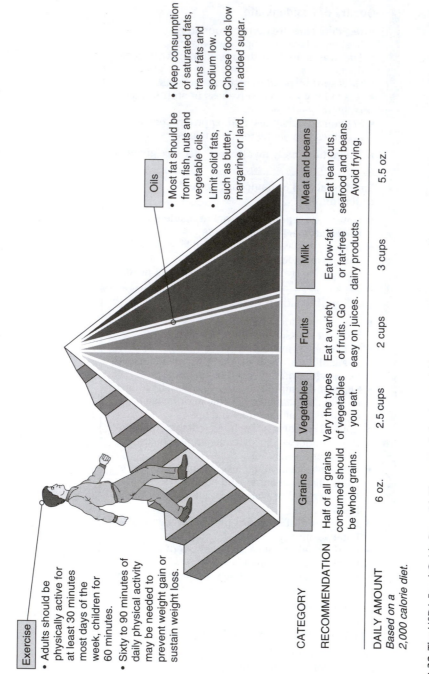

Exercise
- Adults should be physically active for at least 30 minutes most days of the week, children for 60 minutes.
- Sixty to 90 minutes of daily physical activity may be needed to prevent weight gain or sustain weight loss.

Oils
- Most fat should be from fish, nuts and vegetable oils.
- Limit solid fats, such as butter, margarine or lard.
- Keep consumption of saturated fats, trans fats and sodium low.
- Choose foods low in added sugar.

CATEGORY	Grains	Vegetables	Fruits	Milk	Meat and beans
RECOMMENDATION	Half of all grains consumed should be whole grains.	Vary the types of vegetables you eat.	Eat a variety of fruits. Go easy on juices.	Eat low-fat or fat-free dairy products.	Eat lean cuts, seafood and beans. Avoid frying.
DAILY AMOUNT *Based on a 2,000 calorie diet.*	6 oz.	2.5 cups	2 cups	3 cups	5.5 oz.

B-32 The USDA Food Guide Pyramid. The example food pyramid here was published in 2005. It is based on the average, 2000 calorie per day diet. The pyramid was designed to be individualized by each person to maintain a healthy weight. It contains 12 intake levels, ranging from 1,000 calories per day to 3,200 calories per day. This can be easily done by visiting http://www.mypyramid.gov.

Dietary Considerations for Cultural and Religious Groups in the United States

Religion/Group	Food Requirements and Prohibitions
Adventist, Seventh Day	Alcohol, coffee, and tea are prohibited. A vegetarian diet is encouraged.
American Indian	In some tribes, sharing food is customary. Explain to visitors that they should not share the resident's food in the health care facility. After prayer and certain ceremonies, berries, corn, and dried meat are consumed. These foods may be provided by family members or other members of the tribe.
Buddhist	Buddhists do not eat meat.
Catholic	Some residents do not eat meat on Fridays and other holy days. Avoid food for one hour before Communion.
Chinese Americans	Believe in the balance of heat and cold in the body and use food to maintain this balance, as well as to treat disease. Rice and noodles are staples in the diet. Very little meat is eaten. Meat is usually mixed with cooked vegetables. Family members may bring in special foods to treat certain illnesses. Also use herbs and herb preparations to treat illnesses.
Christian Scientist	Alcohol prohibited. Some abstain from coffee and tea.
Church of Jesus Christ of Latter Day Saints (LDS or Mormon)	Alcohol, coffee, and tea not allowed.
Hindu	Most Hindus are vegetarians. A light meal is eaten for breakfast, a heavy meal for lunch, and a light meal for supper. Dietary customs state that the right hand is used for eating and the left hand for toileting and personal hygiene.
Islam	Alcohol, pork, and some shellfish are not allowed.
Jewish	Milk and meat are not eaten together. Predatory fowl, shellfish, and pork are not allowed. Fish with fins and scales are permitted. Other types of fish are not allowed. Some Jewish residents request kosher food, which requires very special preparation.
Mexican American	Prefer fresh, natural ingredients in food preparation. Beans, corn tortillas, and rice are staples of the Mexican American diet. Tomatoes are used extensively in preparation of sauces. Food is highly spiced with onions, cilantro, and chilies. Mexican Americans believe that the properties of some diseases are hot or cold. Foods are served to complement the hot or cold disease state. The terms do not refer to food temperature, but rather to the effect the food has on the body.
Puerto Rican	Some observe traditional coffee time at 10:00 a.m. and 3:00 p.m. Coffee is traditionally prepared with boiled milk and sugar. Rice, beans, and plantains are served with most meals. Do not eat red meat or chicken during certain religious events.

B-33 Dietary considerations for ethnic and religious groups

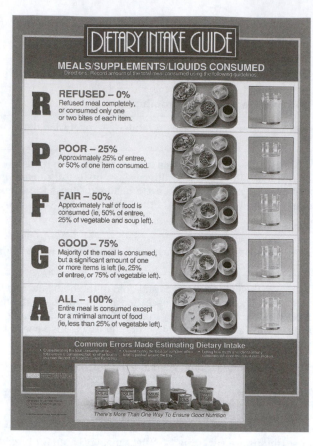

B-34 Accurate documentation of meal intake is an important nursing assistant responsibility. (Used with permission of Ross Products Division, Abbott Laboratories, Columbus, Ohio)

A

Alternate method of documenting meal intake

Breakfast

Egg, cheese or cottage cheese	50%
Hot or cold cereal	30%
Bread	10%
Bacon, ham or sausage	10%
Total	100%

Occasionally, a resident will request no protein foods (eggs, meat, cheese, cottage cheese) at breakfast. Please reassign the percentages to the other items on the tray and document accordingly.

Lunch and Supper

Meat, egg, cheese, or cottage cheese	40%
Starchy vegetable	20%
Vegetable or salad	20%
Bread	10%
Dessert	10%
Total	100%

The meat and starchy vegetables may be combined in some dishes, such as casseroles. If so, add the point values for these items together to total 60%. Sandwiches are also 60% because the two bread slices are the starchy vegetable. An additional bread item such as crackers may also be served at the meal.

B

Alternate method of documenting meal intake

	Food Item	Percentage of Meal
Breakfast		
	eggs	35%
	eggs and bacon	40%
	eggs and sausage	45%
	toast *or* cereal	30%
	milk	20%
	fruit juice	15%
Dinner and Supper	meat group, including eggs, main dish, legumes	50%
	fruit group, including dessert items	15%
	bread or cereal group	10%
	vegetable group	15%
	fluids	10%

B-35 Alternate methods of documenting resident meal intake

Diet _____

CALORIE/PROTEIN SUMMARY

RESIDENT _____   ROOM # _____

DAY 1					DAY 2					DAY 3				
DATE ___ / ___ / ___					DATE ___ / ___ / ___					DATE ___ / ___ / ___				
	% 0–25	% 25–50	% 50–75	% 75–100		% 0–25	% 25–50	% 50–75	% 75–100		% 0–25	% 25–50	% 50–75	% 75–100
Breakfast					**Breakfast**					**Breakfast**				
Meat					Meat					Meat				
Milk					Milk					Milk				
Fruit					Fruit					Fruit				
Starch					Starch					Starch				
Fat					Fat					Fat				
Other					Other					Other				
AM Supp.					AM Supp.					AM Supp.				
Noon Meal					**Noon Meal**					**Noon Meal**				
Meat					Meat					Meat				
Milk					Milk					Milk				
Juice					Juice					Juice				
Starch					Starch					Starch				
Vegetable					Vegetable					Vegetable				
Bread					Bread					Bread				
Fat					Fat					Fat				
Dessert					Dessert					Dessert				
Other					Other					Other				
PM Supp.					PM Supp.					PM Supp.				
Evening Meal					**Evening Meal**					**Evening Meal**				
Meat					Meat					Meat				
Milk					Milk					Milk				
Juice					Juice					Juice				
Starch					Starch					Starch				
Vegetable					Vegetable					Vegetable				
Bread					Bread					Bread				
Fat					Fat					Fat				
Dessert					Dessert					Dessert				
Other					Other					Other				
PM Supp.					PM Supp.					PM Supp.				
Total Kcal					**Total Kcal**					**Total Kcal**				
Total Pro					**Total Pro**					**Total Pro**				
Avg. for 3 days Kcal:					**Avg. Protein for 3 days:**									

PLEASE RETURN COMPLETED FORM TO NUTRITION CARE MANAGER

B-36 The calorie count provides an accurate picture of the resident's calorie and nutrient intake over a three-day period. The information is used to adjust the resident's diet and nutritional plan of care.

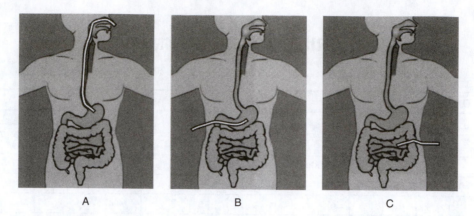

B-37 Enteral feeding methods: (A) Nasogastric feeding (B) Gastrostomy feeding (C) Jejunostomy feeding

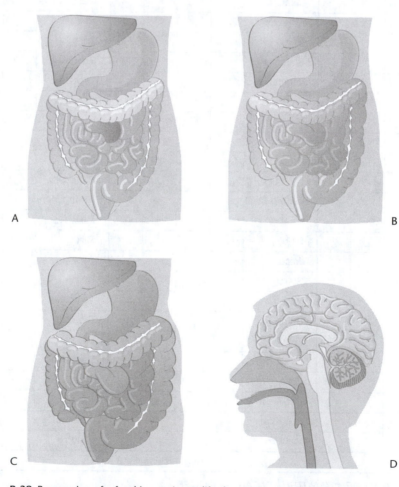

B-38 Progression of a fecal impaction, a life-threatening condition: (A) A fecal impaction blocks the rectum. The rectum and sigmoid colon become enlarged. (B) The colon continues to enlarge. (C) Fecal material gradually fills the colon. Digested and undigested food back up into the small intestines and stomach. The resident has signs and symptoms of acute illness, including lethargy, distention, constipation, and pain that is dull and cramping. (D) The entire system is full, and the resident vomits fecal material. The feces are commonly aspirated into the lungs.

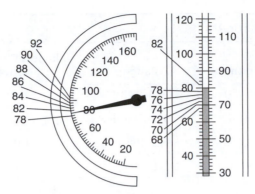

B-39 Read the blood pressure at the closest line. The pressure on both these gauges is 80.

National Heart, Lung, and Blood Institute Blood Pressure Definitions 2003			
	Blood Pressure Level (mm Hg)		
Category	**Systolic**	*****	**Diastolic**
Normal	< 120	and	< 80
Prehypertension	120–139	or	< 80
High Blood Pressure			
Stage I Hypertension	140–159	or	90–99
Stage II Hypertension	≥ 160	or	≥ 100

Legend:
< means less than
≥ means greater than or equal to
Source: National Heart, Lung, and Blood Institute, National Institutes of Health 2003.
For additional information, see
http://www.nhlbi.nih.gov/hbp/index.html

B-40 In 2003, the guidelines for identifying hypertension were revised. A new category called "prehypertension" was added. *Prehypertension* is a condition that means you are likely to develop high blood pressure in the future. In this condition, blood pressure is between 120/80 mm Hg and 139/89 mm Hg. People with prehypertension should take steps to decrease their risk.

Normal Vital Sign Ranges for Adults

Temperature	Normal	Range	Report Changes Above	Report Changes Below
Axillary temperature	97.6°F	96.6–98.6°F	99°F	96°F
Oral temperature	98.6°F	97.6–99.6°F	100°F	97°F
Rectal temperature	99.6°F	98.6–100.6°F	101°F	98°F
Pulse	76	60–100	100	60
Respiration	16	14–20	20	12
Blood pressure	120/80	100/60–140/90	140/90	100/60

B-41 These values are guidelines only. Your instructor will inform you if reporting values are different in your facility. Know and follow facility policies.

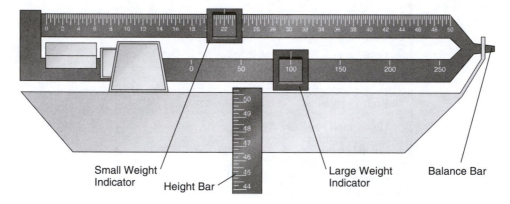

Small Weight Indicator   Height Bar   Large Weight Indicator   Balance Bar

B-42 To weigh a resident on the balance scale, you must understand how to calculate the weight by adding the reading on the two bars. Always balance the scale before beginning. The lower bar is marked with lines every 50 pounds. The upper bar has single pound readings. Even numbers are marked on the bar every two pounds. Each long line indicates an odd-numbered pound. Each short line on the upper bar is 1/4 of a pound. Adjust the weights on each balance bar until the rod hangs free on the end. To obtain the total weight, add the number of pounds on each bar.

Test-Taking Methods and Guidelines

As you know, the Nursing Home Reform Act was passed by Congress in 1987. It says that all people working as nursing assistants before July 1, 1989, must satisfactorily complete a competency evaluation program. Those employed after July 1, 1989, must first enroll in a nursing assistant education program and then successfully complete a competency exam. The competency exam is made up of written questions and performances. In some cases, an oral exam may be given instead of a written exam.

The 13 chapters and appendices in this manual are designed to provide the information and skills needed to complete the competency exam. We want you to become eligible for, or to continue, work as a nursing assistant. *We want you to be successful.*

The material covered in this appendix will help you prepare for the written portion of the competency exam. No one was born knowing how to take a test. Your performance on an exam can be improved by learning some test-taking methods and guidelines. By learning what to expect and by developing test-taking skills, you will know more and be more confident when taking the exam.

THE TEST

Unexpected surprises can make you tense and confused. Avoid this by learning as much as possible about a test in advance.

Standardized Tests

The exam you will be taking is **standardized.** This means that it was planned and written in such a way that everyone who takes the exam will be tested fairly. A test becomes standardized after it has been used, revised, and used again until it shows consistent results. The purpose is to establish an average score on the exam. The average score, called a **norm,** allows the results of one person's performance to be compared with those of many others across the country who have taken the same test.

A standardized test must be given in the same way. The test examiner must follow the same plan, read the same directions, and give only certain kinds of help. The situation at all test sites should be as much alike as possible. Scoring is standardized also. Every answer is scored according to definite rules.

Computerized Testing

Some states use computerized testing. In these states, you will report to a designated testing center and take the written state exam electronically. The program is simple to use, and the test is scored immediately, so you know the results when you leave. Testing programs usually have a tutorial available to familiarize you with the program, and demonstrate how to take the exam. Even if you have no previous computer experience, you should be able to master the program and become comfortable using it quickly.

Overview of the Test

The content of the **Nursing Assistant Test** covers:
Physical care skills

- Activities of daily living
  - hygiene
  - dressing and grooming
  - nutrition and hydration

— elimination

— comfort, rest, and sleep

- Basic nursing skills

  — infection control

  — safety and emergency procedures

  — therapeutic and technical procedures such as bedmaking, taking vital signs, and use of restraints

  — observation, data collection, and reporting

- Restorative skills

  — preventive health care, such as pressure ulcer and contracture prevention

  — promoting self-care and resident independence

Psychosocial care skills

- Emotional and mental health needs, including behavior management, needs of the dying resident, and sexuality needs
- Spiritual and cultural needs

Role of the nursing assistant

- Communication (includes verbal and nonverbal communication, listening, communicating with residents with various conditions)
- Resident rights
- Legal and ethical behavior
- Role and responsibilities of the nursing assistant as a member of the health care team

The test is made up of 50 to 75 multiple-choice questions that are given in a time period ranging from 90 minutes to 2 hours. About one-third of the test is devoted to basic nursing skills.

The questions are not grouped by content area. Questions about basic nursing skills, for instance, appear throughout the test.

You will mark answers to test questions on the test booklet, or enter them directly into the computer, depending on the type of test you are taking. A separate machine-readable information page may be included to collect your name, sex, race, birth date, education level, work experience, and state of residence.

Multiple-Choice Format

Most standardized tests use multiple-choice items. This is because multiple-choice questions can measure a variety of learning outcomes, from simple to complex. They also provide the most consistent results. The multiple-choice item consists of a **stem,**

which presents a problem situation, and four or five possible choices called **alternatives.** The alternatives include the correct answer and several wrong answers called **distractors.** The stem may be a question or an incomplete statement, as shown.

- Question form:

  Q. Which of the following people is responsible for taking care of a resident?

  Ⓐ janitor

  Ⓑ cook

  Ⓒ nurse aide

  Ⓓ dishwasher

- Incomplete-statement form:

  Q. The care of a resident is the responsibility of a

  Ⓐ janitor.

  Ⓑ cook.

  Ⓒ nurse aide.

  Ⓓ dishwasher.

Although worded differently, both stems present the same problem. The alternatives in the examples contain only one correct answer. All distractors are clearly incorrect.

Another type of multiple-choice item is the **best-answer** form. In this form, the alternatives are all partially correct, but one is clearly better than the others. Look at the following example.

- Best-answer form:

  Q. Which of the following ethical behaviors is the MOST important?

  Ⓐ Being polite to coworkers.

  Ⓑ Act as a responsible employee.

  Ⓒ Be courteous to visitors.

  Ⓓ Promote quality of life for each resident.

Other variations of the best-answer form may ask you "what is the first thing to do," the "most helpful action," the "best response," or a similar kind of question. Whether the correct answer or best-answer form is used depends on the information given.

The examples use four alternatives. The chance of getting the correct answer by guessing is only one in four (25 percent).

MANAGING TEST ANXIETY

Test anxiety, or stress, is an emotional and physical response that the body makes to any demand made upon it. Stress may be good or bad. Its symptoms may be mild or severe. Mild stress may include feelings of anxiety, muscle tension, "butterflies" in the stomach, sweating, pounding of heart, dry mouth, and reduced ability to concentrate. You have probably had some of these feelings before.

Most stress, including test anxiety, does not last long. Once the stressful situation has passed, the symptoms disappear. You can learn to cope with stress and anxiety. The following guidelines will help you deal with test anxiety.

Understanding Stress

Two important characteristics to know about stress are that: (1) stress is normal, and (2) stress can be good. If you are anxious about taking a test, you are not alone. Almost everyone has some test anxiety. The person who does not feel anxious about taking a test is usually the abnormal one.

You may be surprised to learn that stress can be good. Studies have shown that mild stress is associated with improved performance in athletes, entertainers, public speakers, and yes, test-takers. Butterflies, breathing faster, sweating, and other symptoms are automatic bodily responses to stressful situations. Stress can sharpen your attention, keep you alert, and give you greater energy.

Controlling Negative Thoughts

Factors that increase test anxiety include negative thoughts and self-doubt. Perhaps you have thought such things as, "I am going to fail the exam," "I won't do well," or "What will my family and co-workers think when I don't pass?" You must stop thinking such thoughts. Instead, say to yourself, "I have done this job successfully for a long time. I know what it takes to be a nursing assistant. I am prepared to take this exam." Think of the exam as a chance to show what you know and can do. Positive thinking comes before positive action and positive results.

Preparing Yourself Physically

Learning information and guidelines help you prepare mentally for an exam. Physical preparation is also important. Some stressful situations cannot be predicted. An exam, however, is known in advance. During the time before the exam, try not to schedule other stressful activities. Eat well and get plenty of rest. Combine studying with exercise and relaxation. Don't stay up late cramming the night before an exam. This is the time for reviewing studied material and getting a good night's sleep.

If you feel stressed during the period before the exam, try this deep-breathing method recommended by a stress management expert. Breathe deeply from your diaphragm. Do not move your chest and shoulders. You should feel your abdominal muscles expand as you breathe in and deflate when you breathe out. As you breathe out, your diaphragm and rib muscles relax, and your body may seem to sink down into the chair. Sixty seconds of deep breathing several times a day can help relieve stress.

GETTING READY FOR THE TEST

To prepare for a test, it is helpful to know whether it will contain **supply-type** or **selection-type** questions. Supply-type items are ones in which the test-taker supplies the answer. Essay and completion items are of this type. Selection-type items are ones in which the test-taker selects the answer from a number of possible answers. True-false, multiple-choice, and matching items are of this type. The exam you will take is a selection-type exam because it is made up of only multiple-choice questions. You must select the correct answer from four different choices.

Studying for a selection-type test is done differently than for a supply-type test. In studying for an essay exam (supply-type), you should be ready to explain major theories, principles, or ideas; look for ways to compare and contrast concepts; list pros and cons of important issues; and provide definitions of basic terms.

Whereas the essay test tends to measure one's ability to organize, integrate, and express ideas, the multiple-choice test more often measures word-for-word memory. The same subject matter should be studied for selection-type items as for supply-type items. For selection-type items, though, concentrate on learning specific facts and information.

Multiple-choice questions are used in standardized tests because they can be used to measure knowledge of facts and information as well as the application of facts and information. Knowledge items deal with such things as specific facts, common terms, methods and procedures, basic concepts and principles. Several examples of knowledge-level items follow.

Q. The most basic human need is for

   ① food.

   ② oxygen.

   ③ water.

   ④ elimination.

Q. Which of the following is NOT a psychological need?

① love

② belonging

③ exercise

④ identity

Application items measure a higher level of understanding. Here the test-taker must show that he or she not only understands the information, but also can apply it to a situation. You must apply facts, concepts, principles, rules, methods, and theories to situations on the job. Following is an example of an application-level question.

Q. The self-actualization needs of a resident can be assisted by

① listening to the resident.

② calling the resident by name.

③ encouraging the resident to be independent.

④ praising accomplishments of the resident.

You should be prepared to answer both knowledge and application-level questions.

Studying and Reviewing

No matter what type of test you take, you must first learn the material. A good way to study for an exam is to use a system of index cards. Thomson Delmar Learning has made this easy for you. The *Nurse Aide Exam Review Cards* and *Nurse Aide Exam Review Cards with Audio CD* are available in both English and Spanish. Using these items to study for your state test will greatly improve your chances of successfully completing the exam.

If you wish to prepare additional study cards of your own, obtain some 3 × 5 index cards or cut sheets of paper into a convenient size. On one side of the card, write down terms, methods and procedures, basic concepts and principles, and other specific facts. On the reverse side of the card, write the answer, definition, explanation, or whatever else is important. Here are several examples.

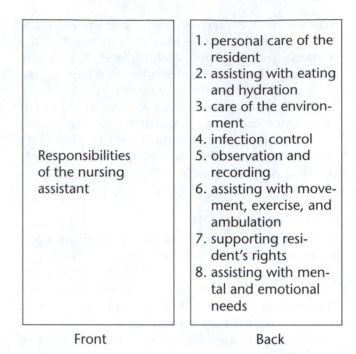

Front | Back

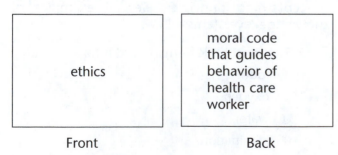

Front | Back

To study, look at the front of the card, and try to remember what is written on the back. Turn the card over to see whether you are correct. After going through all the cards once, shuffle them and review the cards again. You want to be sure you know the information in any order.

As you review the cards, begin to sort them into two piles. One pile will be those you know well and the other pile will be those you are having trouble remembering. Once you have two piles, try to learn the more difficult information. Continue reviewing the cards until you are sure you have learned the material. Review the cards several times a day during the time before the exam.

There are a number of advantages to using this system. First, preparing the cards is a learning experience. Second, the cards are easy to carry with you in a pocket or purse. You can study them during spare moments throughout the day. Another advantage is that you can use the cards with a friend to quiz each other.

Taking the Practice Test

Practicing what is required to get ready for a test is excellent preparation for taking an actual exam. Taking a practice test can get you used to the kinds of directions that are given, the types of questions you will be expected to answer, and the process of marking machine-readable test booklets. It can also help you learn your strengths and weaknesses.

Appendix D contains a practice test that you will take. Treat the practice test as a real test. The practice test will be given under conditions as similar as possible to the real test. Time yourself when taking this practice exam, but avoid feeling pressured or rushing.

Practice working with time limits. Note specifically the average time it takes you to complete a question. If you work at a steady pace, you should have plenty of time to complete the exam in, the time allowed.

After finishing the practice test, you will have an opportunity to score it and discuss specific questions. Use this opportunity to ask questions about questions that you missed. Use the results of the practice test to identify those areas you need to study. The score does not indicate whether you will pass or fail the competency test. Different states use different passing scores.

TAKING THE TEST

To do well on a test, you should be at your best when you start. Eat a good breakfast or lunch. Try to avoid anything that will make you tense. Leave for the test site early enough to arrive on time. Be sure to allow for minor delays. Take a watch and two number two black lead pencils with erasers. Many states require you to bring an identification card with your picture on it to show the examiner. When you arrive, do not allow another person's last-minute questions or comments to disturb you. Follow these general rules for taking the test:

1. You will get verbal instructions before you take the test. You will complete an information page. Listen carefully to what the examiner tells you to do. Remember that the examiner is required to read or give very specific directions. The rules and directions are designed to treat fairly everyone who takes the test.

2. Before the test begins, take a few seconds to pay attention. Close your eyes and take several deep breaths. Remind yourself that you have studied well. Think positive.

3. Once you get the test and are told to begin, carefully read the directions. Look at any sample questions. Make sure that you understand how to mark answers on the test booklet or answer sheet. The test probably will be machine-scored, so be careful in recording answers.

4. You will have 90 minutes to 2 hours to answer 50 to 75 questions. This is a very generous amount of time. If you work at a steady pace you should have no problem finishing the test on time. Pause to check time and make sure that you are working at about the right speed. The examiner will post the time remaining.

5. Read the stem of the question and answer it in your own words without looking at the choices or alternatives. Then search for the alternative that matches your answer. Always read all of the alternatives. Answer "A" may be right, but answer "C" may be a better answer.

6. Some questions may ask you to analyze a situation or use what you have learned to solve a problem. If you do not know the answer immediately, it is often helpful to cross out unnecessary information. Distracting or extra information has been crossed out in the following example.

   Q. A resident ~~who~~ wears a wig ~~understands that the nurse aide will not talk about this information outside the facility~~ because this information is

   ① legal.

   ② confidential.

   ③ negligent.

   ④ cultural.

7. If you do not know an answer, circle the question and move on. You can come back to it later. This will save you time and help prevent the anxiety that comes from trying to remember. More importantly, you may find a clue to the answer somewhere in a later question.

8. If you encounter a very difficult question, do not worry. The rest of the test-takers will probably have trouble with it also. Keep in mind that a perfect score is not expected on a standardized test.

9. Be alert to such words as *not* and *except* that can completely change the intent of the question. Words in the stem are often *italicized,* CAPITALIZED, or are within "quotation marks" or (parentheses). Pay attention to such words. They are usually important to answering the question.

10. Standardized tests are revised several times so that the questions are clearly worded. Do not read more into a question than is asked for. Do not look for trick questions or hidden meanings. If a question seems unclear, read it several times. Pay close attention to how it is worded. Try to relate the question to information and tasks with which you are familiar.

11. Avoid unfamiliar choices or alternatives. An alternative that you do not know, uses difficult words, or seems complicated is probably incorrect.

12. If you do not know an answer, try to determine what the answer is *not.* Begin by crossing out alternatives that you know or feel are incorrect. If you can cross out two choices, you now have

a 50% chance of choosing the correct answer of the remaining two alternatives.

13. Your score on the exam will be based on the number of questions answered correctly. So, be sure and answer all questions. There is no penalty for guessing. This means that for those items that have you completely stumped, you should go ahead and guess. First, however, try to cross out choices that seem wrong.

14. As you near the end of the test, do not worry if some individuals have finished already. Studies have shown that those who complete a test early do not necessarily get better scores than those who finish later.

15. When you get to the end of the test, go back and complete those items that you skipped earlier. You may remember the answer or be able to narrow down the answer.

16. If you answer all of the questions and still have time remaining, review your answers. After rereading a question, you may have second thoughts about the answer. Should you change it? For those who have studied well for an exam, research shows that more of them are helped than hurt by changing answers. Do not change answers without a good reason, but go ahead and change any answers that are based on new insights or recall of new information.

17. Before turning in the test, review how you marked the answers. Check to see that you answered every question, that you marked only one answer per question, that you marked the answer neatly and legibly, and that you completely erased any changes that were made. Erase any other marks you may have made on the test booklet.

Miscellaneous Testing Concerns

- Many states have a practice test and candidate handbook available. Ask your instructor if these tools are available in your state. They will be invaluable in preparing for your state test. Many state nursing assistant registries also maintain websites. If your state registry is online, you may wish to check its website for information about the state test.

- Some states administer oral examinations. Some states administer examinations in languages other than English. These special examinations must be requested from your state testing agency when you register to take the test. If you think you need an oral examination or non-English version of the test, contact your instructor or state testing service for information and instructions.

- Your state will accommodate individuals with certain disabilities during the test. Contact your state testing agency in advance for information on requesting accommodations.

- Your state will have a skills (manual competency) examination portion of the state certification test. You must pass both portions of the test before being entered in the nursing assistant registry. Some states require candidates to pass the written portion of the test before they are allowed to take the skills test, or vice versa. Contact your instructor or state testing agency for information.

- Do not bring children or visitors to the test site. These individuals will not be admitted.

- Do not bring pagers, telephones, or electronic devices to the test site. Use of these items will not be permitted.

Test Security

- The person who is giving the test will answer questions about the mechanics of taking the test, but he or she is not permitted to help you or to clarify questions about content of the test.

- Do not give help to or receive help from anyone during the test. If this occurs, the test will be stopped and your test will not be scored. You may be reported to your state nursing assistant registry for this activity.

- Individuals caught removing a test from the testing site may be prosecuted.

THE SKILLS EXAMINATION

Part of the state test you will take is a skills examination or competency evaluation. This examination is administered differently in each state. Usually, a nurse who has no affiliation with your nursing assistant program will administer the examination. You will be tested on the number of skills required by your state. The pass and fail criteria are also determined by your state. In some states, testing is done in a skills laboratory setting. In other states, testing is done on residents of a nursing facility.

Preparing for the Skills Examination

The only way to adequately prepare for the skills examination is to practice the procedures in sequence. The skills that you will be tested on are randomly chosen from the procedures you learned in class. If your nursing assistant program has a review day or a mock skills examination before you take the test, be sure to attend. This will be very helpful to you in preparing for the test. You should also review your vocabulary terms so that you are familiar with the various names of the procedures. For example, the skills examiner may direct you to "ambulate the resident." From your review of the vocabulary, you know that *ambulate* means *to walk.* When reviewing the procedures, pay attention to the list of equipment and supplies that you will need to gather before you perform the procedure.

There is no way to study for the skills examination except by practicing the procedures you have learned in class. The skills examiner will watch for some things during the examination. Some of these observations are very important and may be the deciding factor on whether you pass or fail a particular skill on the examination.

Observations Made During the Skills Examination

- The skills examiner will observe **handwashing.** He will look at your handwashing technique to be sure that you follow the accepted procedure. The examiner will also observe how often you wash your hands and if you wear gloves when necessary. The examiner may observe how and where you dispose of the gloves.

- You will be observed in how well you **communicate** with the resident. You must introduce yourself and the skills examiner. Explain what you are going to do, even if the resident is confused. You may also be evaluated on whether you talk to the resident while you are performing the procedure.

- The skills examiner will observe how well you practice **safety.** For example, do you put the side rails up on the bed when you are not directly next to it? Do you lock the brakes on the wheelchair before you transfer the resident?

- **Infection control** is another area on which you are evaluated. The skills examiner will observe whether you keep clean items separated from

dirty ones, and how well you practice medical asepsis.

- **Practicing resident rights is important.** Be sure to knock on doors. Use the bath blanket during the bathing procedure. Pull the privacy curtain, close the window curtains, and close the door to the room.

Gather all of the supplies you will need before you take each section of the skills test. If you will be making a bed, stack the linen in the order of use. The test will go more smoothly for you if you are well organized.

If your state uses skills checklists that note the automatic failures on the skills examination, pay close attention to them. For example, in many states if you fail to balance the scale before you weigh the resident, you will fail this skill. If you are assigned to do peri care on a female, and you wash the resident from **back to front,** you will fail the skill. If this information is available in your nursing assistant program, it will be very helpful to you. The automatic failure points on the skills examination are things that could potentially cause harm to a resident, so studying them will do more than help you pass the test. Knowing these things will help you feel more secure that you are providing quality care when you are working with your assigned residents!

AFTER THE TEST

When time is called, you can breathe a sigh of relief. Listen carefully, however, to instructions about what to do with the test booklet. Information may also be given about when and how you will find out the results. The examiner will not be allowed to give you the answers to test questions after the test.

You may have to wait several weeks before you receive the test results. During this time, try not to worry. People tend to underestimate their performance on an exam. Thousands of people will take this exam. Be confident that you probably will score as well as or better than most of them.

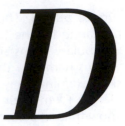

Practice Exam

Choose the best answer for the following questions.

1. The moral code that guides the behavior of the health care worker is called
   - Ⓐ etiquette.
   - Ⓑ ethics.
   - Ⓒ care plan.
   - Ⓓ dignity.

2. When communicating with the resident who is hearing-impaired, it is important to
   - Ⓐ approach the resident from behind.
   - Ⓑ make sure the light source is at your back.
   - Ⓒ yell into the resident's good ear.
   - Ⓓ gently touch the resident to get his attention.

3. When you position a resident in the lateral position, you will use pillows to support
   - Ⓐ the lower arm and leg.
   - Ⓑ the upper arm and hand.
   - Ⓒ the lower foot and leg.
   - Ⓓ the upper arm and leg.

4. Which of the following is a developmental task of the elderly resident?
   - Ⓐ increased social involvement
   - Ⓑ adjusting to losses
   - Ⓒ having a second career
   - Ⓓ adjusting to middle age

5. Which of the following would be considered an example of a pressure-reducing device?
   - Ⓐ quad cane
   - Ⓑ walker
   - Ⓒ gel mattress
   - Ⓓ pulley

6. Before replacing dentures into a resident's mouth,
   - Ⓐ apply gloves.
   - Ⓑ rinse the dentures with mouthwash.
   - Ⓒ store dentures in denture cup.
   - Ⓓ floss the resident's teeth.

7. The electronic thermometer can be used for taking what kind of temperature?
   - Ⓐ oral and tympanic
   - Ⓑ oral, axillary, and tympanic
   - Ⓒ oral and rectal only
   - Ⓓ oral, rectal, axillary, and tympanic

8. When you have completed colostomy care for a resident, you will record any output as
   - Ⓐ urinary output.
   - Ⓑ a bowel movement.
   - Ⓒ an emesis.
   - Ⓓ homeostasis.

9. To properly give a bed bath,
   - Ⓐ cover the resident and bathe the entire body one part at a time.
   - Ⓑ uncover the resident, bathe the entire body, then cover again.
   - Ⓒ cover the resident and bathe face, hands, underarms, back, and genital area, one part at a time.
   - Ⓓ cover the resident and take him or her to the shower in a shower chair.

10. When personal mail is sent to a long-term care facility resident, who has the right to open it first?

    (A) administrator

    (B) director of nurses

    (C) resident

    (D) state inspectors

11. Mrs. Smith is an ambulatory resident. It would be most appropriate in a long-term care facility for her to have lunch in

    (A) her bed.

    (B) her room.

    (C) the dining room.

    (D) the lobby.

12. The nursing assistant is responsible for:

    (A) cutting the fingernails and toenails of all residents.

    (B) keeping the fingernails and toenails of residents clean.

    (C) filing the toenails with a nail file to round the edges.

    (D) calling the podiatrist when a resident needs nails cut.

13. When you are washing your hands, what part of the procedure removes the most germs?

    (A) using warm, running water

    (B) shaking water off your hands

    (C) using friction while scrubbing hands

    (D) using plenty of soap.

14. Safety of residents is the responsibility of

    (A) family members.

    (B) the administrator.

    (C) the maintenance staff.

    (D) all staff.

15. In order for a fire to occur, there must be a spark or flame, oxygen, and material that will burn. In most fire situations, where would the oxygen come from?

    (A) oxygen tanks

    (B) the air itself

    (C) the air conditioning

    (D) the heating system

16. Why is it important to explain lifting procedures to residents before you do them?

    (A) to be polite

    (B) to enlist their cooperation and help

    (C) to prevent any arguments

    (D) to provide therapeutic communication

17. When removing soiled linen from the bed,

    (A) shake linen gently to find lost items.

    (B) roll it into a ball and place it on the floor.

    (C) place the linen into the hamper.

    (D) put it on the overbed table.

18. A resident is waving one arm wildly, grabbing at the throat area and coughing. Your best response is to

    (A) get him a drink of water.

    (B) run and get the nurse.

    (C) stay there and allow him to continue coughing.

    (D) slap his back four times firmly.

19. The nurse asks you to check vital signs on Mrs. Jones. You will check her

    (A) blood pressure, pulse, and weight.

    (B) temperature, pulse, height, and weight.

    (C) temperature, pulse, respirations, and weight.

    (D) blood pressure, temperature, pulse, and respirations.

20. When a resident with a paralyzed side wants to brush his own teeth, you should

    (A) brush his teeth for him anyway.

    (B) set out the supplies and allow him to do it.

    (C) explain that you are happy to help him and do it for him.

    (D) guide his toothbrush through the procedure.

21. Mr. Ronzani is a bedfast resident with a stage IV pressure ulcer. He uses a therapeutic air mattress. The bottom sheet slides around on the mattress and gets bunched up under the resident at least once a day. You should:

    (A) check the sheet and straighten it when needed.

    (B) pin the sheet securely to the mattress.

    (C) tuck the sheet in very tightly.

    (D) tie the sheet to the side rails.

22. When communicating with a resident who has a vision impairment, you should:

    (A) yell loudly in the resident's ear.

    (B) place a bright light behind your back so the resident can see you.

Ⓒ discuss what you see, interesting changes, and what various people are doing.

Ⓓ always use sign language.

23. The correct positioning of the resident's body is called

Ⓐ muscle development.

Ⓑ body mechanics.

Ⓒ body alignment.

Ⓓ range of motion.

24. What kind of problems exist for a resident who needs elastic stockings (TED hose)?

Ⓐ urinary

Ⓑ respiratory

Ⓒ circulatory

Ⓓ digestive

25. The nurse tells you to ambulate Mrs. Black. This means to

Ⓐ sit her in the wheelchair.

Ⓑ sit her on the edge of the bed.

Ⓒ assist her to the bathroom.

Ⓓ walk the resident.

26. To properly wash the eyes while giving a bed bath, you would

Ⓐ wipe from outer side of eye to inner side.

Ⓑ wipe from inner side of eye to outer side.

Ⓒ use a back-and-forth motion.

Ⓓ use plenty of soap and water.

27. An example of meeting the spiritual needs of a resident would be to assist with

Ⓐ eating supper.

Ⓑ going to sleep.

Ⓒ saying prayers.

Ⓓ getting dressed.

28. Microorganisms are completely destroyed by

Ⓐ sterilization.

Ⓑ handwashing.

Ⓒ disinfection.

Ⓓ medical asepsis.

29. When you find a resident who appears to have fallen on the floor, your first action is to

Ⓐ run to get help.

Ⓑ put the resident in bed.

Ⓒ stay with the resident.

Ⓓ call the paramedics.

30. The skin of the elderly resident becomes

Ⓐ thicker.

Ⓑ fatter.

Ⓒ thinner.

Ⓓ brittle.

31. Standard equipment in the resident's unit is the

Ⓐ television, electric bed, and telephone.

Ⓑ wheelchair, stretcher, and mechanical lift.

Ⓒ hopper, sink, table, and work counter.

Ⓓ bedside stand, bed, chair, and overbed table.

32. Your resident's care plan states to check BP q.i.d. This means to check the blood pressure

Ⓐ every day.

Ⓑ four times a day.

Ⓒ every other day.

Ⓓ six times a day.

33. You have taken a resident's rectal temperature and the thermometer reads 100 degrees. From your knowledge about body temperature, the oral temperature on this resident would be

Ⓐ 101.

Ⓑ 99.

Ⓒ 98.

Ⓓ 97.

34. Mrs. Gree is a 70-year-old resident who has been on bedrest with pneumonia for three days. You note a reddened area on her back. Your best response is to

Ⓐ encourage her to get up and move about.

Ⓑ apply a dressing to the area.

Ⓒ massage the area with lotion.

Ⓓ report the area to the nurse.

35. If you are assisting a resident with ADLs, you are helping with

Ⓐ activities of daily living.

Ⓑ activities during leisure.

Ⓒ proper alignment.

Ⓓ AM care.

36. When residents are helpless and lie in one position for too long, there is a risk of developing

Ⓐ range of motion.

Ⓑ vision impairment.

Ⓒ incontinence.

Ⓓ contractures.

37. When you take a resident's pulse, you are using a/an

    Ⓐ artery.

    Ⓑ vein.

    Ⓒ capillary.

    Ⓓ alveoli.

38. You remove the resident's clothes to give her a shower. A dressing falls from her hip onto the floor, revealing a minor open wound. The wound is not bleeding, but there is a small amount of old, dried blood on the dressing. You should:

    Ⓐ pick it up and put it in the open trash can.

    Ⓑ apply gloves and place the dressing in a plastic bag.

    Ⓒ get the nurse in charge at once.

    Ⓓ do nothing, as this is not your responsibility.

39. The strongest muscles you should use for lifting are in your

    Ⓐ buttocks.

    Ⓑ thighs.

    Ⓒ back.

    Ⓓ abdomen.

40. Restraints require a doctor's order and must be released every

    Ⓐ half-hour.

    Ⓑ hour.

    Ⓒ two hours.

    Ⓓ four hours.

41. When residents are admitted to a long-term care facility, they

    Ⓐ no longer have the right to vote.

    Ⓑ can continue to vote in elections.

    Ⓒ cannot leave the facility.

    Ⓓ can keep medicine on the overbed table.

42. Exposing a resident unnecessarily would be a threat to the right to

    Ⓐ privacy.

    Ⓑ security.

    Ⓒ acceptance.

    Ⓓ belonging.

43. Basic human needs are

    Ⓐ different for each person.

    Ⓑ varied in men and women.

    Ⓒ the same for all people.

    Ⓓ different, depending on religion.

44. When a resident has a need for recognition, you can easily provide this by

    Ⓐ calling the resident by name.

    Ⓑ explaining procedures.

    Ⓒ providing privacy.

    Ⓓ turning on the television.

45. A resident who frequently wanders at night, becomes easily agitated, and cannot be calmed down is displaying symptoms of

    Ⓐ mental retardation.

    Ⓑ multiple sclerosis.

    Ⓒ Alzheimer's disease.

    Ⓓ delusions.

46. When giving a bed bath, always obtain clean bathwater after washing the

    Ⓐ abdomen.

    Ⓑ legs and feet.

    Ⓒ armpits.

    Ⓓ face.

47. An example of an adaptive device to help a resident in dressing and grooming tasks would be a

    Ⓐ handroll.

    Ⓑ transfer belt.

    Ⓒ long-handled shoehorn.

    Ⓓ four-pronged cane.

48. Mr. Brown's TPR is 96.8(R)-104-30. Which, if any, are normal?

    Ⓐ temperature

    Ⓑ pulse

    Ⓒ respirations

    Ⓓ none are normal

49. Who is responsible for balancing the scale before taking a resident's weight?

    Ⓐ nurse

    Ⓑ nursing assistant

    Ⓒ maintenance staff

    Ⓓ administrator

50. An occupied bed is made with the

    Ⓐ resident in a chair.

    Ⓑ assistance of the nurse.

Ⓒ resident in the bed.

Ⓓ resident out of the room.

51. The food guide pyramid should be used to:

Ⓐ plan the diet for residents who are receiving tube feedings.

Ⓑ plan well-balanced meals each day.

Ⓒ calculate the resident's height and weight.

Ⓓ ensure that residents who have diabetes receive their snacks.

52. The term *edema* means

Ⓐ abnormal swelling in the tissues.

Ⓑ loss of fluid from the tissues.

Ⓒ instilling fluid into the rectum.

Ⓓ the same as dehydration.

53. When counting a resident's pulse, you notice it is weak and irregular. Proper technique would be to count

Ⓐ for one full minute, report it to the nurse, and record.

Ⓑ for 30 seconds, double that number, and record.

Ⓒ for 15 seconds, multiply by 4, and record.

Ⓓ the pulse in two separate locations.

54. One of your residents wants to see the chaplain immediately, but the chaplain has left for the day. What should you do?

Ⓐ Ignore the request. The chaplain will be back tomorrow.

Ⓑ Tell the resident the chaplain has left for the day.

Ⓒ Ask the resident, "Why do you want to see him?"

Ⓓ Refer the request to the nurse.

55. The nurse informs you that Mrs. White has high blood pressure. Another word for this is

Ⓐ hypotension.

Ⓑ systolic.

Ⓒ hypertension.

Ⓓ diastolic.

56. When you logroll a resident, before placing him on a bedpan, place your hands on the resident's

Ⓐ shoulder and hip.

Ⓑ waist and hip.

Ⓒ hip and leg.

Ⓓ arm and leg.

57. When you take a resident's blood pressure, you are measuring

Ⓐ the volume of blood.

Ⓑ the force of the heart.

Ⓒ how fast the heart is beating.

Ⓓ the rhythm of the pulse.

58. The skin of the geriatric resident produces

Ⓐ more oil.

Ⓑ less oil.

Ⓒ less pigment.

Ⓓ more fat.

59. When a resident expresses a like or dislike for certain foods, it may be because of

Ⓐ the surroundings in which it is served.

Ⓑ your influence on the resident.

Ⓒ family customs and cultural influence.

Ⓓ a decrease in appetite.

60. You are assigned to take blood pressures on four residents. Mr. Keeley is the second resident you have taken vital signs on. Mr. Keeley's vital signs are: T 98.2, P 96, R 18, B/P 202/126. You should:

Ⓐ finish taking the vital signs on the other residents you are assigned to.

Ⓑ go to the nurses' station and record Mr. Keeley's vital signs in the chart.

Ⓒ notify the nurse of Mr. Keeley's abnormal pulse rate.

Ⓓ notify the nurse of Mr. Keeley's blood pressure.

61. During Mrs. Smith's bath, you observe that her face is very flushed and her skin feels warm to the touch. The best way to report this to the nurse is

Ⓐ "Mrs. Smith has a fever."

Ⓑ "I think Mrs. Smith is getting sick."

Ⓒ "You should take Mrs. Smith's temperature."

Ⓓ "Mrs. Smith's face is flushed and her skin feels warm."

62. Effective communication is a very important part of your job as a nursing assistant. When you smile at a resident, what kind of communication are you using?

Ⓐ sign language

Ⓑ body language

Ⓒ oral communication

Ⓓ verbal communication

63. "STAT" means
   - Ⓐ as desired.
   - Ⓑ as necessary.
   - Ⓒ at once.
   - Ⓓ at mealtime.

64. When a resident is on I & O, you will do your recording as
   - Ⓐ ounces and quarts.
   - Ⓑ cups and gallons.
   - Ⓒ cubic centimeters or milliliters.
   - Ⓓ centigrade or Fahrenheit.

65. When you sit a resident up on the edge of the bed and the resident becomes dizzy, your best action is to
   - Ⓐ sit the resident in the chair.
   - Ⓑ lay the resident down and call the nurse.
   - Ⓒ tell the resident it will be okay in a few minutes.
   - Ⓓ put the resident into a wheelchair and take her to the nurse.

66. The extent to which a person is capable of moving a joint is called
   - Ⓐ flexibility.
   - Ⓑ body mechanics.
   - Ⓒ restoration.
   - Ⓓ range of motion.

67. When a resident has died and you are doing postmortem care, the right to privacy is
   - Ⓐ no longer necessary.
   - Ⓑ still protected after death.
   - Ⓒ only for the family.
   - Ⓓ only for the funeral home.

68. When you assist residents to get ready for mealtime, you would also include checking their
   - Ⓐ weight.
   - Ⓑ blood pressure.
   - Ⓒ need to use the toilet.
   - Ⓓ need to say grace.

69. If a resident leaves 1/4 of an 8-ounce glass of milk on the tray, how much would you record as taken?
   - Ⓐ 60 mL.
   - Ⓑ 120 mL.
   - Ⓒ 180 mL.
   - Ⓓ 240 mL.

70. Mrs. Smith's blood pressure is 142/88. You will record the systolic reading as
   - Ⓐ 230.
   - Ⓑ 142.
   - Ⓒ 88.
   - Ⓓ 54.

71. Mr. Jones, a bedridden resident, states he has to move his bowels. You would help him use the
   - Ⓐ bedpan.
   - Ⓑ urinal.
   - Ⓒ commode.
   - Ⓓ colostomy bag.

72. When you communicate to residents in a manner called "therapeutic communication," what specifically are you doing?
   - Ⓐ preparing them for a visit from the doctor
   - Ⓑ healing or improving an existing situation
   - Ⓒ planning to take them to physical therapy
   - Ⓓ encouraging them to get involved in activities

73. Helping residents reach their highest level of ability is the goal of
   - Ⓐ range of motion.
   - Ⓑ disease prevention.
   - Ⓒ rehabilitation.
   - Ⓓ supination.

74. A good ethical practice as a nursing assistant would be to
   - Ⓐ share your problems with the resident.
   - Ⓑ use care with the resident's belongings.
   - Ⓒ discuss the resident's condition at break.
   - Ⓓ borrow items from the resident's dresser.

75. To properly practice what you have been taught about standard precautions, it is best to
   - Ⓐ always wear a mask.
   - Ⓑ dispose of trash first.
   - Ⓒ scrub your hands with a brush.
   - Ⓓ carry gloves at all times.

Note: For practice, use "Practice Exam Answer Sheets (Appendix F)" on page 418.

ANSWERS TO PRACTICE EXAM

1. B	11. C	21. A	31. D	41. B	51. B	61. D	71. A
2. D	12. B	22. C	32. B	42. A	52. A	62. B	72. B
3. D	13. C	23. C	33. B	43. C	53. A	63. C	73. C
4. B	14. D	24. C	34. D	44. A	54. D	64. C	74. B
5. C	15. B	25. D	35. A	45. C	55. C	65. B	75. D
6. A	16. B	26. B	36. D	46. B	56. A	66. D	
7. D	17. C	27. C	37. A	47. C	57. B	67. B	
8. B	18. C	28. A	38. B	48. D	58. B	68. C	
9. A	19. D	29. C	39. B	49. B	59. C	69. C	
10. C	20. B	30. C	40. C	50. C	60. D	70. B	

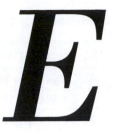

Procedure Review

PERFORMANCE REVIEW CHECKLIST

Procedure ___1___

Procedure <u>Postmortem Care</u>

Name of Nursing Assistant _____ Date of Program _____ to _____

Social Security Number of Nursing Assistant _____

Program Code Number _____

S=Satisfactory Performance
U=Unsatisfactory Performance

Place a full signature to correspond with each set of initials appearing below:

Initials	Corresponding Signature of Instructor	Title

Procedure Guidelines	S/U	Date	Initials	S/U	Date	Initials
1. Wash your hands.						
2. Gather supplies: shroud kit with gown and identification tags, a basin of warm water, soap, washcloth, towels, swabs for oral care, linen, gown, and gloves.						
3. Pull the curtains and close the door for privacy.						
4. Treat the body gently and with respect.						

(continues)

continued

5.	Apply gloves.						
6.	Raise the bed to a comfortable working height.						
7.	Place the resident on her back, with a pillow beneath the head and shoulders in proper body alignment.						
8.	Close the eyes by gently pulling eyelids down.						
9.	Provide mouth care using moistened oral care swabs or sponges.						
10.	Place cleaned dentures in the mouth or in a labeled denture cup. The dentures should be sent to the funeral home with the body.						
11.	Close the mouth. A rolled-up washcloth may be placed under the chin to keep the jaw closed.						
12.	Remove all tubing from the body if this is your facility policy. In most facilities this is done by the nurse.						
13.	Bathe the body, comb hair, and straighten the arms and legs.						
14.	Apply clean dressings to wounds, if necessary.						
15.	Place a disposable pad under the buttocks.						
16.	Put a gown on the body.						
17.	Attach an identification tag to the body as indicated by facility policy.						
18.	Replace soiled linen and cover the body to the shoulders with a sheet.						
19.	Remove gloves and dispose according to facility policy.						
20.	Wash your hands.						
21.	Tidy the unit.						
22.	Wash your hands.						
23.	Provide privacy and allow family members to be alone with the resident.						
24.	Collect all belongings, place them in a bag, and label them correctly. Usually these are given to the family. If no family members are present,						

(continues)

continued

	follow facility policy. Complete and sign the inventory sheet if this is your facility policy.						
25.	After the family leaves, wash your hands and put the shroud on the body. Wear gloves if contact with blood, body fluid, secretions, or excretions is likely.						
26.	Remove gloves, if worn, and dispose according to facility policy.						
27.	Follow facility policy to take the body to the morgue, or close the door until the funeral home staff arrives.						
28.	Notify the nurse when the funeral home staff arrives.						
29.	Assist the funeral home staff to move the body, if necessary.						
30.	Strip and clean the unit according to your facility policy after the body has been removed.						

PERFORMANCE REVIEW CHECKLIST

Procedure ___2___

Procedure <u>Handwashing</u>

Name of Nursing Assistant _____ Date of Program _____ to _____

Social Security Number of Nursing Assistant _____

Program Code Number _____

S=Satisfactory Performance
U=Unsatisfactory Performance

Place a full signature to correspond with each set of initials appearing below:

Initials	Corresponding Signature of Instructor	Title

Procedure Guidelines	S/U	Date	Initials	S/U	Date	Initials
1. Stand away from the sink. Your uniform and hands must not touch the sink. Roll up long sleeves and push your watch up above your wrist.						
2. Turn on warm water. Adjust water to a comfortable temperature.						
3. Wet hands, keeping your fingertips pointed down.						
4. Apply soap over hands and wrists, working it into a lather.						
5. Rub your hands together vigorously to create a lather. Rub the hands together in a circular motion for at least 15 seconds. Rub all surfaces of the hands. Pay particular attention to the area between your fingers. Wash your thumbs well. Keep your fingertips pointed down.						
6. Rub the fingernails against the palm of the opposite hand. Clean the nails with a brush or an orange stick if they are soiled.						
7. Rinse your hands from the wrist to the fingertips. Keep the fingers pointed down.						
8. Do not shake water from hands.						

(continues)

continued

9.	Dry hands with a clean paper towel. Discard paper towel properly.					
10.	Use a clean, dry paper towel to turn off the faucet. Do not touch the faucet handle with your hand.					
11.	Discard the paper towel in the wastebasket.					

PERFORMANCE REVIEW CHECKLIST

Procedure ___3–4___

Procedure <u>Isolation Procedures</u>

Name of Nursing Assistant _____ Date of Program _____ to _____

Social Security Number of Nursing Assistant _____

Program Code Number _____

S=Satisfactory Performance
U=Unsatisfactory Performance

Place a full signature to correspond with each set of initials appearing below:

Initials	Corresponding Signature of Instructor	Title

Procedure Guidelines	S/U	Date	Initials	S/U	Date	Initials
Putting on disposable gown, gloves, goggles, and mask						
1. Remove your watch and place it on a clean paper towel. You will carry your watch with you into the isolation room on the paper towel.						
2. Wash your hands and dry them thoroughly.						
3. Put on a gown. Tie the neck ties.						
4. Tie the waist ties of the gown, making certain the gown is overlapping and covering your uniform.						
5. Put a mask on, and adjust it over your nose and mouth. Tie the mask securely at the back of your head, or slip the elastic straps over your ears.						
6. Position goggles over eyes and adjust to fit.						
7. Put on gloves, covering the cuffs of the gown with the top edge of the glove.						
Removing disposable gown, gloves, goggles, and mask						
1. Make sure that all jobs in the isolation unit are complete and that the resident is comfortable and safe. Place needed personal items and the call signal within the resident's reach.						

(continues)

continued

2.	Remove gloves by turning them inside out and dispose of them in the biohazardous waste receptacle.						
3.	Remove goggles or face shield, handling only by the elastic.						
4.	Untie the waist ties of the gown.						
5.	Untie the neck ties of the gown and loosen the gown at the shoulders.						
6.	Slip the fingers of one hand under the cuff of the gown on the opposite arm. Do not touch the outside of the gown. Pull it down over your hand.						
7.	With your hand inside the gown, pull the gown off the other arm.						
8.	Fold and roll the gown away from your body, with the contaminated side facing in.						
9.	Dispose of the gown in the covered biohazardous waste container.						
10.	Remove the mask by grasping only the ties. Untie the bottom tie first, then the top tie, or slip the elastic straps over your ears.						
11.	Discard the mask in the covered trash container.						
12.	Wash and dry your hands. Turn off the faucet with a clean paper towel.						
13.	Pick up your watch and put it on your wrist.						
14.	Holding the clean upper side of the paper towel, pick up the towel and discard it in the trash.						
15.	Obtain a clean paper towel from the dispenser and use it to open the door of the room.						
16.	Discard the towel inside the room.						
17.	Repeat handwashing if this is your preference or facility policy.						

PERFORMANCE REVIEW CHECKLIST

Procedure __5__

Procedure Applying a Vest Restraint

Name of Nursing Assistant _____ Date of Program _____ to _____

Social Security Number of Nursing Assistant _____

Program Code Number _____

S=Satisfactory Performance
U=Unsatisfactory Performance

Place a full signature to correspond with each set of initials appearing below:

Initials	Corresponding Signature of Instructor	Title

Procedure Guidelines	S/U	Date	Initials	S/U	Date	Initials
1. Obtain a restraint of the proper type and size.						
2. Get help if necessary.						
3. Perform your beginning procedure actions.						
4. Slip the resident's arms through the armholes of the vest.						
5. Make sure that the clothing under the restraint is not wrinkled and that the vest fits smoothly.						
6. Cross the vest in the front and thread the straps through the slots on the sides of the vest. If a vest is used on a female resident, be sure that the breasts are not under the straps.						

(continues)

continued

7. Thread the straps *between* the seat and the armrest if the resident is in a wheelchair. Pull the straps back securely. If the resident is in bed, attach the straps to the moveable part of the bed frame. (This way, if the bed is raised, the resident will not be restricted or strangled by the restraint.) Follow your facility policy for the type of beds used. Many different types of beds are used in health care facilities.						
8. Finish tying the restraint in a slipknot under the chair or to the bed frame. Refer to the specific manufacturer's directions for the restraint you are using.						
9. Insert three fingers under the restraint and check to be sure that it is not too tight.						
10. Perform your procedure completion actions.						

PERFORMANCE REVIEW CHECKLIST

Procedure ___6___

Procedure <u>Applying a Belt Restraint</u>

Name of Nursing Assistant _____ Date of Program _____ to _____

Social Security Number of Nursing Assistant _____

Program Code Number _____

S=Satisfactory Performance
U=Unsatisfactory Performance

Place a full signature to correspond with each set of initials appearing below:

Initials	Corresponding Signature of Instructor	Title

	Procedure Guidelines	S/U	Date	Initials	S/U	Date	Initials
1.	Perform your beginning procedure actions.						
2.	Get help from another nursing assistant, if necessary.						
3.	If the resident is in a wheelchair, move the hips as far back as possible, position the footrests to support the feet, and lock the brakes.						
4.	Place the belt around the waist. Cross the straps through the loops behind the resident.						
5.	After the straps are threaded through the loops, tighten the belt securely around the waist.						
6.	Insert the straps between the seat and armrest, or between the seat and backrest, according to the manufacturer's recommendations for the type of restraint you are using.						

(continues)

continued

7.	Bring the straps down and tie them to the kickspurs of the wheelchair, using a quick-release knot, according to the manufacturer's directions.						
8.	Insert three fingers under the restraint and check to be sure that it is not too tight.						
9.	Perform your procedure completion actions.						

PERFORMANCE REVIEW CHECKLIST

Procedure ___7___

Procedure <u>Clearing an Obstructed Airway (Heimlich Maneuver)</u>

Name of Nursing Assistant _____ Date of Program _____ to _____

Social Security Number of Nursing Assistant _____

Program Code Number _____

S=Satisfactory Performance
U=Unsatisfactory Performance

Place a full signature to correspond with each set of initials appearing below:

Initials	Corresponding Signature of Instructor	Title

Procedure Guidelines	S/U	Date	Initials	S/U	Date	Initials
Clearing an Obstructed Airway in a Conscious Resident						
1. Ask the resident, "Are you choking?" or "Can you speak?" (If so, encourage the resident to try to cough the object out. Stay with the resident and assist if the cough is weak or the resident is in distress.) Call for the nurse immediately.						
2. Tell the resident that you will help. If the resident is sitting or standing, stand behind him.						
3. Wrap your arms around the resident's waist, above the hips.						
4. Make a fist with one hand.						
5. Place the thumb side of your fist against the resident's abdomen, just above the navel and below the tip of the breastbone.						
6. Grasp the fist with the other hand.						
7. Pull inward and upward on the abdomen with a quick thrust.						
8. Repeat the thrusts until the foreign body comes out or the resident loses consciousness. If the resident begins to cough, wait and see if he can expel the object.						

(continues)

continued

Clearing an Obstructed Airway in an Unconscious Resident						
It is important that you know your facility's policy regarding this procedure. This procedure may be the responsibility of the nurse. The procedure is listed here for your general understanding only.						
1. Call for help, but do not leave the resident alone.						
2. Wear gloves during this procedure and apply standard precautions.						
3. Lower the resident to the floor and position him on his back.						
4. Open the airway by doing a head tilt, chin lift maneuver.						
5. Look in the mouth. If you see a foreign body, try to remove it. Take care to avoid pushing the object farther down the throat.						
6. Open the airway again by using the head tilt, chin lift. Attempt to ventilate. If the breath does not go in, reposition the head and attempt to ventilate again. Use a pocket mask or other barrier, according to facility policy.						
7. Check for a pulse and begin CPR.						
8. Assist the nurse, code team, or emergency medical services (EMS), as appropriate.						
9. Discard gloves and face shield, or disinfect reusable ventilation device according to facility policy.						
10. Perform your procedure completion actions.						
11. Observe and report to the nurse: • exact time the choking and unconsciousness started and stopped • the procedures done and the time that you started and stopped • the resident's response • factors related to the cause of choking, if known						

PERFORMANCE REVIEW CHECKLIST

Procedure ___8___

Procedure <u>Making the Unoccupied Bed</u>

Name of Nursing Assistant _____ Date of Program _____ to _____

Social Security Number of Nursing Assistant _____

Program Code Number _____

S=Satisfactory Performance
U=Unsatisfactory Performance

Place a full signature to correspond with each set of initials appearing below:

Initials	Corresponding Signature of Instructor	Title

Procedure Guidelines	S/U	Date	Initials	S/U	Date	Initials
1. Wash your hands. Gather supplies needed: two large sheets (or one flat and one fitted sheet), a linen draw sheet (if used), plastic or rubber draw sheet (if used), pillowcase, laundry bag or hamper, and clean bedspread, if needed. Stack the linen in the order in which it will be used. Obtain disposable gloves if the old linen is soiled with blood or any moist body fluid.						
2. Perform your beginning procedure actions.						
3. Carry the clean linen away from your uniform.						
4. Place the linens on a clean area near the bed in the order of use, from bottom to top.						
5. Elevate the bed to a good working height for you.						
6. Position the bed so that it is flat.						
7. Remove and fold the bedspread if you are reusing it.						

(continues)

continued

8.	Apply gloves if linen to be removed is soiled.						
9.	Remove the linen from the bed by rolling it in a ball. Do not let it touch your uniform.						
10.	Place soiled linen in a laundry bag, or dispose of it according to facility policy. If gloves were used, remove them and dispose of them according to facility policy. Check the mattress to be sure it is in good repair. Wash your hands before handling clean linen, even if gloves were worn.						
11.	Follow your facility policy for wiping the mattress. Some facilities require that the mattress be wiped with disinfectant if the linen was soiled with excretions or secretions. (Wear gloves for this task.)						
12.	Place the bottom sheet on the bed, centering the lengthwise middle fold of the sheet in the middle of the bed.						
13.	Open the sheet.						
14.	Place the sheet with small hem even with the foot edge of the mattress.						
15.	Tuck the top of the sheet under the top of the mattress.						
16.	Miter the corner of the sheet at the head of the bed on the side where you are working. OR Secure upper and lower corners of fitted sheet.						
17.	Tuck in the bottom sheet on the side of the bed, working from head to foot.						
18.	Place the plastic draw sheet, if used, over the middle one-third of the bed.						
19.	Place the linen draw sheet over the plastic sheet, covering the entire plastic sheet.						
20.	Tuck the edge of the plastic sheet and draw sheet under the mattress.						
21.	Place the top sheet on the bed, centering the lengthwise middle fold in the center of the bed.						

(continues)

continued

22.	Position the sheet with the top edge even with the top of the mattress.						
23.	Tuck the bottom of the sheet under the mattress at the foot of the bed.						
24.	Place the bedspread on the bed.						
25.	Position the bedspread about 4 inches above the top edge of the mattress.						
26.	Miter linens at the foot of the bed.						
27.	Move to the other side of the bed.						
28.	Pull and smooth out the bottom sheet.						
29.	Tuck the bottom sheet under the mattress at the head of the bed, pulling tight.						
30.	Miter the corner of the sheet at the head of the bed. OR Secure upper and lower corners of the fitted sheet.						
31.	Pull and tightly tuck the side of the bottom sheet under the mattress.						
32.	Pull the plastic sheet tight.						
33.	Tuck the plastic sheet under the mattress, pulling and tucking from the middle of the plastic sheet first. Then pull and tuck the edges of the sheet.						
34.	Pull the linen draw sheet tight.						
35.	Tuck the linen draw sheet under the mattress, pulling and tucking from the middle of the draw sheet first. Then pull and tuck the edges of the sheet.						
36.	Check the foundation of the bed. Make sure the bed is smooth and wrinkle-free.						
37.	Pull and smooth the top sheet.						
38.	Pull and smooth the spread.						
39.	Tuck the sheet and spread under the foot of the mattress.						
40.	Miter the top linens at the foot of the bed.						
41.	Fold the spread back about 30 inches.						

(continues)

continued

42.	Make a cuff on the top sheet by folding it back about 4 inches at the top edge of the sheet.						
43.	Place the pillow on the bed.						
44.	Fold the pillow in half lengthwise and insert the zippered end of the pillow in the pillowcase toward the closed end. OR Grab the center end of the pillowcase with your dominant hand. Fold it up over your arm. Grab the pillow with this hand. Unfold the pillowcase over the pillow.						
45.	Straighten the pillowcase on the pillow.						
46.	Place the pillow at the head of the bed with the open end facing away from the door.						
47.	Cover the pillow with the bedspread.						
48.	Perform your procedure completion actions.						

PERFORMANCE REVIEW CHECKLIST

Procedure ___9___

Procedure <u>Positioning the Resident in the Supine Position</u>

Name of Nursing Assistant _____ Date of Program _____ to _____

Social Security Number of Nursing Assistant _____

Program Code Number _____

S=Satisfactory Performance
U=Unsatisfactory Performance

Place a full signature to correspond with each set of initials appearing below:

Initials	Corresponding Signature of Instructor	Title

Procedure Guidelines	S/U	Date	Initials	S/U	Date	Initials
1. Perform your beginning procedure actions.						
2. Position the resident so that she is lying on her back.						
3. Place the resident's arms at her sides in a comfortable, functional position, supporting them with pillows if necessary.						
4. Check for good body alignment.						
5. Pad bony prominences of elbows and heels, if indicated.						
6. Elevate the knees slightly for comfort, if desired.						
7. Perform your procedure completion actions.						

PERFORMANCE REVIEW CHECKLIST

Procedure ___10___

Procedure <u>Moving the Resident to the Side of the Bed</u>

Name of Nursing Assistant _____ Date of Program _____ to _____

Social Security Number of Nursing Assistant _____

Program Code Number _____

S=Satisfactory Performance
U=Unsatisfactory Performance

Place a full signature to correspond with each set of initials appearing below:

Initials	Corresponding Signature of Instructor	Title

Procedure Guidelines	S/U	Date	Initials	S/U	Date	Initials
1. Perform your beginning procedure actions.						
2. Stand on the side of the bed opposite from the one on which the resident will lie.						
3. Use proper body mechanics to move the resident.						
4. Place the resident's arms across his chest. Cross the resident's legs at the ankles.						
5. Remove the pillow.						
6. Place one of your arms under the resident's shoulder. Place the other arm under the back.						
7. Move the upper part of the resident's body toward you.						
8. Place one of your arms under the resident's waist and the other arm under the resident's thighs.						
9. Move the resident's midsection toward you.						

(continues)

continued

10.	Move the resident's legs toward you. Uncross the ankles. Straighten the resident's arms.						
11.	Replace the pillow.						
12.	Begin positioning or transferring the resident, or go to the next step of this procedure.						
13.	If the resident is to be left in this position, straighten the linen and raise the side rails.						
14.	Perform your procedure completion actions.						

PERFORMANCE REVIEW CHECKLIST

Procedure ___11___

Procedure <u>Moving the Resident to the Side of the Bed Using a Draw Sheet</u>

Name of Nursing Assistant _____ Date of Program _____ to _____

Social Security Number of Nursing Assistant _____

Program Code Number _____

S=Satisfactory Performance
U=Unsatisfactory Performance

Place a full signature to correspond with each set of initials appearing below:

Initials	Corresponding Signature of Instructor	Title

Procedure Guidelines	S/U	Date	Initials	S/U	Date	Initials
1. Perform your beginning procedure actions.						
2. Use proper body mechanics to move the resident.						
3. Place the resident's arms across her chest. Cross the resident's legs at the ankles.						
4. Remove the pillow.						
5. Roll the sides of the draw sheet toward the resident until they touch the body.						
6. Using an overhand grip, place one hand at the upper end of the draw sheet, by the resident's shoulders. Place the lower hand on the draw sheet in the hip area.						
7. The nursing assistant on the side of the bed to which the resident will be moved does most of the work and calls the signals.						

(continues)

continued

8.	Move one foot about 12 inches forward to give you a broad base of support. Place your weight on this foot.					
9.	Flex your knees and keep your back straight.					
10.	On the count of three, both nursing assistants lift and pull the sheet toward the side of the bed.					
11.	Uncross the resident's ankles and straighten her arms.					
12.	Replace the pillow and unroll the draw sheet.					
13.	Begin positioning or transferring the resident, or go to the next step of this procedure.					
14.	If the resident is to be left in this position, straighten the linen and raise the side rails, if ordered.					
15.	Perform your procedure completion actions.					

PERFORMANCE REVIEW CHECKLIST

Procedure ___12___

Procedure <u>Assisting the Resident to Move Up in Bed</u>

Name of Nursing Assistant _____ Date of Program _____ to _____

Social Security Number of Nursing Assistant _____

Program Code Number _____

S=Satisfactory Performance
U=Unsatisfactory Performance

Place a full signature to correspond with each set of initials appearing below:

Initials	Corresponding Signature of Instructor	Title

Procedure Guidelines	S/U	Date	Initials	S/U	Date	Initials
1. Perform your beginning procedure actions.						
2. Lower the head of the bed.						
3. Remove the pillow and lean it against the headboard.						
4. Stand next to the bed.						
5. Ask the resident to bend her knees and put her feet flat on the mattress.						
6. If the resident is able, ask her to bend her arms at her sides and place her hands on the bed. Ask her to push when told to do so.						
7. Slide one hand and arm under the resident's upper back and shoulders.						
8. Slide the other arm under the resident's hips and buttocks.						
9. Instruct the resident to push with her hands and feet on the count of three.						

(continues)

continued

10. On the count of three, move the resident to the head of the bed. Repeat as necessary until the resident is correctly positioned.						
11. Replace the pillow.						
12. Check to see if the resident is in good alignment.						
13. Perform your procedure completion actions.						

PERFORMANCE REVIEW CHECKLIST

Procedure ___13___

Procedure <u>Moving the Resident to the Head of the Bed Using a Draw Sheet</u>

Name of Nursing Assistant _____ Date of Program _____ to _____

Social Security Number of Nursing Assistant _____

Program Code Number _____

S=Satisfactory Performance
U=Unsatisfactory Performance

Place a full signature to correspond with each set of initials appearing below:

Initials	Corresponding Signature of Instructor	Title

Procedure Guidelines	S/U	Date	Initials	S/U	Date	Initials
1. Perform your beginning procedure actions.						
2. Place the resident's arms across his chest.						
3. Remove the pillow.						
4. Roll the sides of the draw sheet toward the resident until they touch his body.						
5. Using an overhand grip, place one hand at the upper end of the draw sheet, by the resident's shoulders. Place the lower hand on the draw sheet in the hip area.						
6. Both nursing assistants stand with their feet apart, one foot ahead of the other.						
7. Bend your knees and keep your back straight.						

(continues)

continued

8.	On the count of three, both nursing assistants shift their weight from one foot to the other while lifting the draw sheet and moving it toward the head of the bed.					
9.	Straighten the resident's arms.					
10.	Replace the pillow and unroll the draw sheet.					
11.	Straighten the linen and leave the resident comfortable.					
12.	Perform your procedure completion actions.					

PERFORMANCE REVIEW CHECKLIST

Procedure ___14___

Procedure <u>Using a Transfer (Gait) Belt</u>

Name of Nursing Assistant _____ Date of Program _____ to _____

Social Security Number of Nursing Assistant _____

Program Code Number _____

S=Satisfactory Performance
U=Unsatisfactory Performance

Place a full signature to correspond with each set of initials appearing below:

Initials	Corresponding Signature of Instructor	Title

Procedure Guidelines	S/U	Date	Initials	S/U	Date	Initials
1. Perform your beginning procedure actions.						
2. Assist the resident to sit on the side of the bed.						
3. Assist the resident to put on clothing and shoes or other footwear with non-slip soles.						
4. Explain to the resident that the transfer belt is a safety device that will prevent pulling and tugging on the resident. Explain that it will be removed when the resident has been transferred.						
5. Always apply the belt over the resident's clothing.						
6. Place the belt around the resident's waist and buckle it in the front. Take care with female residents to ensure that the breasts are not under the belt.						

(continues)

continued

7.	Thread the belt through the teeth side first. Place the end of the belt through both openings so that it is double-locked.						
8.	The belt should fit snugly, but you should check it by slipping your fingers comfortably underneath to be sure it is not too tight. Monitor female residents to be sure that the breasts are not under the belt.						
9.	Using an underhand grasp, insert your hands under the belt on each side and assist the resident to stand.						
10.	Complete the transfer or ambulation procedure.						
11.	Perform your procedure completion actions.						

APPENDIX E PROCEDURE REVIEW

PERFORMANCE REVIEW CHECKLIST

Procedure ___15___

Procedure _Transferring the Resident from Bed to Wheelchair—One Person_

Name of Nursing Assistant _____ Date of Program _____ to _____

Social Security Number of Nursing Assistant _____

Program Code Number _____

S=Satisfactory Performance
U=Unsatisfactory Performance

Place a full signature to correspond with each set of initials appearing below:

Initials	Corresponding Signature of Instructor	Title

Procedure Guidelines	S/U	Date	Initials	S/U	Date	Initials
1. Perform your beginning procedure actions.						
2. Position the wheelchair so the resident's stronger side will be closest to the wheelchair when the resident is sitting on the edge of the bed. Place the wheelchair within one foot of the bed at a slight angle. Position the large part of the front wheels facing forward.						
3. Raise or remove the wheelchair footrests.						
4. Lock the wheelchair brakes.						
5. Raise the head of the bed.						
6. Lock the wheels of the bed.						
7. Lower the bed to the lowest position. Lower the side rail.						
8. Assist the resident to sit on the side of the bed.						
9. Assist the resident to put on clothing and shoes or other footwear with non-slip soles.						

(continues)

continued

10.	Place the transfer belt around the resident's waist and buckle it in the front.					
11.	Thread the belt through the teeth side first. Place the end of the belt through both openings so that it is double-locked.					
12.	Check the fit of the belt by inserting your fingers underneath it.					
13.	Make sure that the resident's feet are flat on the floor. If not, use the transfer belt to move the resident to the side of the bed until his feet touch the floor.					
14.	Instruct the resident to push off the bed with his hands on the count of three.					
15.	Using an underhand grasp, insert your hands under the belt on each side, count to three, and assist the resident to stand.					
16.	Support the resident's weaker side.					
17.	Pivot and turn the resident with his back to the wheelchair.					
18.	Continue to hold the transfer belt and guide the resident backward until he can feel the edge of the wheelchair seat with the back of his legs.					
19.	Tell the resident to place his hands on the wheelchair arms. Seat the resident in the chair.					
20.	Remove the transfer belt.					
21.	Adjust the wheelchair footrests.					
22.	Cover the resident's lap with a lap blanket or other covering, if needed. Be sure that the blanket does not become caught in the wheels.					
23.	Perform your procedure completion actions.					

PERFORMANCE REVIEW CHECKLIST

Procedure ____16____

Procedure <u>Transferring the Resident from Bed to Wheelchair—Two Persons</u>

Name of Nursing Assistant _____ Date of Program _____ to _____

Social Security Number of Nursing Assistant _____

Program Code Number _____

S=Satisfactory Performance
U=Unsatisfactory Performance

Place a full signature to correspond with each set of initials appearing below:

Initials	Corresponding Signature of Instructor	Title

Procedure Guidelines	S/U	Date	Initials	S/U	Date	Initials
1. Perform your beginning procedure actions.						
2. Position the wheelchair so the resident's stronger side will be closest to the wheelchair when the resident is sitting on the edge of the bed. Place the wheelchair within one foot of the bed at a slight angle. Position the large part of the front wheels facing forward.						
3. Raise or remove the wheelchair footrests.						
4. Lock the wheelchair brakes.						
5. Raise the head of the bed.						
6. Lock the wheels of the bed.						
7. Lower the bed to the lowest position. Lower the side rail.						
8. Assist the resident to sit on the side of the bed.						
9. Assist the resident to put on clothing and shoes or other footwear with non-slip soles.						

(continues)

continued

10.	Place the transfer belt around the resident's waist and buckle it in the front.					
11.	Thread the belt through the teeth side first. Place the end of the belt through both openings so that it is double-locked.					
12.	Check the fit of the belt by inserting your fingers underneath it.					
13.	Use the transfer belt to move the resident to the edge of the bed until his feet are flat on the floor. Each nursing assistant places the hand closest to the resident at the back of the belt and the other hand at the front of the belt and slides the resident forward.					
14.	On the count of three, both nursing assistants move the resident at the same time. Coordination of movement is very important.					
15.	Each nursing assistant places the hand closest to the resident through the belt with an underhand grasp behind the resident.					
16.	The nursing assistant closest to the chair, on the resident's stronger side, stands in a position so that she can pivot and move away, allowing the resident access to the chair. This nursing assistant should stand with the left leg further back than the right leg.					
17.	The other nursing assistant should use her left knee to support the resident's weaker leg. This nursing assistant's right leg is positioned further back than the left one.					
18.	Instruct the resident to lean forward and push off the bed, using the palms of his hands, on the count of three.					
19.	The resident's knees should be spread apart. Tell the resident to put both feet back, with the stronger foot behind the weaker foot.					
20.	Both nursing assistants should bend their knees, squat slightly, and spread their feet to provide a broad base of support.					

(continues)

continued

#							
21.	On the count of three, the resident stands. The nursing assistants pivot the resident slowly and smoothly by pivoting their feet, legs, and hips toward the chair until the resident can feel the wheelchair with the back of his legs.						
22.	Tell the resident to place both hands on the armrests of the chair and lean forward slightly.						
23.	Both nursing assistants bend their knees and lower the resident into the chair.						
24.	Remove the transfer belt.						
25.	Adjust the wheelchair footrests.						
26.	Cover the resident's lap with a lap blanket or other covering, if needed. Be sure that the blanket does not become caught in the wheels.						
27.	Perform your procedure completion actions.						

PERFORMANCE REVIEW CHECKLIST

Procedure ___17___

Procedure <u>Ambulating the Resident with a Gait Belt</u>

Name of Nursing Assistant _____ Date of Program _____ to _____

Social Security Number of Nursing Assistant _____

Program Code Number _____

S=Satisfactory Performance
U=Unsatisfactory Performance

Place a full signature to correspond with each set of initials appearing below:

Initials	Corresponding Signature of Instructor	Title

Procedure Guidelines	S/U	Date	Initials	S/U	Date	Initials
1. Perform your beginning procedure actions.						
2. Assist the resident to sit on the side of the bed.						
3. Assist the resident to put on shoes or other footwear with nonslip soles.						
4. Explain to the resident that the gait belt is a safety device that will prevent pulling and tugging on the resident. It allows you to guide and support the resident during the ambulation procedure.						
5. Always apply the belt over the resident's clothing.						
6. Place the belt around the resident's waist and buckle it in the front.						
7. Thread the belt through the teeth side first. Place the end of the belt through both openings so that it is double-locked.						

(continues)

continued

8.	The belt should fit snugly, but you should check it by slipping your fingers comfortably underneath to be sure it is not too tight. Monitor female residents to be sure that the breasts are not under the belt.						
9.	Using an underhand grasp, insert your hands under the belt on each side and assist the resident to stand.						
10.	Walk behind and slightly to one side of the resident during ambulation. Maintain a firm, underhand grasp at the center back of the gait belt.						
11.	Encourage the resident to use handrails in the hallway.						
12.	Walk the distance recommended by the care plan or the nurse's instructions.						
13.	Monitor the resident for signs of fatigue. If this occurs, assist the resident to sit in a chair.						
14.	After ambulating the resident, return to the resident's room.						
15.	Assist the resident to sit in the chair or return to bed.						
16.	Remove the gait belt.						
17.	Perform your procedure completion actions.						

PERFORMANCE REVIEW CHECKLIST

Procedure ___18___

Procedure <u>Ambulating the Resident with a Cane or Walker</u>

Name of Nursing Assistant _____ Date of Program _____ to _____

Social Security Number of Nursing Assistant _____

Program Code Number _____

S=Satisfactory Performance
U=Unsatisfactory Performance

Place a full signature to correspond with each set of initials appearing below:

Initials	Corresponding Signature of Instructor	Title

Procedure Guidelines	S/U	Date	Initials	S/U	Date	Initials
1. Perform your beginning procedure actions.						
2. Assist the resident to sit on the side of the bed.						
3. Assist the resident to put on shoes or other footwear with nonslip soles.						
4. Check the tips of the cane or walker for safety.						
5. Place the gait belt around the resident's waist and check the fit.						
6. Place the cane in the resident's hand or the walker in front of the resident.						
7. Help the resident stand. Grasp the gait belt underhand at the resident's sides.						
8. When the resident is standing and is balanced, ask if she feels dizzy or weak.						
9. Walk behind and slightly to one side of the resident during ambulation. Maintain a firm, underhand grasp at the center back of the gait belt.						

(continues)

continued

10.	Walk the distance recommended by the care plan or the nurse's instructions.					
11.	Monitor the resident for signs of fatigue. If this occurs, assist the resident to sit in a chair.					
12.	After ambulating the resident, return to the resident's room.					
13.	Assist the resident to sit in the chair or return to bed.					
14.	Remove the gait belt.					
15.	Perform your procedure completion actions.					

PERFORMANCE REVIEW CHECKLIST

Procedure ___19___

Procedure <u>Transferring the Resident from Wheelchair to Toilet</u>

Name of Nursing Assistant _____ Date of Program _____ to _____

Social Security Number of Nursing Assistant _____

Program Code Number _____

S=Satisfactory Performance
U=Unsatisfactory Performance

Place a full signature to correspond with each set of initials appearing below:

Initials	Corresponding Signature of Instructor	Title

	Procedure Guidelines	S/U	Date	Initials	S/U	Date	Initials
1.	Perform your beginning procedure actions.						
2.	Make sure the bathroom is empty.						
3.	Bring the resident in a wheelchair to the bathroom.						
4.	Close the bathroom door.						
5.	Position the wheelchair at right angles to the toilet.						
6.	Place the transfer belt around the resident's waist.						
7.	Lock the wheelchair brakes.						
8.	Tell the resident to push up from the wheelchair while you lift her with the transfer belt. Count to three to match movements.						
9.	Ask the resident to hold the bathroom grab bar.						
10.	Help the resident stand, giving her time to get balanced.						

(continues)

continued

11. Pivot the resident so that she is standing in front of the toilet, facing you.						
12. Lower the resident's underwear.						
13. Help the resident sit on the toilet.						
14. Be sure the call signal is close to the resident. Instruct the resident to call when she is finished.						
15. Wash your hands and leave the bathroom if doing so is safe for the resident. Close the door behind you.						
16. Return when the resident calls.						
17. Put on gloves if helping the resident wipe excess urine or bowel movement is necessary.						
18. Remove the gloves and discard according to facility policy.						
19. Wash your hands.						
20. Assist the resident to stand by using the gait belt. Tell the resident to hold onto the bathroom grab bar and pull herself up. Match movements on the count of three.						
21. Pull the resident's underwear up.						
22. Smooth the resident's clothing.						
23. Pivot and seat the resident in the locked wheelchair. Flush the toilet. If abnormalities are noted in the urine or stool, do not flush. Save the specimen for the nurse to see.						
24. Help the resident wash her hands.						
25. Remove the resident from the bathroom.						
26. Remove the transfer belt.						
27. Perform your procedure completion actions.						

PERFORMANCE REVIEW CHECKLIST

Procedure ___20___

Procedure <u>Transferring the Resident Using a Mechanical Lift</u>

Name of Nursing Assistant _____ Date of Program _____ to _____

Social Security Number of Nursing Assistant _____

Program Code Number _____

S=Satisfactory Performance
U=Unsatisfactory Performance

Place a full signature to correspond with each set of initials appearing below:

Initials	Corresponding Signature of Instructor	Title

	Procedure Guidelines	S/U	Date	Initials	S/U	Date	Initials
1.	Perform your beginning procedure actions.						
2.	Place the wheelchair at right angles to the foot of the bed, facing the head. Lock the wheelchair and elevate or remove the footrests.						
3.	Elevate the bed to a good working height for you. Lock the wheels of the bed.						
4.	Lower the side rail on the side nearest you.						
5.	Roll the resident on her side.						
6.	Position the lift seat under the resident's body so that it supports the resident's shoulders, buttocks, and thighs. Smooth out the sling.						
7.	Roll the resident back onto the sling and properly position it on the other side.						

(continues)

continued

8. Position the frame of the lift over the bed. Spread the legs of the lift to the widest open position to maintain a broad base of support.						
9. Attach the suspension straps or chains to the sling. The "S" hooks should face *away* from the resident's body, to prevent injury.						
10. Position the resident's arms comfortably inside the sling.						
11. Attach the straps or chains to the lift frame.						
12. While talking to and reassuring the resident, slowly raise the boom of the lift until the resident is above the bed.						
13. Slowly guide the lift away from the bed.						
14. Position the lift over the chair.						
15. The second nursing assistant holds the sling and helps lower the resident slowly into the chair, keeping the hips back, while the first nursing assistant slowly lowers the lift.						
16. Monitor the location of the resident's feet and arms to prevent injury.						
17. Unhook the straps or chains and remove the lift.						
18. Support the resident's feet with footrests.						
19. Perform your procedure completion actions.						

PERFORMANCE REVIEW CHECKLIST

Procedure ___21___

Procedure <u>Giving Passive Range-of-Motion Exercises</u>

Name of Nursing Assistant _____ Date of Program _____ to _____

Social Security Number of Nursing Assistant _____

Program Code Number _____

S=Satisfactory Performance
U=Unsatisfactory Performance

Place a full signature to correspond with each set of initials appearing below:

Initials	Corresponding Signature of Instructor	Title

Procedure Guidelines		S/U	Date	Initials	S/U	Date	Initials
1.	Perform your beginning procedure actions.						
2.	Position the resident in the supine position.						
3.	Exercise the extremities as indicated on the care plan, supporting the extremity at the closest joints.						
	Head and neck. Perform range of motion in this area only if it is your facility policy or if you have a physician's order.						
1.	Lean the head forward, bringing the chin to the chest.						
2.	Lean the head backward, with the chin up.						
3.	Turn the head from side to side.						
4.	Turn the head back and forth in a circular motion.						

(continues)

continued

Shoulders, arms, and elbows						
1. Move the arm over the head, with arm touching the top of the head.						
2. Return the arm to the side.						
3. Move the arm across the chest.						
4. Return the arm to the side.						
5. Move the arm straight up.						
6. Return the arm to the side.						
7. Bring the arm away from the body at the side to the shoulder level.						
8. Return the arm to the side.						
9. With the arm straight out at the side, bend at the elbow and rotate the shoulder.						
10. Return the arm to the side.						
11. Bend at the elbow and bring hand to chin.						
12. Return the arm to the side.						
Wrists, fingers, and forearms						
1. Bend the hand backward at the wrist.						
2. Bend the hand forward at the wrist.						
3. Clench the fingers and thumb slightly, as if making a fist.						
4. Extend the fingers and thumb.						
5. Move fingers and thumb together and then apart.						
6. Flex and extend joints in the thumb and fingers.						
7. Move each finger in a circular motion.						
8. Extend the arm along the side of the body with the palm facing upward.						
9. Rotate the forearm with the palm facing upward, then downward.						
Legs, hips, and knees						
1. Stretch the leg out from the body. Return the leg to the other leg, crossing over the other leg only at the ankle.						
2. Bend and straighten the knee.						

(continues)

continued

3. Roll the knees inward and outward.						
Ankles, feet, and toes						
1. With one leg straight on the bed, push foot and toes toward the front of the leg.						
2. Push the foot and toes out straight. Point toward the foot of the bed.						
3. With the leg straight, turn the foot and ankle from side to side.						
4. Curl toes downward and upward.						
5. Spread the toes and move each toe away from the second toe, then toward the second toe.						
6. Repeat each exercise as indicated on the care plan.						
7. Note the resident's response to exercise.						
8. Perform your procedure completion actions.						

PERFORMANCE REVIEW CHECKLIST

Procedure ___22___

Procedure <u>Brushing the Resident's Teeth</u>

Name of Nursing Assistant _____ Date of Program _____ to _____

Social Security Number of Nursing Assistant _____

Program Code Number _____

S=Satisfactory Performance
U=Unsatisfactory Performance

Place a full signature to correspond with each set of initials appearing below:

Initials	Corresponding Signature of Instructor	Title

Procedure Guidelines	S/U	Date	Initials	S/U	Date	Initials
1. Perform your beginning procedure actions.						
2. Place a towel across the resident's chest.						
3. Help the resident in self-care, if possible.						
4. Moisten the toothbrush. Apply toothpaste.						
5. Brush the resident's teeth using a circular motion on all surfaces. Brush gums, tongue, sides, and roof of the mouth.						
6. Let the resident rinse the mouth with water or mouthwash.						
7. Hold the emesis basin while the resident spits.						
8. Wipe the mouth with a towel.						
9. Check the mouth for sores, redness, or irritation.						
10. Perform your procedure completion actions.						

PERFORMANCE REVIEW CHECKLIST

Procedure ___23___

Procedure <u>Special Oral Hygiene</u>

Name of Nursing Assistant _____ Date of Program _____ to _____

Social Security Number of Nursing Assistant _____

Program Code Number _____

S=Satisfactory Performance
U=Unsatisfactory Performance

Place a full signature to correspond with each set of initials appearing below:

Initials	Corresponding Signature of Instructor	Title

	Procedure Guidelines	S/U	Date	Initials	S/U	Date	Initials
1.	Perform your beginning procedure actions.						
2.	Cover the pillow with a towel and turn the resident's head to the side. Position the head forward so that any fluid and secretions will not run down the resident's throat.						
3.	Place the emesis basin against the resident's chin.						
4.	Gently open the resident's mouth.						
5.	Dip the premoistened applicators into water, mouthwash, or solution used by the facility. Press the applicator against the inside of a glass to remove excess liquid.						
6.	Wipe the gums, teeth, and inside of the mouth with applicators.						
7.	Discard the used applicators in the plastic bag.						
8.	Apply lubricant to the resident's lips.						
9.	Perform your procedure completion actions.						

PERFORMANCE REVIEW CHECKLIST

Procedure <u> 24 </u>

Procedure <u>Denture Care</u>

Name of Nursing Assistant _____ Date of Program _____ to _____

Social Security Number of Nursing Assistant _____

Program Code Number _____

S=Satisfactory Performance
U=Unsatisfactory Performance

Place a full signature to correspond with each set of initials appearing below:

Initials	Corresponding Signature of Instructor	Title

Procedure Guidelines	S/U	Date	Initials	S/U	Date	Initials
1. Perform your beginning procedure actions.						
2. Drape the towel across the resident's chest.						
3. Line the emesis basin with paper towels.						
4. Ask the resident to remove the dentures, if able, and place them in the emesis basin.						
5. Offer the resident a tissue to wipe her mouth after removing the dentures.						
6. If the resident is unable to remove the dentures, cover your gloved fingers with a gauze sponge. Grasp the center of the upper denture with your thumb and index finger. Gently move the denture up and down to break the seal. Pull the denture out of the mouth and place it in the emesis basin. Discard the gauze sponge in the plastic bag.						

(continues)

continued

7.	To remove the lower denture, cover your gloved fingers with a gauze sponge. Gently grasp it with your thumb and index finger. Turn it to the side slightly and lift it from the mouth. Place it in the emesis basin. Discard the gauze sponge in the plastic bag.					
8.	Line the bottom of the sink with paper towels and fill the sink half full of cool water so the dentures will not break if they drop.					
9.	Rinse the dentures well under cool running water to remove food particles and other debris.					
10.	Wet the toothbrush and apply the denture paste or powder.					
11.	Hold the dentures securely and brush all surfaces.					
12.	Rinse the dentures well under cool running water. Place them in the denture cup.					
13.	Return to the bedside.					
14.	Let the resident brush her gums and tongue, then clean and rinse her mouth with a solution of equal parts water and mouthwash before replacing dentures.					
15.	Hold the emesis basin under the chin and allow the resident to spit out the solution.					
16.	Hand the resident the denture cup and ask her to insert the dentures, if able. Some residents may ask for denture paste or powder to hold the dentures in place. Apply it according to the directions on the package.					
17.	If the resident is unable to insert the dentures, grasp the middle front of the upper denture firmly with your thumb and index finger. Raise the upper lip with your other hand and slide the denture into the mouth. Place both index fingers in the mouth on each side of the upper denture and press firmly to ensure that the denture is in place.					

(continues)

continued

18.	Grasp the middle front of the lower denture securely with your thumb and index finger. With your other hand, pull the lower lip down and slide the denture into the mouth. Place both index fingers in the mouth on each side of the denture and press firmly to ensure that is in place.					
19.	Remove the towel and discard according to facility policy.					
20.	Rinse and dry the denture cup and return it, with your other supplies, to the top drawer of the bedside stand. If the resident does not want the dentures in the mouth, they are stored in the cup in the bedside stand. Some dentures are stored dry, but most should be kept moist. Ask the resident how the dentures should be stored. If in doubt, fill the cup with clean, cool water and place the dentures in it. Cover the cup and place it in the bedside stand.					
21.	Perform your procedure completion actions.					

PERFORMANCE REVIEW CHECKLIST

Procedure ___25___

Procedure <u>Giving a Bed Bath</u>

Name of Nursing Assistant _____ Date of Program _____ to _____

Social Security Number of Nursing Assistant _____

Program Code Number _____

S=Satisfactory Performance
U=Unsatisfactory Performance

Place a full signature to correspond with each set of initials appearing below:

Initials	Corresponding Signature of Instructor	Title

	Procedure Guidelines	S/U	Date	Initials	S/U	Date	Initials
1.	Perform your beginning procedure actions.						
2.	Remove the bedspread and blanket. Fold them and place on the chair.						
3.	Place the bath blanket over the top sheet. Remove the sheet without exposing the resident. Place the soiled sheet in the hamper or dispose of it according to facility policy.						
4.	Remove the resident's gown.						
5.	Raise the side rail.						
6.	Fill the basin with warm water. Check the temperature with a thermometer. It should be 105°F. Changing the water during the procedure may be necessary. Add more hot water if it becomes too cool.						
7.	Return to the bedside and lower the side rail.						
8.	Place a towel under the resident's chin.						

(continues)

continued

9.	Offer the resident the washcloth to wash his own face, if possible.					
10.	Make a mitten by folding the wash-cloth around your hand.					
11.	Wash the resident's eyelids from the inner side of the eye to the outer side of the eye, using plain water without soap. The eyes have a mucous membrane, so you should wear gloves during this part of the procedure.					
12.	Rinse the washcloth.					
13.	Dry the washed area.					
14.	Wash the remainder of the resident's face, neck, and ears. Ask the resident if he prefers to use soap. Some elderly residents do not use soap on the face.					
15.	Place a towel under the resident's arm farthest from you.					
16.	Hold the resident's arm up. Wash the whole arm from the shoulder to the wrist and fingertips.					
17.	Rinse and dry the arm.					
18.	Wash, rinse, and dry the axilla, or armpit.					
19.	Repeat for the other arm.					
20.	If possible, place the resident's hands in water. Wash, rinse, and dry hands, fingers, and nails.					
21.	Place the towel across the chest. Pull the bath blanket down to the abdomen.					
22.	Move the towel to expose half of the chest.					
23.	Wash, rinse, and dry the chest. In the female resident, dry the area under the breasts well. Repeat for the other side of the chest.					
24.	Cover the chest with the towel.					
25.	Pull the bath blanket down to expose the abdomen.					
26.	Wash, rinse, and dry the abdomen.					
27.	Return the bath blanket to the resident's shoulders.					

(continues)

continued

28.	Remove the towel from under the blanket.						
29.	Uncover the leg farthest from you. Place the towel under the leg.						
30.	Wash, rinse, and dry the leg from the groin area to the toes.						
31.	Repeat for the other leg.						
32.	If possible, place feet in the basin one at a time.						
33.	Wash, rinse, and dry the feet. Make sure that you dry well between the toes.						
34.	Cover the legs with the bath blanket.						
35.	Raise the side rail.						
36.	Empty the basin and refill with clean water.						
37.	Lower the side rail.						
38.	Ask the resident to turn with his back toward you. Assist if necessary.						
39.	Wash, rinse, and dry the back.						
40.	Put lotion on back, massaging the entire back.						
41.	Use gloves to wash the genital area. Wash from the front of the genital area to the rectal area.						
42.	Dispose of soiled linen according to facility policy.						
43.	Remove gloves and dispose of them according to facility policy.						
44.	Put the side rail up.						
45.	Wash your hands.						
46.	Return to the bedside and put the side rail down.						
47.	Help the resident into a clean gown or other clothing of choice.						
48.	Comb the resident's hair. Help with other grooming requests.						
49.	Replace bed linens, if indicated, or straighten the bed.						
50.	Perform your procedure completion actions.						

PERFORMANCE REVIEW CHECKLIST

Procedure ___26___

Procedure <u>Giving a Partial Bath</u>

Name of Nursing Assistant _____ Date of Program _____ to _____

Social Security Number of Nursing Assistant _____

Program Code Number _____

S=Satisfactory Performance
U=Unsatisfactory Performance

Place a full signature to correspond with each set of initials appearing below:

Initials	Corresponding Signature of Instructor	Title

Procedure Guidelines	S/U	Date	Initials	S/U	Date	Initials
1. Perform your beginning procedure actions.						
2. Place a towel under the resident's chin.						
3. Offer the resident the washcloth to wash her own face, if possible.						
4. Make a mitten by folding the washcloth around your hand.						
5. Wash the resident's eyelids from the inner side of the eye to the outer side of the eye, using plain water without soap. Wash the eye on the opposite side first, then the eye closest to you. The eyes have mucous membranes, so you should wear gloves for this part of the procedure.						
6. Rinse the washcloth.						
7. Dry the washed area.						
8. Wash the remainder of the resident's face, neck, and ears. Ask the resident if she prefers to use soap. Some elderly residents do not use soap on the face.						

(continues)

continued

9.	Dry the washed area.					
10.	Place the towel under the hand farthest from you.					
11.	If possible, place the resident's hand in the basin. Wash, rinse, and dry hand.					
12.	Repeat for the other hand.					
13.	Wash, rinse, and dry axilla (armpit).					
14.	Repeat for the other axilla.					
15.	Ask the resident to turn with her back toward you. Assist if necessary.					
16.	Wash, rinse, and dry the back.					
17.	Put lotion on back, massaging the entire back lightly.					
18.	Use gloves when washing the genital area. Wash from the front of the genital area to the rectal area.					
19.	Put side rail up.					
20.	Remove gloves and dispose of them according to facility policy.					
21.	Wash your hands.					
22.	Return to the bedside and put side rail down.					
23.	Help the resident into a clean gown or other clothing of choice.					
24.	Comb the resident's hair. Help with other grooming requests.					
25.	Replace bed linens, if indicated, or straighten the bed.					
26.	Perform your procedure completion actions.					

PERFORMANCE REVIEW CHECKLIST

Procedure   __27__

Procedure <u>Female Perineal Care</u>

Name of Nursing Assistant _____ Date of Program _____ to _____

Social Security Number of Nursing Assistant _____

Program Code Number _____

S=Satisfactory Performance
U=Unsatisfactory Performance

Place a full signature to correspond with each set of initials appearing below:

Initials	Corresponding Signature of Instructor	Title

Procedure Guidelines	S/U	Date	Initials	S/U	Date	Initials
1. Perform your beginning procedure actions.						
2. Remove the bedspread and blanket. Fold them and place on the chair.						
3. Place the bath blanket over the top sheet. Fanfold the sheet to the foot of the bed without exposing the resident. If the sheet is soiled, dispose of it according to facility policy.						
4. Ask the resident to raise her hips while you place a bed protector under her buttocks. Remove the soiled bed protector, if present. (Apply the principles of standard precautions during this activity.)						
5. Raise the side rail.						
6. Fill the basin with warm water.						
7. Return to the bedside and lower the side rail.						
8. Position the bath blanket so that only the area between the legs is exposed.						

(continues)

continued

9.	Ask the resident to separate and bend her knees.					
10.	Put on disposable gloves.					
11.	Wet the washcloth and make a mitten out of it.					
12.	Apply soap to the washcloth. Use caution. Too much soap can be irritating.					
13.	With one hand, separate the labia.					
14.	With the other hand:					
	a. Wash the far side of the labia from top to bottom, using a single downward stroke.					
	b. Rinse and turn the washcloth.					
	c. Wash the near side of the labia from top to bottom, using a single downward stroke.					
	d. Rinse and turn the washcloth.					
	e. Wash the center of the labia from top to bottom, using a single downward stroke.					
	f. Turn the washcloth. Rinse the area well with the washcloth.					
	g. Gently pat the area dry with a towel.					
15.	Turn the resident away from you. Flex the upper leg slightly, if possible.					
16.	Wet the washcloth and make a mitt. Apply soap.					
17.	Expose the anus.					
18.	Wash the area, stroking from the perineum to the coccyx.					
19.	Rinse the area well with the washcloth.					
20.	Gently dry the area with a towel.					
21.	Return the resident to her back.					
22.	Remove and dispose of the bed protector according to facility policy.					
23.	Raise the side rail.					
24.	Dispose of soiled linen according to facility policy.					
25.	Remove gloves and dispose of them according to facility policy.					

(continues)

continued

26.	Wash your hands.						
27.	Lower the side rail. Replace the top covers and remove the bath blanket.						
28.	Help the resident into a clean gown or other clothing of choice.						
29.	Perform your procedure completion actions.						

PERFORMANCE REVIEW CHECKLIST

Procedure ___28___

Procedure <u>Male Perineal Care</u>

Name of Nursing Assistant _____ Date of Program _____ to _____

Social Security Number of Nursing Assistant _____

Program Code Number _____

S=Satisfactory Performance
U=Unsatisfactory Performance

Place a full signature to correspond with each set of initials appearing below:

Initials	Corresponding Signature of Instructor	Title

	Procedure Guidelines	S/U	Date	Initials	S/U	Date	Initials
1.	Perform your beginning procedure actions.						
2.	Remove the bedspread and blanket. Fold them and place on the chair.						
3.	Place the bath blanket over the top sheet. Fanfold the sheet to the foot of the bed without exposing the resident. If the sheet is soiled, dispose of it according to facility policy.						
4.	Ask the resident to raise his hips while you place a bed protector under his buttocks. Remove the soiled bed protector, if present. Apply the principles of standard precautions during this activity.						
5.	Raise the side rail.						
6.	Fill the basin with warm water.						
7.	Return to the bedside and lower the side rail.						

(continues)

continued

8.	Position the bath blanket so that only the area between the legs is exposed.					
9.	Ask the resident to separate and bend his knees.					
10.	Put on disposable gloves.					
11.	Wet the washcloth and make a mitten out of it.					
12.	Apply soap to the washcloth. Use caution. Too much soap can be irritating.					
13.	With one hand, grasp the penis gently and wash. Begin washing at the urinary meatus and wash the penis in a circular motion toward the base of the penis.					
14.	If the resident is not circumcised, pull the foreskin back to wash it. Rinse the penis, dry, and replace the retracted foreskin.					
15.	Wash the scrotum, then gently lift it and wash the perineum.					
16.	Rinse the washcloth, make a mitten, and rinse the entire area, beginning with the penis.					
17.	Gently dry the area with a towel.					
18.	Ask the resident to turn so his back is facing you. Assist if necessary.					
19.	Expose the anus.					
20.	Wash the area, stroking from the perineum to the coccyx.					
21.	Rinse the area well with the washcloth.					
22.	Gently dry the area with a towel.					
23.	Return the resident to his back.					
24.	Remove and dispose of the bed protector according to facility policy.					
25.	Raise the side rail.					
26.	Dispose of soiled linen according to facility policy.					
27.	Remove gloves and dispose of them according to facility policy.					
28.	Wash your hands.					
29.	Return to the bedside and lower the side rail.					

(continues)

continued

30.	Replace the top covers and remove the bath blanket.					
31.	Help the resident into a clean gown or other clothing of choice.					
32.	Perform your procedure completion actions.					

PERFORMANCE REVIEW CHECKLIST

Procedure ___29___

Procedure Giving a Back Rub

Name of Nursing Assistant _____ Date of Program _____ to _____

Social Security Number of Nursing Assistant _____

Program Code Number _____

S=Satisfactory Performance
U=Unsatisfactory Performance

Place a full signature to correspond with each set of initials appearing below:

Initials	Corresponding Signature of Instructor	Title

Procedure Guidelines	S/U	Date	Initials	S/U	Date	Initials
1. Perform your beginning procedure actions.						
2. Place the bottle of lotion in the basin of water to warm it.						
3. Expose the resident's back and upper buttocks.						
4. Wash, rinse, and dry.						
5. Pour a small amount of lotion into one hand.						
6. Warm the lotion by rubbing it between your hands, if necessary.						
7. Apply lotion to the resident's back.						
8. Rub the back with gentle but firm strokes with both hands in a circular motion from buttocks to shoulders:						
a. Begin at the base of the spine and rub up the center of the back with long, soothing strokes.						

(continues)

continued

	b. Use a circular motion with your hands as you bring them down from the shoulders back to the buttocks.					
	c. Repeat this procedure for three to five minutes.					
9.	Remove excess lotion from the back.					
10.	Straighten and tighten the bottom sheet and draw sheet.					
11.	Change the resident's gown, if necessary.					
12.	Perform your procedure completion actions.					

PERFORMANCE REVIEW CHECKLIST

Procedure ___30___

Procedure <u>Combing the Resident's Hair</u>

Name of Nursing Assistant _____ Date of Program _____ to _____

Social Security Number of Nursing Assistant _____

Program Code Number _____

S=Satisfactory Performance
U=Unsatisfactory Performance

Place a full signature to correspond with each set of initials appearing below:

Initials	Corresponding Signature of Instructor	Title

	Procedure Guidelines	S/U	Date	Initials	S/U	Date	Initials
1.	Perform your beginning procedure actions.						
2.	Cover the pillow with a towel. If the resident is sitting in a chair, place the towel over the shoulders.						
3.	Section the resident's hair with one hand between the scalp and the ends of the hair.						
4.	Brush the hair thoroughly.						
5.	Have the resident turn so that you can comb and brush the back of the hair.						
6.	If the hair is tangled, use the comb to separate it. Take a small section of hair. Beginning at the end, comb downward. Support the hair above where you are combing with the fingers of your other hand so that you do not pull on the resident's scalp. Continue working upward until you reach the scalp.						

(continues)

continued

7.	Ask the resident how she wants the hair styled, or arrange the hair attractively and in a style appropriate for the resident's age. If the resident has long hair, consider braiding it or putting it up. Coarse, tightly curled hair may require special treatment.						
8.	Perform your procedure completion actions.						

PERFORMANCE REVIEW CHECKLIST

Procedure ___31___

Procedure Shaving the Resident

Name of Nursing Assistant _____ Date of Program _____ to _____

Social Security Number of Nursing Assistant _____

Program Code Number _____

S=Satisfactory Performance
U=Unsatisfactory Performance

Place a full signature to correspond with each set of initials appearing below:

Initials	Corresponding Signature of Instructor	Title

Procedure Guidelines	S/U	Date	Initials	S/U	Date	Initials
1. Perform your beginning procedure actions.						
2. Cover the resident's chest with the towel.						
3. Soften the resident's beard by placing a warm washcloth over it for 2 to 3 minutes. Moisten the face with water and apply shaving cream.						
4. Put on disposable gloves.						
5. Beginning in front of the ear, hold the skin taut.						
6. Bring the razor down from the cheek to the chin in one-half- to one-inch increments. Continue until the entire cheek has been shaved. Rinse the razor between strokes.						
7. Repeat with the other cheek.						
8. Ask the resident to tighten his upper lip. Shave from the nose to the upper lip in short, downward strokes.						

(continues)

continued

9.	Ask the resident to tighten his chin. Shave the chin in downward strokes in one-half- to one-inch increments.						
10.	Ask the resident to tip his head back.						
11.	Apply shaving cream to the neck area.						
12.	Hold the skin taut. Shave the neck area in smooth, upward strokes in one-half- to one-inch increments.						
13.	Wash the resident's face and neck. Dry the area well.						
14.	Apply aftershave lotion if resident prefers.						
15.	Perform your procedure completion actions.						

PERFORMANCE REVIEW CHECKLIST

Procedure ___32___

Procedure <u>Hand and Fingernail Care</u>

Name of Nursing Assistant _____ Date of Program _____ to _____

Social Security Number of Nursing Assistant _____

Program Code Number _____

S=Satisfactory Performance
U=Unsatisfactory Performance

Place a full signature to correspond with each set of initials appearing below:

Initials	Corresponding Signature of Instructor	Title

Procedure Guidelines	S/U	Date	Initials	S/U	Date	Initials
1. Perform your beginning procedure actions.						
2. Adjust the height of the overbed table and place it in front of the resident. Cover the overbed table with the bed protector.						
3. Place the basin of water on the table.						
4. Instruct the resident to place hands in the water.						
5. Soak the hands for approximately 10 minutes. Cover the resident's hands and the basin with a towel to keep the water warm. Add more warm water if necessary.						
6. Wash the resident's hands. Push the cuticles back gently with the washcloth or an orange stick.						
7. Lift the resident's hands out of the water and dry them with the towel.						

(continues)

continued

8.	Clip the nails if permitted by facility policy.					
	• Cut the nails straight across.					
	• Do not trim the nails below the fingertips.					
	• Keep the nail clippings on the bed protector to be discarded later.					
9.	Shape the nails with the nail file or emery board. Apply fingernail polish if requested by a female resident.					
10.	Pour a small amount of lotion into your hands and rub it into the resident's hands.					
11.	Perform your procedure completion actions.					
12.	Disinfect the clippers according to facility policy after each use.					

PERFORMANCE REVIEW CHECKLIST

Procedure ___33___

Procedure <u>Applying Support Hosiery</u>

Name of Nursing Assistant _____ Date of Program _____ to _____

Social Security Number of Nursing Assistant _____

Program Code Number _____

S=Satisfactory Performance
U=Unsatisfactory Performance

Place a full signature to correspond with each set of initials appearing below:

Initials	Corresponding Signature of Instructor	Title

Procedure Guidelines	S/U	Date	Initials	S/U	Date	Initials
1. Perform your beginning procedure actions.						
2. Expose one leg at a time.						
3. Grasp the stocking with both hands at the top opening and roll or gather toward the toe end.						
4. Apply the stocking to the leg by rolling or pulling upward over the leg.						
5. Make sure the stocking is on evenly. Be sure there are no wrinkles.						
6. Expose the other leg.						
7. Grasp the stocking with both hands at the top opening and roll or gather toward the toe end.						
8. Apply the stocking to the leg by rolling or pulling upward over the leg.						
9. Make sure the stocking is on evenly. Be sure there are no wrinkles.						
10. Perform your procedure completion actions.						

PERFORMANCE REVIEW CHECKLIST

Procedure ___34___

Procedure <u>Making the Occupied Bed</u>

Name of Nursing Assistant _____ Date of Program _____ to _____

Social Security Number of Nursing Assistant _____

Program Code Number _____

S=Satisfactory Performance
U=Unsatisfactory Performance

Place a full signature to correspond with each set of initials appearing below:

Initials	Corresponding Signature of Instructor	Title

	Procedure Guidelines	S/U	Date	Initials	S/U	Date	Initials
1.	Perform your beginning procedure actions.						
2.	Remove the bedspread and blanket. Fold them and place on the chair.						
3.	Place the bath blanket over the top sheet. Remove the sheet without exposing the resident. Place the soiled sheet in the hamper, or dispose of it according to facility policy.						
4.	Help the resident to turn on the side away from you.						
5.	Loosen bottom linens.						
6.	Roll the soiled draw sheet and rubber sheet, and tuck along the resident's back.						
7.	Place the clean sheet on the bed with the center fold at the center of the bed.						
8.	Unfold one-half of the sheet.						

(continues)

continued

9. Place the bottom hem of the sheet even with the edge of the mattress, or fit the corner of the fitted sheet.						
10. Tuck the top of the sheet under half of the head end of the mattress.						
11. Miter the corner.						
12. Tuck the sheet under the side of the entire mattress, working from the head to the foot of the bed.						
13. Roll the remaining half sheet and tuck it under the soiled sheet.						
14. Place the rubber draw sheet in the middle of the bed. Tuck in at the side.						
15. Place a clean linen draw sheet over the rubber draw sheet. Tuck in at the side. If a bed protector is used, place it on top of the draw sheet and roll it inside the draw sheet.						
16. Roll the remaining halves of draw sheets and tuck them along resident's back under the soiled sheets.						
17. Help the resident roll over the linen pile on his side facing you.						
18. Raise the side rail.						
19. Go to the other side of the bed.						
20. Lower the side rail.						
21. Loosen and remove soiled linens from under the mattress.						
22. Raise the side rail if leaving the bedside.						
23. Dispose of soiled linens according to facility policy. *Do not put soiled linen on the floor. Hold soiled linen away from your uniform.*						
24. Remove gloves and dispose according to facility policy.						
25. Wash your hands.						
26. Return to the bedside and lower the side rail.						
27. Pull the clean bottom sheet over the mattress.						
28. Tuck the bottom sheet tightly under the head of the mattress.						

(continues)

continued

29.	Miter the corner of the sheet at the head of the bed, or fit the corner of the fitted sheet.					
30.	Pull the bottom sheet tight and tuck under the side of the mattress, working from head to foot.					
31.	Pull the rubber sheet tight and tuck over the bottom sheet at the side of the mattress.					
32.	Pull the draw sheet tight and tuck over the rubber sheet at the side of the mattress. If a bed protector is used, smooth and straighten it.					
33.	Help the resident to roll on his back. Cover the resident with the bath blanket.					
34.	Place the clean sheet over the bath blanket, centering the center fold of the sheet.					
35.	Pull the bath blanket from under the clean sheet.					
36.	Place the blanket and bedspread over the sheet.					
37.	Fold the top sheet over the edge of the blanket. Spread to make a cuff with the sheet.					
38.	Tuck the top linens under the foot of the mattress, allowing room for the resident's toes. Follow the care plan instructions for special devices, such as bed cradles and footboards.					
39.	Miter the corner of top linens at the foot of the bed.					
40.	Raise the side rail.					
41.	Go to the other side of the bed.					
42.	Lower the side rail.					
43.	Miter the corner of the top linens at the foot of the bed.					
44.	Remove the pillow and soiled pillowcase.					
45.	Place a clean pillowcase on the pillow.					
46.	Perform your procedure completion actions.					

PERFORMANCE REVIEW CHECKLIST

Procedure ___35___

Procedure <u>Feeding the Resident</u>

Name of Nursing Assistant _____ Date of Program _____ to _____

Social Security Number of Nursing Assistant _____

Program Code Number _____

S=Satisfactory Performance
U=Unsatisfactory Performance

Place a full signature to correspond with each set of initials appearing below:

Initials	Corresponding Signature of Instructor	Title

Procedure Guidelines	S/U	Date	Initials	S/U	Date	Initials
1. Perform your beginning procedure actions.						
2. Check the name on the tray and the diet served.						
3. Check the meal tray for utensils and spilled foods.						
4. Place the tray on the table. Remove food covers.						
5. Sit near the resident.						
6. Explain what is on the tray.						
7. Ask the resident what foods she would like to eat first.						
8. Encourage the resident to feed herself, if able, by using finger foods or adaptive equipment.						
9. Use hand-over-hand technique to help the resident feed herself, if consistent with the care plan.						

(continues)

continued

10.	Fill the fork or spoon only half full or less, according to the resident's ability to swallow.					
11.	Use a straw for liquids.					
12.	Encourage the resident to eat. Talk pleasantly. Do not rush.					
13.	Wipe the resident's mouth.					
14.	Offer liquids between bites of solid food.					
15.	Remove the tray when the resident is finished.					
16.	Wash the resident's hands, if necessary.					
17.	Perform your procedure completion actions.					

PERFORMANCE REVIEW CHECKLIST

Procedure ___36___

Procedure <u>Recording Intake and Output</u>

Name of Nursing Assistant _____ Date of Program _____ to _____

Social Security Number of Nursing Assistant _____

Program Code Number _____

S=Satisfactory Performance
U=Unsatisfactory Performance

Place a full signature to correspond with each set of initials appearing below:

Initials	Corresponding Signature of Instructor	Title

	Procedure Guidelines	S/U	Date	Initials	S/U	Date	Initials
1.	Perform your beginning procedure actions.						
2.	Check to identify equivalents used in your facility.						
3.	Identify foods considered to be liquid as taken by the resident.						
4.	Estimate liquid food taken.						
5.	Record how much liquid is taken by the resident in cubic centimeters (cc) or milliliters (mL), according to facility policy.						
6.	Record amounts under the intake column.						
7.	Apply the principles of standard precautions when measuring output.						
8.	Measure output by pouring the contents of the bedpan, urinal, or emesis basin into the graduate. Remove one glove. Flush contents down the toilet after they are measured by holding graduate with gloved hand and pushing flush lever on toilet with ungloved hand.						

(continues)

continued

9.	Rinse and disinfect the graduate and bedpan, urinal, or emesis basin according to facility policy.					
10.	Record the elimination in the *output* column.					
11.	Perform your procedure completion actions.					

PERFORMANCE REVIEW CHECKLIST

Procedure ___37___

Procedure <u>Giving a Bedpan</u>

Name of Nursing Assistant _____ Date of Program _____ to _____

Social Security Number of Nursing Assistant _____

Program Code Number _____

S=Satisfactory Performance
U=Unsatisfactory Performance

Place a full signature to correspond with each set of initials appearing below:

Initials	Corresponding Signature of Instructor	Title

Procedure Guidelines	S/U	Date	Initials	S/U	Date	Initials
1. Perform your beginning procedure actions.						
2. Ask the resident to flex the knees and rest weight on the heels, if able.						
3. Help the resident to raise the buttocks:						
a. Put one hand under the small of the resident's back, and gently lift while the resident pushes with the feet.						
b. With the other hand, insert the bed protector under the resident.						
4. If the resident is unable to lift the buttocks:						
a. Help the resident to turn on the side, with his back toward you.						
b. Place the bed protector on the bed.						
c. Place the bedpan flat against the resident's buttocks.						
d. Roll the resident on his back while holding the bedpan in place.						

(continues)

continued

5.	Cover the resident with the top sheet.						
6.	Raise the head of the bed slightly for comfort.						
7.	Remove the disposable gloves.						
8.	Raise the side rail.						
9.	Dispose of gloves according to facility policy.						
10.	Wash your hands.						
11.	Give the resident the call signal and toilet tissue. Instruct him to use the signal when he is done. Leave the room.						
12.	Return immediately when the resident calls.						
13.	Put on disposable gloves.						
14.	Lower the side rail.						
15.	Remove the bedpan by asking the resident to raise his hips.						
16.	If the resident is unable to raise his hips, hold the bedpan securely while the resident rolls to his side with back facing you. Remove the bedpan. Cover the pan with a bedpan cover or other cover according to facility policy.						
17.	Place the bedpan on a bed protector on the chair in the room, or according to facility policy. It is usually not placed on the overbed table or bedside stand.						
18.	Fill the washbasin with water (105°F). Help the resident to clean his perineal area, if necessary. Dispose of toilet tissue in the bedpan. Cover the bedpan.						
19.	Wash the resident's perineal area with soap and water. Rinse and dry.						
20.	Remove one glove and raise the side rail with the ungloved hand.						
21.	Take the covered bedpan to the bathroom. Empty and disinfect it according to facility policy. Use the ungloved hand to turn on faucets and flush the toilet. Store the bedpan in its proper location.						
22.	Remove the other glove and dispose according to facility policy.						

(continues)

continued

#							
23.	Wash your hands.						
24.	Help the resident to wash his hands. Clean and return the basin to its proper location.						
25.	Perform your procedure completion actions.						

PERFORMANCE REVIEW CHECKLIST

Procedure ___38___

Procedure <u>Giving a Urinal</u>

Name of Nursing Assistant _____ Date of Program _____ to _____

Social Security Number of Nursing Assistant _____

Program Code Number _____

S=Satisfactory Performance
U=Unsatisfactory Performance

Place a full signature to correspond with each set of initials appearing below:

Initials	Corresponding Signature of Instructor	Title

1.	Perform your beginning procedure actions.						
2.	Lift the top covers and hand the resident the urinal under the covers. If the resident is unable to take the urinal, place the urinal in the bed and insert the resident's penis into the opening.						
3.	Remove the disposable gloves and dispose according to facility policy.						
4.	Raise the side rail.						
5.	Wash your hands.						
6.	Give the resident the call signal and instruct him to use it when he is done. Leave the room.						
7.	Return immediately when the resident calls.						
8.	Put on one disposable glove.						

(continues)

continued

9.	Ask the resident to hand you the urinal. Remove it if he is unable.					
10.	Take the urinal to the bathroom, and empty and disinfect it according to facility policy. Use the ungloved hand to turn on faucets and flush the toilet. Store the urinal in its proper location.					
11.	Remove the glove and dispose according to facility policy.					
12.	Wash your hands.					
13.	Fill the washbasin with water (105°F).					
14.	Lower the side rail.					
15.	Help the resident to wash his hands.					
16.	Raise the side rail.					
17.	Lower the height of the bed.					
18.	Clean and return the basin to its proper location.					
19.	Perform your procedure completion actions.					

PERFORMANCE REVIEW CHECKLIST

Procedure ___39___

Procedure <u>Giving Catheter Care</u>

Name of Nursing Assistant _____ Date of Program _____ to _____

Social Security Number of Nursing Assistant _____

Program Code Number _____

S=Satisfactory Performance
U=Unsatisfactory Performance

Place a full signature to correspond with each set of initials appearing below:

Initials	Corresponding Signature of Instructor	Title

	Procedure Guidelines	S/U	Date	Initials	S/U	Date	Initials
1.	Perform your beginning procedure actions.						
2.	Cover the resident with a bath blanket.						
3.	Fanfold the upper linen down to the foot of the bed.						
4.	Ask the resident to raise hips and place the bed protector under the resident.						
5.	Position the bath blanket to expose the resident's catheter.						
6.	Wash the urethra area around the catheter entrance.						
7.	Using a clean washcloth, wash the catheter for 3 inches from the insertion site into the body. Begin washing at the urinary meatus and wash downward. Avoid rubbing back and forth on the tubing.						
8.	Wash the genital area from front to back. Rinse well.						

(continues)

continued

9.	Dry the area well.					
10.	Secure the catheter with a catheter strap or tape.					
11.	Place the drainage tubing over the resident's leg.					
12.	Place the rubber band around the tubing and pin it to the sheet at the edge of the mattress to make sure that the tubing stays on the bed.					
13.	Cover the resident. Replace the bedding and remove the bath blanket.					
14.	Perform your procedure completion actions.					

PERFORMANCE REVIEW CHECKLIST

Procedure ___40___

Procedure <u>Emptying a Catheter Bag</u>

Name of Nursing Assistant _____ Date of Program _____ to _____

Social Security Number of Nursing Assistant _____

Program Code Number _____

S=Satisfactory Performance
U=Unsatisfactory Performance

Place a full signature to correspond with each set of initials appearing below:

Initials	Corresponding Signature of Instructor	Title

	Procedure Guidelines	S/U	Date	Initials	S/U	Date	Initials
1.	Perform your beginning procedure actions.						
2.	Place a paper towel on the floor and place the graduate on top of it.						
3.	Remove the drainage spout from the bag and center it over the graduate. Be careful not to touch the tip of the drainage spout. Do not let the tip or the sides of the drainage spout touch the graduate.						
4.	Open the clamp on the drainage spout and allow the urine to drain into the graduate.						
5.	After the urine has drained into the graduate, wipe the spout with the alcohol sponge, if this is your facility policy. Some facilities do not wipe the tip of the spout unless it has contacted your hands or the graduate.						

(continues)

continued

6.	Replace the drainage spout into the holder on the side of the catheter bag. Pick up the graduate. Dispose of the paper towel.						
7.	Note the amount, color, and character of urine.						
8.	Discard urine and disinfect the graduate according to facility policy. Store the graduate in its proper location.						
9.	Perform your procedure completion actions.						

PERFORMANCE REVIEW CHECKLIST

Procedure ___41___

Procedure <u>Measuring an Oral Temperature</u>

Name of Nursing Assistant _____ Date of Program _____ to _____

Social Security Number of Nursing Assistant _____

Program Code Number _____

S=Satisfactory Performance
U=Unsatisfactory Performance

Place a full signature to correspond with each set of initials appearing below:

Initials	Corresponding Signature of Instructor	Title

Procedure Guidelines	S/U	Date	Initials	S/U	Date	Initials
1. Perform your beginning procedure actions.						
2. If using a glass thermometer, rinse off the disinfectant and dry the thermometer.						
3. Shake the glass thermometer down to 96°.						
4. Cover the thermometer with a plastic sheath or probe cover.						
5. Apply gloves, if this is facility policy.						
6. Place the bulb or tip of the probe under the resident's tongue and instruct the resident to close the lips.						
7. Leave the thermometer in place for 3 minutes, or until the thermometer alarm sounds, according to facility policy and the type of thermometer used.						
8. Remove the thermometer from the resident's mouth.						
9. Discard the sheath or probe cover according to facility policy.						

(continues)

continued

10.	Hold the glass thermometer at eye level and read the mercury column. OR Read the digital display of the electronic thermometer. Note the reading.						
11.	Shake the glass thermometer down to 96°. Place the thermometer in the container for used thermometers, or disinfect it according to facility policy. Place the probe for the electronic thermometer in the probe holder.						
12.	Remove your gloves and discard according to facility policy.						
13.	Record the temperature reading.						
14.	Perform your procedure completion actions.						

PERFORMANCE REVIEW CHECKLIST

Procedure ___42___

Procedure <u>Measuring a Rectal Temperature</u>

Name of Nursing Assistant _____ Date of Program _____ to _____

Social Security Number of Nursing Assistant _____

Program Code Number _____

S=Satisfactory Performance
U=Unsatisfactory Performance

Place a full signature to correspond with each set of initials appearing below:

Initials	Corresponding Signature of Instructor	Title

	Procedure Guidelines	S/U	Date	Initials	S/U	Date	Initials
1.	Perform your beginning procedure actions.						
2.	If using a glass thermometer, rinse off the disinfectant and dry the thermometer. Shake the glass thermometer down to 96°F.						
3.	Cover the thermometer with a plastic sheath or probe cover.						
4.	Position the resident in the Sims' position.						
5.	Apply gloves.						
6.	Place a small amount of lubricant on a tissue or paper towel. Use the tissue to lubricate the bulb of the thermometer. (*Note:* Some plastic sheaths are pre-lubricated.)						
7.	Separate the resident's buttocks with one hand.						

(continues)

continued

8.	Insert the bulb of the glass thermometer into the rectum one inch. If using an electronic thermometer, insert the probe into the rectum half an inch, or according to facility policy.						
9.	Hold the thermometer in place for 3 minutes, or until the alarm sounds on the electronic thermometer.						
10.	Remove the thermometer from the resident's anus.						
11.	Discard the sheath or probe cover according to facility policy.						
12.	Hold the glass thermometer at eye level and read the mercury column. OR Read the digital display of the electronic thermometer. Note the reading.						
13.	Shake the glass thermometer down to 96°F. Place the thermometer in the container for used thermometers or disinfect it according to facility policy. OR Place the probe for the electronic thermometer in the probe holder.						
14.	Remove your gloves and discard according to facility policy.						
15.	Record the temperature reading.						
16.	Perform your procedure completion actions.						

PERFORMANCE REVIEW CHECKLIST

Procedure __43__

Procedure <u>Measuring an Axillary Temperature</u>

Name of Nursing Assistant _____ Date of Program _____ to _____

Social Security Number of Nursing Assistant _____

Program Code Number _____

S=Satisfactory Performance
U=Unsatisfactory Performance

Place a full signature to correspond with each set of initials appearing below:

Initials	Corresponding Signature of Instructor	Title

Procedure Guidelines	S/U	Date	Initials	S/U	Date	Initials
1. Perform your beginning procedure actions.						
2. If using a glass thermometer, rinse off the disinfectant and dry the thermometer. Shake the glass thermometer down to 96°.						
3. Cover the thermometer with a plastic sheath or probe cover.						
4. Apply gloves, if this is your facility policy.						
5. Dry the axilla with a towel.						
6. Insert the thermometer into the center of the axilla, then lower the resident's arm and bend it across the abdomen. Hold the thermometer in place, if this is your facility policy.						
7. Leave the thermometer in place for 10 full minutes or until the thermometer alarm sounds.						
8. Remove the thermometer from the resident's axilla.						

(continues)

continued

9.	Discard the sheath or probe cover according to facility policy.						
10.	Hold the glass thermometer at eye level and read the mercury column. OR Read the digital display of the electronic thermometer. Note the reading.						
11.	Shake the glass thermometer down to 96°F. Place the thermometer in the container for used thermometers or disinfect it according to facility policy. OR Place the probe for the electronic thermometer in the probe holder.						
12.	Remove your gloves and discard according to facility policy.						
13.	Record the temperature reading.						
14.	Perform your procedure completion actions.						

PERFORMANCE REVIEW CHECKLIST

Procedure ___44___

Procedure <u>Measuring a Tympanic Temperature</u>

Name of Nursing Assistant _____ Date of Program _____ to _____

Social Security Number of Nursing Assistant _____

Program Code Number _____

S=Satisfactory Performance
U=Unsatisfactory Performance

Place a full signature to correspond with each set of initials appearing below:

Initials	Corresponding Signature of Instructor	Title

	Procedure Guidelines	S/U	Date	Initials	S/U	Date	Initials
1.	Perform your beginning procedure actions.						
2.	Check the lens of the thermometer to make sure it is clean.						
3.	Cover the thermometer lens with a clean probe cover.						
4.	Select the appropriate mode (oral or rectal) on the thermometer.						
5.	Gently pull the ear up and back to straighten the ear canal.						
6.	Insert the thermometer, aiming it toward the tympanic membrane (eardrum). Insert until the tip seals in the ear canal. Rotate the probe handle slightly until it is aligned with the jaw, as if it were a telephone receiver.						
7.	Press the activation (scan) button. Hold the thermometer in place until the display flashes or the thermometer indicates that there is a reading.						

(continues)

continued

8.	Remove the thermometer from the resident's ear and discard the probe cover according to facility policy.						
9.	Record the temperature reading.						
10.	Perform your procedure completion actions.						

PERFORMANCE REVIEW CHECKLIST

Procedure ___45___

Procedure <u>Taking the Radial Pulse</u>

Name of Nursing Assistant _____ Date of Program _____ to _____

Social Security Number of Nursing Assistant _____

Program Code Number _____

S=Satisfactory Performance
U=Unsatisfactory Performance

Place a full signature to correspond with each set of initials appearing below:

Initials	Corresponding Signature of Instructor	Title

Procedure Guidelines	S/U	Date	Initials	S/U	Date	Initials
1. Perform your beginning procedure actions.						
2. Locate the radial pulse and place the first three fingers of your hand on it.						
3. Look at your watch and begin counting.						
4. Count the number of pulse beats for 60 seconds. (Count for 30 seconds and multiply by 2, if permitted by your state laws and facility policies.) Always count for one full minute if the pulse is irregular.						
5. Record the pulse rate.						
6. If you are taking respirations, leave your fingers on the pulse.						
7. If you are not counting respirations, perform your procedure completion actions.						

PERFORMANCE REVIEW CHECKLIST

Procedure __46__

Procedure <u>Counting Respirations</u>

Name of Nursing Assistant _____ Date of Program _____ to _____

Social Security Number of Nursing Assistant _____

Program Code Number _____

S=Satisfactory Performance
U=Unsatisfactory Performance

Place a full signature to correspond with each set of initials appearing below:

Initials	Corresponding Signature of Instructor	Title

	Procedure Guidelines	S/U	Date	Initials	S/U	Date	Initials
1.	Perform your beginning procedure actions.						
2.	Count the resident's pulse and remember the number.						
3.	After you have counted the pulse, glance at the resident's chest while continuing to look at your watch.						
4.	Count one inhalation and one exhalation as one respiration.						
5.	Count the number of respirations in one minute (60 seconds). (Count for 30 seconds and multiply by 2, if permitted by your state laws and facility policies.) Always count for one full minute if the respirations are gasping or irregular.						
6.	Record the respiration rate.						
7.	Record the resident's pulse and respirations on your note pad.						
8.	Perform your procedure completion actions.						

PERFORMANCE REVIEW CHECKLIST

Procedure __47__

Procedure <u>Measuring the Blood Pressure (Two-Step Procedure)</u>

Name of Nursing Assistant _____ Date of Program _____ to _____

Social Security Number of Nursing Assistant _____

Program Code Number _____

S=Satisfactory Performance
U=Unsatisfactory Performance

Place a full signature to correspond with each set of initials appearing below:

Initials	Corresponding Signature of Instructor	Title

Procedure Guidelines	S/U	Date	Initials	S/U	Date	Initials
1. Perform your beginning procedure actions.						
2. Wipe the earpieces and diaphragm of the stethoscope with the alcohol sponge.						
3. Push the resident's sleeve up at least 5 inches above the elbow.						
4. Extend the resident's arm and rest it on the arm of the chair, the bed, or the resident's lap, with the palm upward.						
5. Unroll the cuff and open the valve on the bulb. Squeeze the cuff to deflate the cuff completely.						
6. Locate the brachial artery, on the thumb side of the inner upper arm, by palpating with two or three fingers.						
7. Wrap the cuff around the resident's arm, centering the bladder over the brachial artery. The cuff should be one inch above the artery in the antecubital space, in front of the elbow.						

(continues)

continued

8.	Locate the radial pulse on the thumb side of the wrist. Keep your fingers on it.					
9.	Close the screw on the handset and inflate the bulb until you can no longer feel the radial pulse. This is known as the palpated pressure. Mentally add 30 to this number.					
10.	Open the screw and deflate the cuff.					
11.	Wait 30 seconds.					
12.	Place the stethoscope in your ears. Place the diaphragm of the stethoscope over the brachial artery.					
13.	Close the screw and inflate the cuff to 30 points higher than where the radial pulse was last palpated.					
14.	Slowly release the screw so the pressure in the cuff falls by increments of 2 mm Hg.					
15.	Listen for a sound. When you hear it, note the closest number on the gauge.					
16.	Continue to listen until the sound stops. Note the closest number on the gauge. Continue to listen for 10 to 20 mm Hg below this sound.					
17.	Open the screw completely and deflate the cuff.					
18.	Remove the stethoscope from your ears.					
19.	Remove the cuff from the resident's arm.					
20.	Record the blood pressure on your note pad as a fraction, with the systolic reading first, followed by the diastolic reading.					
21.	If you are unsure of the blood pressure, wait one to two minutes, then check it again.					
22.	Wipe the earpieces and diaphragm of the stethoscope with the alcohol sponge.					
23.	Perform your procedure completion actions.					
24.	Report blood pressure over 140/90 or under 100/60 to the nurse immediately, or according to facility policy.					

PERFORMANCE REVIEW CHECKLIST

Procedure __48__

Procedure <u>Measuring the Blood Pressure (One-Step Procedure)</u>

Name of Nursing Assistant _____ Date of Program _____ to _____

Social Security Number of Nursing Assistant _____

Program Code Number _____

S=Satisfactory Performance
U=Unsatisfactory Performance

Place a full signature to correspond with each set of initials appearing below:

Initials	Corresponding Signature of Instructor	Title

Procedure Guidelines	S/U	Date	Initials	S/U	Date	Initials
1. Wipe the earpieces and diaphragm of the stethoscope with alcohol pads.						
2. Perform your beginning procedure actions. The resident may be lying down or seated in a chair for this procedure.						
3. Push the resident's sleeve up at least 5 inches above the elbow.						
4. Extend the resident's arm and rest it on the arm of the chair, the bed, or the resident's lap, with the palm upward.						
5. Unroll the cuff and open the valve on the bulb. Squeeze the cuff to deflate the cuff completely.						
6. Locate the brachial artery, on the thumb side of the inner elbow, by palpating with two or three fingers.						
7. Wrap the cuff snugly around the resident's arm, centering the bladder over the brachial artery. The cuff should be one inch above the artery in the antecubital space, in front of the elbow.						

(continues)

continued

8.	Position the gauge so you can see the numbers clearly.						
9.	Confirm the location of the brachial artery.						
10.	Place the earpieces of the stethoscope in your ears. Position the diaphragm to the stethoscope over the brachial artery. The diaphragm should not be touching the blood pressure cuff. Hold the diaphragm in place with the fingers of your nondominant hand.						
11.	With your dominant hand, tighten the thumbscrew on the valve (turn clockwise) to close it. Do not tighten it so much that you will have difficulty releasing it.						
12.	Pump the bulb to inflate the cuff until the gauge reaches 160, or according to facility policy.						
13.	Slowly open the valve by turning the thumbscrew counterclockwise. Allow the air to escape slowly.						
14.	Listen for the sound of the pulse in the stethoscope. A few seconds will pass without sound. If you hear pulse sounds immediately, deflate the cuff. Wait a minute, then repeat the procedure, this time inflating the cuff to 200.						
15.	Note the number on the gauge when you hear the first sound.						
16.	Continue listening as the air escapes slowly from the cuff. You will hear a continuous pulse sound. Note the number on the gauge when the sounds disappear completely.						
17.	After the sounds disappear entirely, open the thumbscrew completely to deflate the cuff.						
18.	Remove the stethoscope from your ears.						
19.	Remove the cuff from the resident's arm.						
20.	Record the blood pressure on your note pad. Blood pressure is recorded as a fraction, with the systolic reading first, followed by the diastolic reading.						

(continues)

continued

21.	Roll the blood pressure cuff over the gauge and return it to the case.					
22.	Wipe the earpieces and diaphragm of the stethoscope with an alcohol sponge. If the stethoscope tubing came in contact with the bed linen, wipe it as well.					
23.	Perform your procedure completion actions.					
24.	Report blood pressure over 140/90 or under 100/60 to the nurse immediately, or according to facility policy.					

PERFORMANCE REVIEW CHECKLIST

Procedure ___49___

Procedure <u>Measuring Weight and Height</u>

Name of Nursing Assistant _____ Date of Program _____ to _____

Social Security Number of Nursing Assistant _____

Program Code Number _____

S=Satisfactory Performance
U=Unsatisfactory Performance

Place a full signature to correspond with each set of initials appearing below:

Initials	Corresponding Signature of Instructor	Title

Procedure Guidelines	S/U	Date	Initials	S/U	Date	Initials
1. Perform your beginning procedure actions.						
2. Standing scale:						
a. Balance the scale.						
b. Place a paper towel on the scale platform.						
c. Assist the resident to remove shoes and stand on the platform.						
d. Adjust the weights on the scale until the bar hangs freely on the end.						
e. Add the weight on the two bars to determine the weight. Write this down on your note pad or remember it.						
f. Assist the resident to turn around, facing away from the scale.						
g. Raise the height bar until it is level with the top of the head.						
h. Record the measurement in the center of the height bar.						

(continues)

continued

i. Help the resident down from the scale and assist to put on shoes, if necessary.						
j. Remove and discard the paper towel.						
3. Chair scale						
a. Balance the scale.						
b. Assist the resident to transfer from the wheelchair to the chair scale.						
c. Place the resident's feet on the footrest of the chair.						
d. Move the weights until the balance bar hangs freely, or read the electronic display screen. Remember this number or write it down on your note pad.						
e. Transfer the resident back to the wheelchair.						
4. Wheelchair scale						
a. Balance the scale.						
b. Obtain a wheelchair and take it to the scale and weigh it. Write down the weight.						
• If the resident uses a lap tray on the wheelchair, remove the tray before weighing the resident. If the tray cannot be removed, weigh the tray and the wheelchair together during the first step of the procedure, then subtract the combined weight from the total.						
c. Take the wheelchair to the resident's room and assist the resident to transfer into it.						
d. Take the resident to the scale. Roll the wheelchair up the ramp and lock the brakes.						
e. Adjust the weights until the balance bar hangs freely on the end. Write down this number on your note pad.						
f. Unlock the brakes and slowly guide the wheelchair down the ramp.						

(continues)

continued

g. Return to the resident's room and assist the resident to transfer out of the wheelchair.					
h. Subtract the weight of the empty wheelchair from the total weight of the resident and chair and record this number.					
5. Bed scale (follow the guidelines in Procedure 20 for assisting the resident into the lift seat or sling).					
a. Balance the scale. The scale should be balanced with the canvas seat, chains, or straps attached.					
b. Remove the sling from the scale and position the resident on the sling.					
c. Connect the straps and elevate the lift above the level of the bed. Raise the sling so the resident's body and the sling hang freely over the bed.					
d. Adjust the weights until the balance bar hangs freely on the end, or read the electronic display screen. Remember this number or write it on your note pad.					
e. Lower the resident back into the bed and remove the sling.					
6. Perform your procedure completion actions.					

Procedure Guidelines	S/U	Date	Initials	S/U	Date	Initials

_____   _____

Instructor Signature   Date

_____   _____

Student Signature   Date

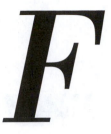

Practice Exam Answer Sheets

Sheet 1 — Left section

#	A B C D	#	A B C D
1.	Ⓐ Ⓑ Ⓒ Ⓓ	41.	Ⓐ Ⓑ Ⓒ Ⓓ
2.	Ⓐ Ⓑ Ⓒ Ⓓ	42.	Ⓐ Ⓑ Ⓒ Ⓓ
3.	Ⓐ Ⓑ Ⓒ Ⓓ	43.	Ⓐ Ⓑ Ⓒ Ⓓ
4.	Ⓐ Ⓑ Ⓒ Ⓓ	44.	Ⓐ Ⓑ Ⓒ Ⓓ
5.	Ⓐ Ⓑ Ⓒ Ⓓ	45.	Ⓐ Ⓑ Ⓒ Ⓓ
6.	Ⓐ Ⓑ Ⓒ Ⓓ	46.	Ⓐ Ⓑ Ⓒ Ⓓ
7.	Ⓐ Ⓑ Ⓒ Ⓓ	47.	Ⓐ Ⓑ Ⓒ Ⓓ
8.	Ⓐ Ⓑ Ⓒ Ⓓ	48.	Ⓐ Ⓑ Ⓒ Ⓓ
9.	Ⓐ Ⓑ Ⓒ Ⓓ	49.	Ⓐ Ⓑ Ⓒ Ⓓ
10.	Ⓐ Ⓑ Ⓒ Ⓓ	50.	Ⓐ Ⓑ Ⓒ Ⓓ
11.	Ⓐ Ⓑ Ⓒ Ⓓ	51.	Ⓐ Ⓑ Ⓒ Ⓓ
12.	Ⓐ Ⓑ Ⓒ Ⓓ	52.	Ⓐ Ⓑ Ⓒ Ⓓ
13.	Ⓐ Ⓑ Ⓒ Ⓓ	53.	Ⓐ Ⓑ Ⓒ Ⓓ
14.	Ⓐ Ⓑ Ⓒ Ⓓ	54.	Ⓐ Ⓑ Ⓒ Ⓓ
15.	Ⓐ Ⓑ Ⓒ Ⓓ	55.	Ⓐ Ⓑ Ⓒ Ⓓ
16.	Ⓐ Ⓑ Ⓒ Ⓓ	56.	Ⓐ Ⓑ Ⓒ Ⓓ
17.	Ⓐ Ⓑ Ⓒ Ⓓ	57.	Ⓐ Ⓑ Ⓒ Ⓓ
18.	Ⓐ Ⓑ Ⓒ Ⓓ	58.	Ⓐ Ⓑ Ⓒ Ⓓ
19.	Ⓐ Ⓑ Ⓒ Ⓓ	59.	Ⓐ Ⓑ Ⓒ Ⓓ
20.	Ⓐ Ⓑ Ⓒ Ⓓ	60.	Ⓐ Ⓑ Ⓒ Ⓓ
21.	Ⓐ Ⓑ Ⓒ Ⓓ	61.	Ⓐ Ⓑ Ⓒ Ⓓ
22.	Ⓐ Ⓑ Ⓒ Ⓓ	62.	Ⓐ Ⓑ Ⓒ Ⓓ
23.	Ⓐ Ⓑ Ⓒ Ⓓ	63.	Ⓐ Ⓑ Ⓒ Ⓓ
24.	Ⓐ Ⓑ Ⓒ Ⓓ	64.	Ⓐ Ⓑ Ⓒ Ⓓ
25.	Ⓐ Ⓑ Ⓒ Ⓓ	65.	Ⓐ Ⓑ Ⓒ Ⓓ
26.	Ⓐ Ⓑ Ⓒ Ⓓ	66.	Ⓐ Ⓑ Ⓒ Ⓓ
27.	Ⓐ Ⓑ Ⓒ Ⓓ	67.	Ⓐ Ⓑ Ⓒ Ⓓ
28.	Ⓐ Ⓑ Ⓒ Ⓓ	68.	Ⓐ Ⓑ Ⓒ Ⓓ
29.	Ⓐ Ⓑ Ⓒ Ⓓ	69.	Ⓐ Ⓑ Ⓒ Ⓓ
30.	Ⓐ Ⓑ Ⓒ Ⓓ	70.	Ⓐ Ⓑ Ⓒ Ⓓ
31.	Ⓐ Ⓑ Ⓒ Ⓓ	71.	Ⓐ Ⓑ Ⓒ Ⓓ
32.	Ⓐ Ⓑ Ⓒ Ⓓ	72.	Ⓐ Ⓑ Ⓒ Ⓓ
33.	Ⓐ Ⓑ Ⓒ Ⓓ	73.	Ⓐ Ⓑ Ⓒ Ⓓ
34.	Ⓐ Ⓑ Ⓒ Ⓓ	74.	Ⓐ Ⓑ Ⓒ Ⓓ
35.	Ⓐ Ⓑ Ⓒ Ⓓ	75.	Ⓐ Ⓑ Ⓒ Ⓓ
36.	Ⓐ Ⓑ Ⓒ Ⓓ		
37.	Ⓐ Ⓑ Ⓒ Ⓓ		
38.	Ⓐ Ⓑ Ⓒ Ⓓ		
39.	Ⓐ Ⓑ Ⓒ Ⓓ		
40.	Ⓐ Ⓑ Ⓒ Ⓓ		

Sheet 2 — Right section

#	A B C D	#	A B C D
1.	Ⓐ Ⓑ Ⓒ Ⓓ	41.	Ⓐ Ⓑ Ⓒ Ⓓ
2.	Ⓐ Ⓑ Ⓒ Ⓓ	42.	Ⓐ Ⓑ Ⓒ Ⓓ
3.	Ⓐ Ⓑ Ⓒ Ⓓ	43.	Ⓐ Ⓑ Ⓒ Ⓓ
4.	Ⓐ Ⓑ Ⓒ Ⓓ	44.	Ⓐ Ⓑ Ⓒ Ⓓ
5.	Ⓐ Ⓑ Ⓒ Ⓓ	45.	Ⓐ Ⓑ Ⓒ Ⓓ
6.	Ⓐ Ⓑ Ⓒ Ⓓ	46.	Ⓐ Ⓑ Ⓒ Ⓓ
7.	Ⓐ Ⓑ Ⓒ Ⓓ	47.	Ⓐ Ⓑ Ⓒ Ⓓ
8.	Ⓐ Ⓑ Ⓒ Ⓓ	48.	Ⓐ Ⓑ Ⓒ Ⓓ
9.	Ⓐ Ⓑ Ⓒ Ⓓ	49.	Ⓐ Ⓑ Ⓒ Ⓓ
10.	Ⓐ Ⓑ Ⓒ Ⓓ	50.	Ⓐ Ⓑ Ⓒ Ⓓ
11.	Ⓐ Ⓑ Ⓒ Ⓓ	51.	Ⓐ Ⓑ Ⓒ Ⓓ
12.	Ⓐ Ⓑ Ⓒ Ⓓ	52.	Ⓐ Ⓑ Ⓒ Ⓓ
13.	Ⓐ Ⓑ Ⓒ Ⓓ	53.	Ⓐ Ⓑ Ⓒ Ⓓ
14.	Ⓐ Ⓑ Ⓒ Ⓓ	54.	Ⓐ Ⓑ Ⓒ Ⓓ
15.	Ⓐ Ⓑ Ⓒ Ⓓ	55.	Ⓐ Ⓑ Ⓒ Ⓓ
16.	Ⓐ Ⓑ Ⓒ Ⓓ	56.	Ⓐ Ⓑ Ⓒ Ⓓ
17.	Ⓐ Ⓑ Ⓒ Ⓓ	57.	Ⓐ Ⓑ Ⓒ Ⓓ
18.	Ⓐ Ⓑ Ⓒ Ⓓ	58.	Ⓐ Ⓑ Ⓒ Ⓓ
19.	Ⓐ Ⓑ Ⓒ Ⓓ	59.	Ⓐ Ⓑ Ⓒ Ⓓ
20.	Ⓐ Ⓑ Ⓒ Ⓓ	60.	Ⓐ Ⓑ Ⓒ Ⓓ
21.	Ⓐ Ⓑ Ⓒ Ⓓ	61.	Ⓐ Ⓑ Ⓒ Ⓓ
22.	Ⓐ Ⓑ Ⓒ Ⓓ	62.	Ⓐ Ⓑ Ⓒ Ⓓ
23.	Ⓐ Ⓑ Ⓒ Ⓓ	63.	Ⓐ Ⓑ Ⓒ Ⓓ
24.	Ⓐ Ⓑ Ⓒ Ⓓ	64.	Ⓐ Ⓑ Ⓒ Ⓓ
25.	Ⓐ Ⓑ Ⓒ Ⓓ	65.	Ⓐ Ⓑ Ⓒ Ⓓ
26.	Ⓐ Ⓑ Ⓒ Ⓓ	66.	Ⓐ Ⓑ Ⓒ Ⓓ
27.	Ⓐ Ⓑ Ⓒ Ⓓ	67.	Ⓐ Ⓑ Ⓒ Ⓓ
28.	Ⓐ Ⓑ Ⓒ Ⓓ	68.	Ⓐ Ⓑ Ⓒ Ⓓ
29.	Ⓐ Ⓑ Ⓒ Ⓓ	69.	Ⓐ Ⓑ Ⓒ Ⓓ
30.	Ⓐ Ⓑ Ⓒ Ⓓ	70.	Ⓐ Ⓑ Ⓒ Ⓓ
31.	Ⓐ Ⓑ Ⓒ Ⓓ	71.	Ⓐ Ⓑ Ⓒ Ⓓ
32.	Ⓐ Ⓑ Ⓒ Ⓓ	72.	Ⓐ Ⓑ Ⓒ Ⓓ
33.	Ⓐ Ⓑ Ⓒ Ⓓ	73.	Ⓐ Ⓑ Ⓒ Ⓓ
34.	Ⓐ Ⓑ Ⓒ Ⓓ	74.	Ⓐ Ⓑ Ⓒ Ⓓ
35.	Ⓐ Ⓑ Ⓒ Ⓓ	75.	Ⓐ Ⓑ Ⓒ Ⓓ
36.	Ⓐ Ⓑ Ⓒ Ⓓ		
37.	Ⓐ Ⓑ Ⓒ Ⓓ		
38.	Ⓐ Ⓑ Ⓒ Ⓓ		
39.	Ⓐ Ⓑ Ⓒ Ⓓ		
40.	Ⓐ Ⓑ Ⓒ Ⓓ		

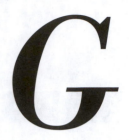

Answer Keys to Chapter Review Quizzes and Crossword Puzzles

CHAPTER 1 KEY

1. b	6. d	10. d	14. a	18. d
2. c	7. a	11. a	15. c	19. c
3. d	8. c	12. d	16. b	20. b
4. a	9. c	13. b	17. c	21. c
5. b				

CHAPTER 1 PUZZLE SOLUTION

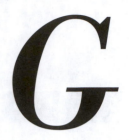

CHAPTER 2 KEY

1. a	6. c	10. d	14. d	18. a
2. b	7. a	11. a	15. b	19. d
3. d	8. c	12. b	16. b	20. b
4. b	9. b	13. c	17. c	21. c
5. a				

CHAPTER 2
PUZZLE SOLUTION

CHAPTER 3 KEY

1. c	7. a	12. b	17. b	22. a
2. d	8. b	13. a	18. c	23. c
3. a	9. c	14. d	19. d	24. b
4. c	10. d	15. a	20. a	25. a
5. b	11. c	16. c	21. d	26. d
6. d				

CHAPTER 3
PUZZLE SOLUTION

Solution words:

CHOICES, PRIVACY, DIGNITY, NAME, ADAPTIVE, COMMUNICATION, PRIVATE, PROTECT, VOTE, ABUSE, RIGHTS, CONFIDENTIALITY, ACTIVITIES, CRIMINAL, COUNCILS, GRIEVANCE, RESTRAINT, EXERCISE, LAW, REFUSE, SELF, REPRISAL, NEGLECT, EXPLAIN, SURVEY

CHAPTER 4 KEY

1. b	5. b	9. c	13. a	17. d
2. a	6. d	10. d	14. c	18. a
3. a	7. b	11. a	15. d	19. b
4. c	8. a	12. c	16. b	20. c

CHAPTER 4
PUZZLE SOLUTION

CHAPTER 5 KEY

1. b	7. c	13. d	19. b	25. b
2. d	8. a	14. a	20. a	26. c
3. a	9. c	15. d	21. a	27. a
4. d	10. b	16. b	22. a	28. b
5. b	11. c	17. d	23. b	29. a
6. d	12. c	18. c	24. c	

CHAPTER 5
PUZZLE SOLUTION

CHAPTER 6 KEY

1. c	7. a	13. b	19. d	25. d
2. a	8. c	14. d	20. b	26. c
3. c	9. a	15. b	21. c	27. b
4. a	10. b	16. c	22. b	
5. b	11. c	17. d	23. c	
6. d	12. d	18. a	24. a	

CHAPTER 6
PUZZLE SOLUTION

Crossword solution grid — words appearing:

HEPA, SCABIES, INDIRECT, CONTACT, VIRUS, MICROORGANISM, BIOHAZARDOUS, GOWN, CONTAMINATED, TRANSMISSION, STERILE, HIV, DISINFECTION, GLOVES, DROPLET, COMMUNICABLE, GERMS, SWEAT, PORTAL, SOURCE, RESERVOIR, MASK, PATHOGEN, PROTECTION, ISOLATION, HANDWASHING

CHAPTER 7 KEY

1. d
2. c
3. b
4. a
5. a
6. d
7. b
8. a
9. c
10. b
11. a
12. b
13. c
14. c
15. a
16. d
17. d
18. b
19. d
20. b

CHAPTER 7 PUZZLE SOLUTION

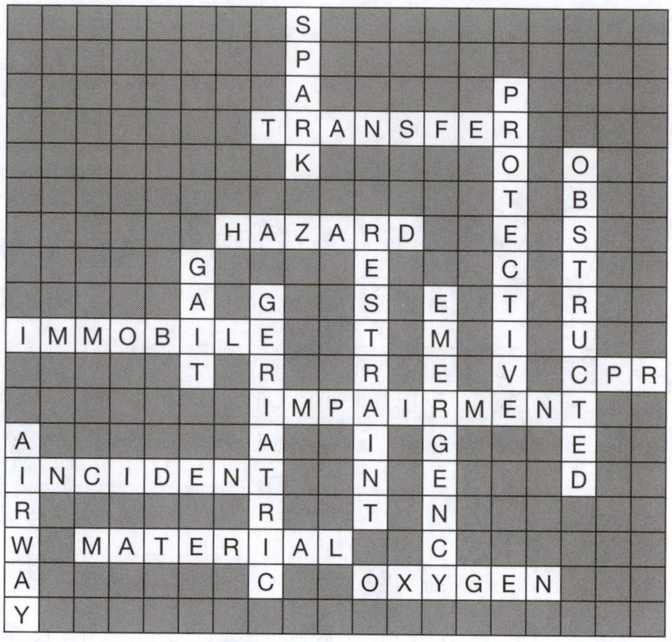
SPARK
TRANSFER
PROTECTIVE
OBSTRUCTED
HAZARD
GAIT
GERIATRIC
RESTRAINT
EMERGENCY
IMMOBILE
CPR
IMPAIRMENT
AIRWAY
INCIDENT
MATERIAL
OXYGEN

CHAPTER 8 KEY

1. c
2. d
3. a
4. b
5. b
6. a
7. c
8. d
9. c
10. a
11. c
12. d

CHAPTER 8 PUZZLE SOLUTION

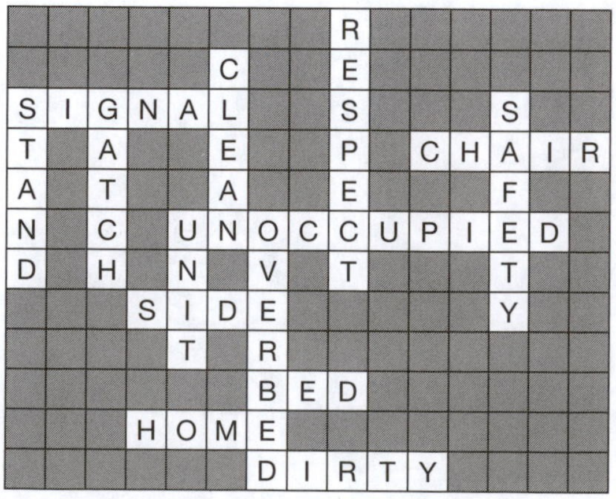
RESPECT
CLEAN
SIGNAL
STAND
GATCH
SAFETY
CHAIR
UNOCCUPIED
UNIT
OVERBED
SIDE
BED
HOME
DIRTY

CHAPTER 9 KEY

1. b	6. a	11. a	16. a	21. b
2. c	7. d	12. d	17. d	22. c
3. d	8. b	13. b	18. c	23. d
4. c	9. b	14. a	19. c	24. c
5. a	10. c	15. b	20. b	25. b

CHAPTER 9
PUZZLE SOLUTION

CHAPTER 10 KEY

1. a	5. b	9. d	13. b	17. b
2. b	6. a	10. b	14. c	18. c
3. c	7. b	11. a	15. b	19. a
4. b	8. c	12. c	16. c	20. b

CHAPTER 10
PUZZLE SOLUTION

```
                              G
            P R E S S U R E   E
                              N
                      A X I L L A
    P E R I N E A L   N       T   B
            N         U       A   R
      D E C U B I T U S   L   L   A
            O               N     S
P R O S T H E S I S         I     I
            T               N     O
    U       I               E     N
    L   E M B O L I S M      N
    C   N
  D E N T U R E S
    R
```

CHAPTER 11 KEY

1. a	5. b	9. b	13. d	17. c
2. c	6. a	10. c	14. c	18. a
3. b	7. d	11. a	15. b	19. d
4. c	8. b	12. b	16. b	20. b

CHAPTER 11
PUZZLE SOLUTION

```
                    I
                    N
        O           F
        U           U           F
        N           S   R       O
    A   C E N T I M E T E R     R C E
    S   E       I   S       F   R C E
    P   G       O   T           E     P
    I N T A K E     N   M I L L I L I T E R
    R   S           D   C               Y
    A   T           E   C               R
    T H E R A P E U T I C               A
    I   O           H   N               M
    O   S           Y   T               I
    N   T           D   G R A D U A T E D
        O           R   A
    E D E M A       A   V
        Y           T   E
                    I   N U T R I E N T S
D I G E S T I O N   O   O
    M               N O U T P U T
    E                   S
    S
    I
    S
```

CHAPTER 12 KEY

1. c	5. a	9. b	13. b	17. d
2. b	6. c	10. a	14. c	18. b
3. a	7. c	11. c	15. b	19. a
4. b	8. d	12. a	16. c	20. c

CHAPTER 12
PUZZLE SOLUTION

Across and down answers:

COMMODE
URINAL
COD
BOWEL
CATHETER
VOID
COLON
STOOL
IMPACTION
ENEMA
DIVERTICULOSIS
HOMEOSTASIS
OSTOMY
INVOLUNTARY
DEFECATE
FECES
BEDPAN
STOMA
URETHRA
ANUS

CHAPTER 13 KEY

1. b	5. c	9. a	13. c	17. d
2. d	6. b	10. b	14. b	18. a
3. a	7. c	11. c	15. a	19. d
4. b	8. d	12. a	16. c	20. a

CHAPTER 13
PUZZLE SOLUTION

Index